Genetic Differences in Chemical Carcinogenesis

Editor

Richard E. Kouri
Director of Research
Microbiological Associates
Bethesda, Maryland

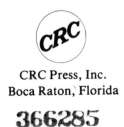

CRC Press, Inc.
Boca Raton, Florida

Library of Congress Cataloging in Publication Data

Main entry under title:

Genetic differences in chemical carcinogenesis.
  Bibliography: p.
  Includes index.
  1. Carcinogenesis. 2. Cancer—Genetic aspects.
3. Carcinogens. I. Kouri, Richard E.
[DNLM: 1. Carcinogens. 2. Genetics, Biochemical.
3. Neoplasms—Chemically induced. 4. RNA viruses—
Genetics. QZ202.3 G328]
RC268.5.G44   616.9'94'071   79-16133
ISBN O-8493-5285-1

Direct all inquiries to CRC Press, 2000 N.W. 24th Street, Boca Raton, Florida, 33431.

© 1980 by CRC Press, Inc.

International Standard Book Number 0-8493-5285-1

Library of Congress Card Number 79-16133
Printed in the United States

DEDICATION

To Pauline, whose patience I wish I possessed.

January, 1979

PREFACE

The process of chemically induced cancers involves a series of complex stages, each of which is capable of determining the rate of progression of this disease (see Stages in Carcinogenesis). At virtually every step, there are naturally-occurring variations among both individuals and groups of individuals which are controlled or regulated by host genes. It would seem that a specific genotype or, more likely, a certain set of gene combinations ultimately define which individuals are susceptible to chemically induced cancers.

The first stage in the disease process entails exposure, uptake and distribution of chemical carcinogens within an individual (Chapter 1). Although exposure levels normally determine uptake, the assimilation and distribution of many chemical carcinogens seem to depend upon the presence of cytoplasmic receptor molecules. Moreover, the degree of expression of these receptor molecules may be regulated by host genes. Since most chemical carcinogens are relatively inert, they would remain within cells forever if not for specific enzyme systems that metabolize them to polar end products for bodily excretion. This metabolic process is highly complex, is host gene regulated, and controls not only this metabolic alteration to water-soluble forms, but also controls the production of intermediates that may be much more biologically active than the parent compounds (Chapter 2). These active intermediates can be detoxified and removed from cells; may bind to cellular macromolecules resulting in no appreciable damage; or can bind in a specific manner to macromolecular DNA, forming DNA adducts. DNA adducts, recognized as such by DNA repair enzymes, are either repaired, nonrepaired or misrepaired (Chapter 3). The latter two alternatives result in a stable DNA effect. Upon expression of this DNA sequence either naturally via normal endogenous factors, e.g., hormones or viruses (Chapters 4 and 5) or after exposure to exogenous chemicals (Chapter 6), this defect can be transformed into a stable cellular genotype. Proliferation of this stable genotype by exogenous promoters seems to be the major method by which transformation to the cancer cell phenotype occurs. These cancer cells may remain quiescent, may express a specific phenotype that is recognized by the immune system for removal from the body, or may proliferate into a palpable tumor (Chapter 6).

Each of these stages can be, in certain instances, under host genetic control. Variations in the level of expression of these stages can determine susceptibility to chemically induced cancers. The determination of the cancer prone genotype(s) is a very viable approach to the understanding and eventual control of cancer in humans (Chapter 7).

This book is an attempt to present the state-of-the-art of genetic control of chemical carcinogenesis. The authors hope that this book will provide some insight into the intricacies of the chemical carcinogenic process and present some logical methods for the understanding and subsequent control of this disease.

Richard E. Kouri

STAGES IN CARCINOGENESIS

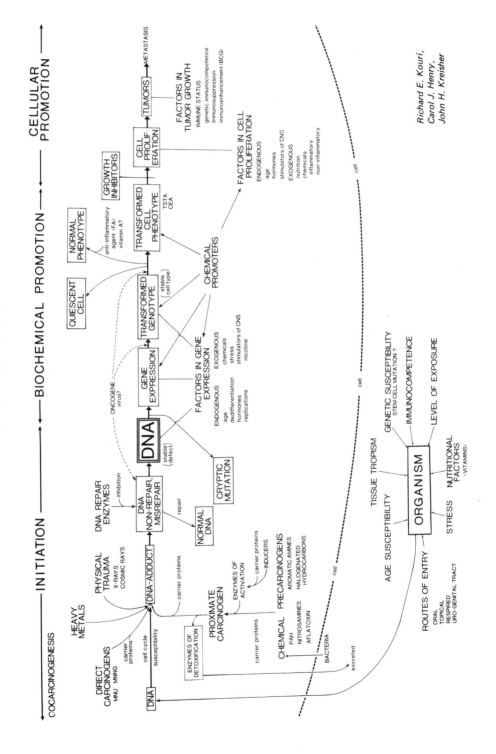

THE EDITOR

Dr. Richard E. Kouri is Director of Research and Head of the Department of Biochemical Oncology at Microbiological Associates, Bethesda, Maryland.

Dr. Kouri received his B.S. degree in Microbiology at Ohio State University in 1965, his M.S. and Ph.D. in 1968 and 1970 at the University of Tennessee in Radiation Biology. From 1970—1971 he was a postdoctoral fellow at the Roche Institute of Molecular Biology. Since 1971 he has been at Microbiological Associates, first as an Associate jinvestigator, 1971—1972; then Co-Project Director, 1972—1974; and to the present as Head, Department of Biochemical Oncology. He was made Director of Research in June 1977.

His research interests have included: in vivo and in vitro toxicological bioassays, carcinogen metabolism, genetic regulation of cancer susceptibility, and the molecular basis for chemically induced mutagenesis and carcinogenesis.

Dr. Kouri has authored over 80 publications in these various fields and has presented these results as a participant/lecturer at 37 major international symposia, workshops, conferences, round tables and seminars.

CONTRIBUTORS

Darwin O. Chee
Department of Clinical Immunology
City of Hope National Medical
Center
Duarte, California

Hoda A. Guirgis
Department of Community and
Environmental Medicine
University of California
Irvine, California

Rishab K. Gupta
Division of Oncology
Department of Surgery
University of California
at Los Angeles
Medical School
Los Angeles, California

Carol J. Henry
Department of Experimental
Oncology
Microbiological Associates
Bethesda, Maryland

Richard E. Kouri
Department of Biochemical
Oncology
Microbiological Associates
Bethesda, Maryland

Henry T. Lynch
Department of Preventative
Medicine and Public Health
Creighton University
School of Medicine
Omaha, Nebraska

Patrick M. Lynch
Department of Preventative
Medicine and Public Health
Creighton University
School of Medicine
Omaha, Nebraska

Sukdeb Mondal
Department of Pathology LAC/USC
Cancer Research Center
Los Angeles, California

Kunjuraman T. Nayar
Department of Biochemical
Oncology
Microbiological Associates
Bethesda, Maryland

Daniel W. Nebert
Developmental Pharmacology
Branch
National Institute of Child Health
and Human Development
National Institutes of Health
Bethesda, Maryland

Barbara O'Neill
Department of Biochemical
Oncology
Microbiological Associates
Bethesda, Maryland

Ronald E. Rasmussen
Department of Community and
Environmental Medicine
California College of Medicine
University of California
Irvine, California

Leonard M. Schechtman
Department of Biochemical
Oncology
Microbiological Associates
Bethesda, Maryland

TABLE OF CONTENTS

Chapter 1

EXPOSURE, UPTAKE AND DISTRIBUTION OF CHEMICAL CARCINOGENS

Leonard M. Schechtman, Carol J. Henry, and Richard E. Kouri

TABLE OF CONTENTS

I. INTRODUCTION

Carcinogenesis is a multistep, highly complex process. Manifestation of the carcinogenic process is dependent upon the interaction of such factors as environmental exposure to carcinogens and/or adventitious agents, genetic susceptibility to carcinogenesis, host modifying factors (e.g., diet, metabolic capacity, hormonal effects, immune responses and age), co-carcinogenic interactions, as well as other intrinsic and extrinsic determinants.

Control of chemical carcinogenesis can hypothetically be excercised at any one of the many steps involved in the carcinogenic process. The role played by genetics in this process and the genetic regulation of carcinogenesis will be the subject of succeeding chapters in this book. The subject of this chapter will be human exposure to chemical carcinogens and control of this exposure to potentially carcinogenic environmental factors.

II. ENVIRONMENTAL EXPOSURE TO CHEMICAL CARCINOGENS

The first step that is amenable to control of carcinogenesis is at the level of exposure.[1] In its simplest sense, a decrease in the level of exposure to carcinogenic agents should result in a decreased risk. Whereas there is firm genetic influence on other steps in carcinogenesis (see ensuing chapters), few such obvious genetic controls exist at the level of exposure, uptake or distribution of chemical carcinogens.

Exposure to chemical carcinogens is itself not a genetically controlled occurrence and should be at random. However, there is some evidence which suggests that cellular uptake of chemical agents is under genetic control and that this genetic control occurs via the binding of chemicals to macromolecules in mammalian cells. Poland et al.[2] have examined the binding affinity of various halogenated dibenzo-p-dioxins, dibenzofurans and polycyclic hydrocarbons by hepatic cytosol and have proposed that hepatic uptake of such agents may be genetically regulated. Wilding et al.[3] have also shown that drug binding may be under genetic control in man.

Genetics could also play other more subtle roles in certain aspects related to exposure, uptake, and distribution of chemical carcinogens through such factors as ethnic background, personal preferences, and some psychological and physiological influences such as alcoholism and/or smoking.[4] However, the genetic factors that control, regulate, or influence these characteristics have not as yet been thoroughly defined, due mainly to the limitation of good model systems by which to study such characteristics. Thus, in view of such limitations, it is difficult to discriminate genetic from nongenetic influences.

It has been estimated that approximately 85% of all human cancers result directly or indirectly from environmental influences.[5] Evidence in support of this contention has evolved slowly over roughly the last 200 years, which were marked initially by the discovery of Sir Percivall Pott in 1775 that scrotal cancer among chimney sweeps was attributable to occupational exposure to soot.[6]

One of the prime evidences in support of the major role played by the environment in the incidence of human cancers is that cancer morbidity and mortality in the human population show marked geographical pattern differences.[7-13] The examination of the wide variety of cancers and their incidences relative to geographical distribution has provided information regarding the role of both the environment and genetic determinants in the etiology of cancer. The National Cancer Institute has compiled a publication tabulating the cancer mortality rates by individual county in the continental United States for the period 1950-1969,[11] as well as an atlas depicting the geographical

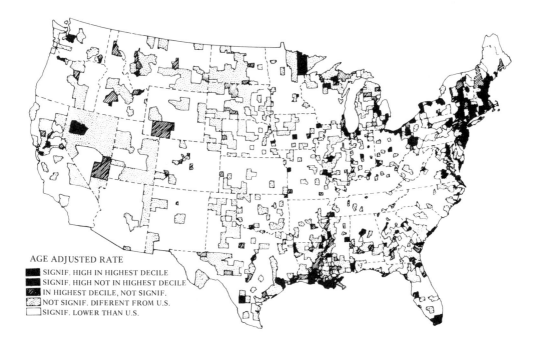

AGE ADJUSTED RATE

■ SIGNIF. HIGH IN HIGHEST DECILE
■ SIGNIF. HIGH NOT IN HIGHEST DECILE
▨ IN HIGHEST DECILE, NOT SIGNIF.
▦ NOT SIGNIF. DIFERENT FROM U.S.
□ SIGNIF. LOWER THAN U.S.

FIGURE 1.   Cancer Mortality, 1950—1969, by county, all sites combined white males. Symbols shown on figure. (Taken from Mason, T. J., McKay, F. W., Hoover, R., Blot, W. J., and Fraumeni, J. F., Jr., Atlas of Cancer Mortality for U.S. Counties: 1950—1969, DHEW Publ. No. (NIH) 75-780, U.S. Government Printing Office, Washington, D.C., 1975. With permission.)

patterns of these cancer mortalities per county over the same 20 year period.[12] Two cancer mortality maps from the atlas depicting age-adjusted rates for 35 anatomic sites of cancer for white males and females are presented in Figures 1 and 2, respectively. A similar analysis was performed for The Danish Cancer Registry for the period 1943-1972.[13] Such analyses serve to identify locales with elevated cancer death rates, geographical clustering of specific kinds of cancers, and high-risk communities; they serve to provide information regarding ethnic influences, and contributory effects of occupational and other environmental factors; and they serve to provide a means for relating the cancer mortality patterns with human risk factors. Epidemiologic evaluations of this kind have also furnished data regarding the influence of such parameters as sex, age, urbanization, socioeconomic status, cultural factors, air pollution levels, and geographic relocation of migrant workers. For example, it has been determined that cancer incidences in the offspring of migrants more often reflect those of the new environs rather than those of the geographical locale from which they originated.[14]

Today human contact with physical and chemical carcinogenic agents through occupational exposure is considered to be one of, if not the major, environmental factor(s) which contribute to the high incidence of this enigmatic and ubiquitous disorder.[15] A comprehensive list of environmental agents which have been associated with occupational, iatrogenic, and other environmental cancers has been tabulated by R. Doll,[16] reproduced here (Tables 1, 2, and 3) with permission. From these and other data it becomes obvious that the influential role of physical agents, industrial products and by-products, drugs, diet, cigarette smoking, and adventitious agents take on a great deal of importance in terms of their total impact on human cancer.

By-products of cigarette smoking have been recognized as important environmental factors which play a role in human carcinogenesis. Cigarette smoke and specific subfractions of tobacco smoke condensate have been implicated as both mutagens and

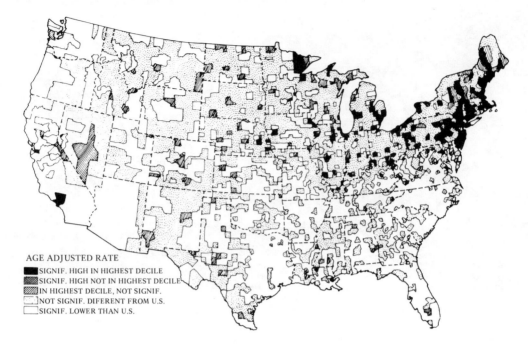

FIGURE 2.   Cancer Mortality, 1950—1969, by county, all sites combined white females. Symbols shown on figure. Taken from Mason, T. J., McKay, F. W., Hoover, R., Blot, W. J., and Fraumeni, J. F., Jr., Mortality for U.S. Counties: 1950—1969, DHEW Publ. No. (NIH) 75-780, U.S. Government Printing Office, Washington, D.C., 1975. With permission.)

carcinogens, and are currently being examined as potential initiators and/or promoters of pulmonary carcinogenesis see Reference 17 for review). It has been reported that cigarette smoking is a major factor contributing to cancer in the United States, with lung cancer accounting for >25% of all cancer deaths in the U.S. in 1975, and approximately 25% of the total cancer mortality in the United Kingdom.[18]

It is not within the scope of this chapter to discuss the individual roles of cigarette smoke, adventitious agents (such as viruses), diet, metabolism, genetic factors (such as genetic predisposition, familial incidence, race, sex, etc.), and systemic factors (such as humoral influences, immunosurveillance, aging, etc.). Some of these will be dealt with further in this volume as they relate to chemically-induced carcinogenesis; others have been discussed previously elsewhere (see Reference 19 for review).

III. SOURCES AND ROUTES OF EXPOSURE IN HUMAN CARCINOGENESIS

A. Carcinogenesis by Physical Agents

The major routes of exposure to carcinogenic agents to which humans are subjected include dermal exposure, exposure through inhalation, and exposure by ingestion. Epidermal exposures to carcinogens are mainly attributed to physical agents such as ultraviolet (UV) radiation and ionizing radiation (X- and gamma rays, alpha and beta particles, neutrons and protons). Data to date suggest that changes in the levels of exposure to UV radiation as a function of geographical locale (e.g., degrees north latitude), time, weather patterns, etc., influence the incidence of skin cancer in man.[20] A similar correlation has been found with respect to ionizing radiation. Differences in exposure levels to ionizing radiation from naturally occurring sources are also dependent upon geographical locale (radioactivity differences in different parts of the earth's

TABLE 1

Occupational Cancers

Agent	Occupation	Site of cancer
Ionizing radiations		
Radon	Certain underground miners (uranium, fluorspar, hematite)	Bronchus
X-rays, radium	Radiologists, radiographers	Skin
Radium	Luminous dial painters	Bone
Ultraviolet light	Farmers, sailors	Skin
Polycyclic hydrocarbons in soot, tar, oil	Chimney sweepers	Scrotum
	Manufacturers of coal gas	Skin
	Many other groups of exposed industrial workers	Bronchus
2-Naphthylamine; 1-naphthylamine	Chemical workers; rubber workers; manufacturers of coal gas	Bladder
Benzidine; 4-aminobiphenyl	Chemical workers	Bladder
Asbestos	Asbestos workers; shipyard and insulation workers	Bronchus pleura and peritoneum
Arsenic	Sheep dip manufacturers; gold miners; some vineyard workers and ore smelters	Skin and bronchus
Bis(chloromethyl)ether	Makers of ion-exchange resins	Bronchus
Benzene	Workers with glues, varnishes, etc.	Marrow (leukemia)
Mustard gas	Poison gas makers	Bronchus; larynx; nasal sinuses
Vinyl chloride	PVC manufacturers	Liver (angiosarcoma)
(Chrome ores)	Chromate manufacturers	Bronchus
(Nickel ore)	Nickel refiners	Bronchus; nasal sinuses
(Isopropyl oil)	Isopropylene manufacturers	Nasal sinuses
Specific agent not identified	Hardwood furniture makers	Nasal sinuses
Specific agent not identified	Leather workers	Nasal sinuses

surface, exposure to cosmic rays as a function of altitude).[20] Upton has suggested that cancers attributable to low-level ionizing radiation may follow a "linear, nonthreshold dose-incidence relationship" and in this respect, could account for up to 1% of naturally occurring induced cancer.[20] On the other hand, medical technological sources of radiation (e.g., medical X-ray and fluoroscopy equipment, in vivo deposition of radioisotopic tracers) account for only a fractional amount of total physically-induced cancers.[20, 21] That UV radiation is a prime cause of skin cancer in man is supported by a multiplicity of facts relating the incidence of skin cancer to (1) the amount and intensity of UV radiation from the sun, (2) the levels of pigmentation among races, (3) the extent of exposure of various body parts, (4) exposure of laboratory animals to UV radiation, and (5) the capacity to repair UV-damaged DNA.[22]

B. Chemically Induced Carcinogenesis

Carcinogenesis attributable to ingestive exposures result mainly from food, water, and drug consumption, while cancers attributable to inhalation exposure result mainly from polluted air, aerosolized environmental and occupationally related carcinogens, and cigarette smoking. The passive consumption of materials other than proximate or ultimate carcinogens associated with these products is generally not considered the direct cause of human cancers, but generally results from an interaction of these with

TABLE 2

Iatrogenic Cancers

Agent	Site of cancer
Diagnostic or therapeutic X-rays	All sites
Thorium	Bone
Thorotrast	R.E. system (liver, spleen)
Polycyclic hydrocarbons	
In coal tar ointments	Skin
In liquid paraffin (?)	Stomach, colon, rectum
Alkylating agents	
Melphalan, cyclophosphamide	Myeloid leukemia
Estrogens	Corpus uteri, breast ♀ (?)
Stilbestrol	Vagina, breast ♂
Steroid contraceptives	Liver
Androgens (anabolic steroids)	Liver
Arsenic	Skin, lung
Chlornaphazine	Bladder
Phenacetin	Renal pelvis
Immunosuppressive drugs	Reticulosarcoma
SV40 virus contaminating polio vaccine (transplacental) (?)	Central nervous system

TABLE 3

Other Environmental Cancers

Agent	Site of cancer
Sunlight	Exposed skin (rodent ulcer, squamous carcinoma, melanoma [?])
Use of "kangri" and "dhoti"	Skin of abdomen and thigh
Chewing betel, tobacco, lime	Mouth
Reverse smoking	Palate
Smoking	Mouth, pharynx, larnyx, bronchus, esophagus, bladder
Alcoholic drinks	Mouth, pharnyx, larynx, esophagus
Aspect of sexual intercourse (? virus)	Cervix uteri
Infectious mononucleosis (?)	Hodgkin's disease
Aflatoxin	Liver
Shistosomiasis	Bladder

such factors as flora associated with the gastro-intestinal tract and endogenous cellular enzymes which can metabolically activate (and inactivate) procarcinogens.

The role that nutritional factors play in human cancers has been reviewed elsewhere.[23-26] Aside from the possibility that certain foods may be carcinogenic, it has been suggested that foods, food components, and food additives can alter the levels of enzymes which metabolize carcinogens in vivo.[27,28] These alterations can be manifest as enzyme induction or repression and can ultimately affect activation, inactivation and endogenous metabolic generation of carcinogenic metabolites. Dietary constituents have been implicated in most forms of gastro-intestinal and peripherally associated organ cancers, such as stomach, colonic, esophageal, hepatic, and pancreatic cancers, and have been associated with certain cancers of organs and tissues under endocrine control, such as breast, ovarian, endometrial, and prostatic cancers (see Reference 25 for review). In addition, approximately 20 organic chemical carcinogens which are naturally occurring have been identified in foods, mainly as metabolites of fungi and green plants.[29-31] Some of those associated with green plants include cycasin (methylazoxymethanol-β-glucoxide), nitrosamines and nitrosamides, pyrrolizidine alkaloids, allyl and propenyl benzene derivatives (e.g., safrole), brachen fern, trace amounts of polycyclic aromatic hydrocarbons and thiourea.[29] Some carcinogens associated with fungi include aflatoxins, sterigmatocystin, yellow rice toxins (eg., the fungal metabolites luteoskyrin and cyclochlorotine), and griseofulvin.[29] Other carcinogenic substances of biological origin have been associated with *Streptomyces* bacteria (e.g., actinomycin D, mitomycin C, streptozotocin and elaiomycin), *Escherichia coli* (e.g., ethionine), and other bacteria (e.g., nitrosamines).[29]

Exposure to carcinogens by ingestion is further complicated by the contribution of marine and fresh water foods exposed to aquatic pollutants. These pollutants are derived from effluents from industry and sewage, erosion of land treated with pesticides, insecticides and other agricultural chemicals, dumping and discharges by ships at sea, offshore crude oil drilling sites, exchange of pollutants between the atmosphere and waterways, seepage of oil and polycyclic aromatic hydrocarbons from the ocean floor, and introduction of chlorinated hydrocarbons and chlorinated phenols through attempts to disinfect water via chlorination.[32,33] That contamination of the aquatic environment is not an oversimplification is emphasized by the current estimates of marine polycyclic hydrocarbon pollution which amount to $0.2—6 \times 10^6$ metric tons per year,[32] and of chlorinated organic contaminants from sewage treatment plants approximating >1000 tons per year.[34] As of 1975, 423 organic chemicals had been identified in the aquatic environment; of these, 325 were determined to be present in treated drinking water, a significant proportion of which are potentially carcinogenic or toxic.[34] Aquatic animals exhibit neoplasms as a result of exposure to chemical pollutants in their environment,[35,36] but in addition, as a major part of the food chain, marine and fresh water life can serve as carriers of carcinogenic pollutants.[37,38] Industrial wastes expelled into municipal and coastal waterways which find their way to more widespread bodies of water including lakes, streams, estuaries, and the sea can thus be consumed by humans via consumption of marine and fresh water plants and animals, as well as consumption of drinking water (see Reference 35 for review).

Drugs, such as certain immunosuppressive agents,[39] estrogens,[40] oral contraceptives,[41] antineoplastic agents,[42] schistosomicides,[43] trichomonicides,[44] diethylstilbestrol,[45] and other commonly used drugs[46] have also been associated with the development of human cancer. It is estimated that drug-induced cancers amount to less than 1% of all human cancers;[46] however, this figure may rise with the current increased rate of introduction of new drugs if not prescreened through the available in vitro and in vivo bioassays for their mutagenic and carcinogenic potentials.

Human exposure to chemical carcinogens by inhalation originates mainly from three major sources, i.e., tobacco smoke, air pollution, and occupational exposure. Among those cancers associated with cigarette smoking are cancers of the lung, lip, mouth, tongue, esophagus, pharynx, larynx, and urinary bladder.[47] Of these, the incidence of lung cancer surpasses the others by a wide margin. Similarly, lung cancer is one of the most prevalent neoplasms associated with job-related exposure and air pollution exposure to carcinogens. Nearly 13% of all deaths among individuals >45 years old are attributable to lung cancer,[48] although statistics vary with geographical locale, sex, and (possibly) genetic predisposition. Sawicki[49] has tabulated the constituents of the gaseous, vapor and particulate phases of ambient air in terms of background levels, urban levels and levels of high pollution, and has indicated the presence of a wide variety of

TABLE 4

Influence of Occupational and Other Factors Upon BaP Intake

Factor	BaP intake (μg/day)	Cigarette equivalents (packs/day)
Smoking one pack of cigarettes each day	0.4	1.0
Coke oven workers		
Top side exposures	180.0	450.0
Side and bench exposure	70.0	175.0
Coal tar pitch worker	750.0	1875.0
Airplane pilots		
Transatlantic flights	0.93	2.3
Domestic cross country	1.38	3.5
Employee in restaurant	0.8	2.0
Person living near expressway 24 hr/day (adverse meteorology)	0.02	0.05
Commuter on an expressway 2 hr/day (adverse meteorology)	0.04	0.10
Exposure to ambient BaP levels 8 hr/day	0.02	0.05

From Bridbord, K., Finklea, J. F., Wagoner, J. K., Moran, J. B., and Caplan, P., in *Carcinogenesis, Polynuclear Aromatic Hydrocarbons: Chemistry, Metabolism, and Carcinogenesis,* Vol. 1, Freudenthal, R. I. and Jones, P. W., Eds., Raven Press, New York, 1976, 319. With permission.

known carcinogens, co-carcinogens, carcinogen precursors, and potential carcinogens. These include nitrous compounds, alkenes, alkeneoxides, sulfur dioxide, ozone, formaldehyde and other aldehydes, halocarbon compounds (e.g., fluorinated gases, vinyl chloride), hydrocarbons, phenols, nitrosamines and their precursors, chloroalkylethers, para-dioxane and aza arenes, sulfates, aromatic amines, sulfites, unsaturated compounds (e.g., olefinic hydrocarbons), polycyclic aromatic hydrocarbons, and asbestos.[49]

Among these chemical agents, polycyclic aromatic hydrocarbons (PAH) have been studied quite extensively. PAH are combustion products of compounds composed of carbon and hydrogen and generally result from the incomplete combustion of organic matter. They are omnipresent in the environment (aquatic and atmospheric)[35, 50] and are derived from a number of sources including cigarette smoke, heat and power generation, fossil fuel combustion, refuse burning, motor vehicle emissions, coke production, and industrial contaminants.[25,49,51-58] Gross[54] reported on the identification of more than 40 PAH associated with auto exhaust emissions; a number of these are probable human carcinogens. At least as many PAH are likely to be associated with the other environmental sources.

Generally, benzo(a)pyrene (BaP) is accepted as the model PAH. To date, more is known about BaP than that of all other PAH. BaP has been identified as an atmospheric pollutant, comprising 3 to 5% of motor vehicle emissions, as a by-product of char-broiling foods, as an occupational risk factor (e.g., in coal for pitch, in sidewalk and roofing tar), and as a constitutent of cigarette smoke.[51] Measurements of human exposure to PAH generally employ BaP as an index compound.[51] Bridbord et al.[51] have tabulated the relative daily BaP intake of various ambient and occupational exposures and have related these to the number of cigarettes that would have to be consumed per day to obtain an equivalent exposure to BaP by smoking; the data is reproduced here (Table 4). From these data the authors concluded that (1) PAH levels can

TABLE 5

Analysis of the Evaluations Made by Working Groups for Substances Included in *IARC Monographs on the Evaluation of Carcinogenic Risk of Chemicals to Man*

Number of chemicals evaluated	222
Number of chemicals carcinogenic to man	19
Number of chemicals definitely carcinogenic in experimental animals only	111
Number of chemicals producing some carcinogenic effect in experimental animals	42
Number of chemicals for which the data were inadequate for evaluation	32
Number of chemicals for which the available data did not reveal a carcinogenic effect	18

From Preussmann, R., *Oncology*, 33, 51, 1976. With permission.

TABLE 6

Chemicals for Which There Is Unquestionable Evidence of Carcinogenicity in Experimental Animals

Number of chemicals carcinogenic in experimental animals only	111
Human exposure known for	106
Occupational exposure known for	95[a]
Medicinal exposure known for	29
General environmental exposure known for	52[a]

[a] Including 11 to 15 polycyclic aromatic hydrocarbons which occur in soot and tars.

From Preussmann, R., *Oncology*, 33, 51, 1976. With permission.

be attributed to both outdoor as well as indoor exposure with the latter source surprisingly high, (2) the greatest exposure to BaP for smokers is cigarettes, (3) occupational exposure to BaP can amount to exposure levels several orders of magnitude higher than that for tobacco smokers, and (4) motor vehicle emissions are an important source of BaP, although relatively small compared to other sources listed.

Many of the identified job-related carcinogens have yet to be defined with respect to their biologically relevant routes of exposure, although cutaneous, ingestion, and inhalation constitute the main routes and the latter is most likely the primary entry route of many such agents. Occupationally related chemical carcinogens and potential carcinogens include (among others) vinyl chloride,[59-61] bis(chloromethyl)ether,[62-64] certain inhalation anesthetics[65] such as trichloroethylene (which is structurally similar to vinyl chloride, which itself at one time was considered for possible use as an anesthetic for humans), and isoflurane (which is structurally similar to the carcinogenic halogenated ethers bis[chloromethyl]ether and chloromethyl methyl ether), benzoyl chloride,[66] chloroprene (a monomer in manufacture of synthetic rubber),[67,68] and other ingredients employed in rubber manufacture (e.g., β-napthylamine, benzene, asbestos, and certain nitrosamines),[69] coke by-products,[70] BaP,[51,71] benzene,[72] metals (such as copper, aluminum, nickel, lead, cadmium, uranium, arsenic, beryllium, and chromium),[73-79] agricultural chemicals such as certain chlorinated hydrocarbon pesticides[80] (e.g., DDT, aldrin, dieldrin, chlordane, heptachlor, and kepone), and various industrial compounds such as polychlorinated biphenyls,[81] asbestos,[82-86] and fibrous glass.[87]

A number of agents, including several of those discussed above, have been evaluated for carcinogenic risk under the auspices of the International Agency for Research on Cancer (IARC). For summarial purposes, the information available up through 1975 published by IARC[88] is shown in Tables 5, 6, and 7, as presented by Preussmann.[57] In addition, a further detailed breakdown of 94 of the chemical agents examined under the IARC program has been presented by Tomatis[89] and are reproduced here (Tables 8, 9, and 10). It should be noted that some of the studies to date have reported equivocal results and are therefore subject to various interpretations. As time progresses and the data base increases more of these problems should be resolved.

TABLE 7

Chemicals for Which Carcinogenicity to Man or a Strong Suspicion of Carcinogenicity to Man Has Been Found

Chemical	Type of Exposure	Target organ(s)	Route of exposure	Exposure level
Aflatoxin	Dietary	Liver	Oral	5—15 μg/kg body weight/day
4-Aminobiphenyl	Occupational	Bladder	Inhalation, oral	Unknown
Arsenic compounds	Occupational, medicinal	Skin, lung	Oral, inhalation	Unknown
Asbestos (crocidolite, amosite and chrysotile)	Occupational	Lung, pleural cavity, gastrointestinal tract	Inhalation, oral	Unknown
Auramine	Occupational	Bladder	Oral, inhalation, skin	Unknown
Benzene	Occupational	Bone marrow	Inhalation, skin	Unknown
Benzidine	Occupational	Bladder	Inhalation, oral, skin	Unknown
N,N-Bis(2-chloroethyl) 2-naphthylamine	Medicinal	Bladder	Oral	4-350 g (total dose)
Bis(chloromethyl) ether	Occupational	Lung	Inhalation	Unknown
Cadmium oxide	Occupational	Prostate	Inhalation, oral	Unknown
Chromium (chromate-producing industries)	Occupational	Lung	Inhalation	Unknown
Haematite (mining)	Occupational	Lung	Inhalation	Unknown
Melphalan	Medicinal	Bone marrow	Oral	1.2—12 g (total dose)
Mustard gas	Occupational	Lung	Inhalation, skin	0.5—0.7 mg/1
2-Naphthylamine	Occupational	Bladder	Inhalation, oral	Unknown
Nickel (refining)	Occupational	Nasal cavity, lung	Inhalation	Unknown
Soot and tars	Occupational, environmental	Lung skin (scrotom)	Inhalation skin contact	? 320 μg BaP/hr unknown
Stilboestrol	Medicinal	Vagina, uterus	Oral	1.5—150 mg/day
Vinyl chloride	Occupational	Liver, brain, lung	Inhalation, skin	50—3000 ppm

From Preussmann, R., *Oncology*, 33, 51, 1976. With permission.

TABLE 8

94 Chemicals Carcinogenic in Experimental Animals Only

Human exposure known	89
Occupational exposure known	78[a]
Medicinal exposure known	16
General environmental exposure known	49[a]

[a]   Including 15 polycyclic aromatic hydrocarbons present in soot, tar and exhaust fumes.

From Tomatis, L., *Ann. N.Y. Acad. Sci.*, 271, 396, 1976. With permission.

TABLE 9

Chemicals Carcinogenic in Experimental Animals Only

Compound	Unknown	Occupational	Medicinal	General environmental
1. Acetamide		+		
2. 2-Amino-5-(5-nitro-2-furyl)-1,3,4-thiadiazole		+	+	
3. Amitrole		+		+
4. Aramite®		+		+ ?
5. Benz(c)acridine[a]		+		+
6. Benz(a)anthracene[a]		+		+
7. Benzo(b)fluoranthrene[a]		+		+
8. Benzo(j)fluoranthene		+		+
9. Benzo(a)pyrene[a]		+		+
10. Benzo(e)pyrene[a]		+		+
11. Beryl ore		+		
12. Beryllium		+		
13. Beryllium oxide		+		
14. Beryllium phosphate		+		
15. Beryllium sulphate		+		
16. BHC (technical grades)		+		+
17. Cadmium chloride		+		
18. Carbon tetrachloride		+		+
19. Chlorobenzilate		+		+ ?
20. Chrysene[a]		+		+
21. Cycasin				+
22. DDD		+	+	+
23. DDE		+		+
24. DDT		+		+
25. Diazomethane		+		
26. Dibenz(a,h)acridine[a]		+		+
27. Dibenz(a,j)acridine[a]		+		+
28. Dibenz(a,h)anthracene[a]		+		+
29. 7H-Dibenzo(c,g)carbazole[a]				+
30. Dibenzo(a,e)pyrene[a]				+
31. Dibenzo(a,h)pyrene[a]				+
32. Dibenzo(a,i)pyrene[a]				+
33. 3,3′-Dichlorobenzidine		+		
34. Dieldrin		+		+
35. 1,2-diethylhydrazine		+		
36. Diethyl sulphate		+		
37. Dihydrosafrole		+		+
38. 3,3′-Dimethoxybenzidine (o-Dianisidine)		+		
39. trans-2[(Dimethylamino)methylimino]-5-[2-(5-nitro-2-furyl)vinyl]-1,3,4-oxadiazole	+			
40. 3,3′-Dimethylbenzidine (o-Tolidine)		+		
41. 1,1-Dimethylhydrazine		+		
42. 1,2-Dimethylhydrazine		+ ?		
43. Dimethyl sulphate		+		
44. Ethinyloestradiol		+	+	
45. Ethyl methanesulphonate	+			
46. 2-(2-Formylhydrazino)-4-(5-nitro-2-furyl)thiazole	+ ?			
47. Hydrazine		+		
48. Indeno(1,2,3-cd)pyrene[a]		+		+
49. Isonicotinic acid hydrazide		+	+	

TABLE 9 (continued)

Chemicals Carcinogenic in Experimental Animals Only

	Exposure			
Compound	Unknown	Occupational	Medicinal	General environmental
50. Isosafrole		+		+
51. Lead acetate		+		+
52. Lead phosphate		+		
53. Lead subacetate		+		
54. Lindane		+		+
55. Mestranol		+	+	
56. Methylazoxymethanol acetate				+
57. 4,4′-Methylene bis(2-chloro-aniline)		+		
58. 4,4′-Methylene bis(2-methyl-aniline)		+		
59. Methyl methanesulphonate			+	
60. N-Methyl-N′-nitro-N-nitroso-guanidine		+		+
61. Mirex		+	+	
62. 5-(Morpholinomethyl)-3-[(5-nitro-furfurylidine)-amino]-2-oxazoli-dinone		+	+	
63. 4-Nitrobiphenyl		+		
64. 1[5-Nitrofurfurylidene)-amino]-2-imidazolidinone		+	+	
65. N-[4-(5-Nitro-2-furyl)-2-thiazolyl]acetamide		+	+	
66. N-Nitroso-di-n-butylamine	+			
67. N-Nitrosodiethylamine				+
68. N-Nitrosodimethylamine				+
69. Nitrosoethylurea		+		
70. Nitrosomethylurea			+	
71. N-Nitroso-N-methylurethane	+			
72. Oestradiol-17β		+	+	
73. Oestrone		+	+	
74. Polychlorinated biphenyls		+		+
75. 1,3-Propane sultone		+		
76. β-Propiolactone		+		
77. Safrole		+		+
78. Sterigmatocystin				+ ?
79. Streptozotocin		+	+	
80. Thioacetamide		+		
81. Thiourea		+	+	+
82. Urethane		+	+	+
83. para- Aminoazobenzene		+		+
84. ortho-Aminoazotoluene		+		+
85. Chrysoidine		+		+
86. Citrus Red No. 2		+		+
87. para-Dimethylaminoazobenzene		+		+
88. Evans blue		+ ?		
89. Oil Orange SS		+		+
90. Ponceau 3R		+		+
91. Ponceau MX		+		+
92. Sudan I		+		+
93. Trypan Blue		+		+
94. Ethylene thiourea		+		+

a   Present in soot and tars.

From Tomatis, L., *Ann. N. Y. Acad. Sci.*, 271, 396, 1976. With permission.

TABLE 10

41 Chemicals with Limited Carcinogenic Activity in Experimental Animals Only

Human exposure known	35
Occupational exposure known	34
Medicinal exposure known	17
General environmental exposure known	7

From Tomatis, L., *Ann. N. Y. Acad. Sci.*, 271, 396, 1976. With permission.

IV. IDENTIFICATION OF CHEMICAL CARCINOGENS

Obviously, in order to gain insight into the etiology of cancer, it is necessary to make estimations of cancer incidences using retrospective analyses.[11-13,90] However, to limit the influence of the environment on the etiology of human cancer, it is also necessary to identify and eliminate potentially carcinogenic environmental agents which are continually being introduced into the environment, or at the very least, control the degree of human exposure. To accomplish this task it has become necessary to design testing procedures by which to assign a specific biological risk associated with specific chemicals or classes of chemicals. During the last decade a number of in vitro and in vivo short-term tests have been developed by which to screen for such environmental carcinogens (and mutagens).[91-95] Advances continually being made in this approach make it a "state-of-the-art" situation, which is constantly being updated.

Of the available in vitro bioassay systems, bacterial and mammalian cell systems are among the most widely used short-term procedures by which to evaluate the potential adverse effects of chemicals. A correlation between bacterial mutagenicity and mammalian carcinogenicity has been reported.[96-99] If this correlation proves to be valid and if these tests can detect carcinogens as mutagens, then the task of identifying and regulating these agents will be simplified. In this respect, it would seem feasible to prescreen potential carcinogens for their mutagenicity prior to assessing the neoplastic potential in mammalian systems. This approach would afford a rational basis for the selection of compounds to be tested in the latter systems. Those compounds which prove to be mutagenic for bacteria in the prescreen could be evaluated for their potential mutagenic and/or carcinogenic effects to mammalian cells in culture (see References 100-102 for reviews). Nevertheless, a negative result in the bacterial mutagenicity test may only reflect the limitations of the test system. Therefore, to rely on any single test as *the* indicator of the safe or hazardous nature of an agent is not recommended. The general consensus among those actively involved in the screening program is that a battery of tests (consisting mainly of short-term bioassays — both in vitro and in vivo) can help rapidly identify agents which may be potentially biohazardous and those which may require detailed analysis in long-term in vivo studies. This approach is useful not only in the examination of substances to which the population is currently exposed, but also in the early developmental stages of new agents prior to introduction into the environment. It is unreasonable to assume that all such evaluations can be performed only in long-term animal test systems, and consequently the need has arisen for sensitive, reproducible, reliable, rapid and more economical in vitro tests and short-term in vivo tests. It is also important to recognize other biological consequences associated with chemical agents (e.g., toxic and teratogenic effects) and thus the endpoints of such bioassays cannot be limited to mutagenicity and carcinogenicity alone.

Of course, results obtained from such bioassays are necessarily limited by the sensitivity each offers as a means to identify potentially biohazardous materials. Bioassay systems must be judiciously selected with regard to sensitivity, reliability, metabolic and macromolecular target similarities to humans, exposure requirements (dose and time), and economy. The utility of such bioassays will rest mainly in the confidence to extrapolate test results to man for human risk assessment.

V. ROLE OF GOVERNMENT AGENCIES IN THE CONTROL OF EXPOSURE TO CHEMICAL CARCINOGENS

Results collected by various procedures including epidemiologic studies, short-term and long-term in vitro and in vivo bioassays, as well as investigations into the molecular mechanisms of carcinogenesis, have established a data base which should be helpful in ascertaining the etiology of cancer. However, there is still much information to be obtained regarding (1) those multifactorial interactions (e.g., risk and host factors) which influence cancer susceptibility, (2) identification of occupationally-related and other environmental carcinogenic agents, and (3) populations at risk to chemically-induced cancer. Nevertheless, the scientific knowledge gathered thus far has enabled regulatory agencies to begin formulating guidelines for the identification of hazardous substances, evaluation of risk vs. benefit factors, determination of "acceptable" levels of exposure and defining those agents which should be banned from use.

Passage of Public Law 94-469 on October 11, 1976 created a job of staggering proportions for a large segment of American industry. Known as the Toxic Substances Control Act (TOSCA), the law authorized the Government to prescribe standards for the development of test data and to require the testing of chemical substances (or mixtures) which by their manufacture, distribution, processing, use or disposal, could present an unreasonable risk of injury to health or to the environment.

No one really knows how many chemical substances in common use could be affected by this legislation. However, in November 1977, Chemical Abstracts Service registry of chemicals contained 4,039,907 distinct entities, with an average growth rate of 6,000 chemicals per week. Recent EPA estimates indicate that safety determinations could be required for as many as 63,000 commonly used chemicals. This number will continue to grow rapidly as new products are developed.

One of the most important categories of chemicals to be tested are the pesticides, as regulated by the Federal Insecticide, Fungicide and Rodenticide Act (FIFRA), Amended. Approximately 3,500 active pesticide ingredients need to be reregistered. Nearly 70% of these need additional long-term evaluation in one or more species, and 85 to 90% need data on possible teratogenic effects of these chemicals. Of those compounds for which inhalation studies are applicable, 90% will have to be studied by this mode of application. In addition to these active ingredients requiring long-term biological studies for carcinogenicity and soon-to-be published required studies for mutagenicity, there are some 35,000 final formulations, all of which require the same types of studies as indicated above.

Several Federal Government research and development and regulatory and enforcement branches including National Cancer Institute (NCI), Department of Defense (DOD), Department of Transportation (DOT), Department of Energy (DOE), Environmental Protection Agency — Office of Toxic Substances (EPA-OTS), Food and Drug Administration (FDA), National Institute of Occupational Safety and Health Administration (OSHA); and Drug Enforcement Administration (DEA) have already experienced difficulties in finding qualified contractors to perform their required studies. One NCI program alone, the Carcinogenesis Bioassay Program, is funded at approximately $47 million and is actively searching for new subcontractors.

Also within the EPA, the OTS is charged with administering and implementing TOSCA and will have jurisdiction over the safety of some 500,000 chemicals, approximately 15,000 of which have proven toxicity of some form. Biological test data have not been generated for most of these chemicals. In addition, approximately 1000 new chemicals are introduced into the environment each year with little or no knowledge of the effects to man or the environment.

The FDA is taking a hard look at the GRAS list (Generally Recognized as Safe) of which there are approximately 800 compounds with little or no long-term data, approximately 2600 food additives with little or no long-term data, innumerable dyes of which currently only a small number are under test, and at least 10,000 other agents such as flavors, cosmetics and toiletries, none of which have been tested in long-term animal studies.

The number of compounds requiring testing by OSHA, DOT, DOD, DOE, etc., is staggering even by conservative estimates, with respect to environmental substances. Many of these, if not all, will require eye and dermal irritation studies. Almost all of them require some form of long-term animal studies, mutagenicity assays, and a good proportion of them will require inhalation studies.

The number of facilities currently available to undertake the herculean task of performing studies on the toxic, carcinogenic, mutagenic, teratogenic, behavioral and synergistic effects of these compounds cannot begin to meet the demand from Government and industry. The funds available for such testing in the United States during fiscal year 1979 alone are only approximately $100 million and in Europe, approximately $50 million.

With regard to the regulatory requirements for product safety evaluation and the future legislation which will mandate testing, there are currently no known federal regulations at this time which require either mutagenicity, carcinogenicity, or short-term testing. EPA's guidelines for pesticides, under FIFRA are expected to be published shortly. TOSCA remains to be implemented. OSHA's carcinogen standards are not yet finalized. The Consumer Product Safety Commission has published their recommendations for this testing in the *Federal Register*, but these were not preferred as requirements. DOT and DOD have made suggestions but no formal requirements, and Section 3001 of the Resources, Recovery and Conservation Act (RECRA) must be rewritten.

VI. CONCLUSIONS

From the foregoing discussion it is obvious that man is exposed to innumerable biohazardous agents which can register their effects at many different levels (e.g., molecular, cellular, tissue, organ, and organism). These effects can be registered as various biological events including cytotoxic, mutagenic, carcinogenic, and teratogenic effects. The ubiquitous nature of chemical carcinogens makes controlling them a complex and major task. Federal regulatory agencies are making attempts to govern human subjection to such agents at the level of environmental exposure; as yet insufficient information is available for imposing control at the biological level. The development of reliable in vitro and in vivo bioassays will allow educated decisions to be made regarding the safe or hazardous nature of an agent, and how best to limit man's exposure to those agents considered deleterious. It remains to be determined the extent to which man can cope with the exposure levels of such agents to which he is subjected. Ongoing studies in various laboratories dealing with uptake, exposure, and distribution of chemical carcinogens, the influence of genetic factors on chemical carcinogenesis, the role of metabolism in chemical carcinogenesis and the identification of potentially carcinogenic agents through use of both short-term and long-term in vitro and in vivo bioassays, should shed some light on both the mechanism of chemical carcinogenesis and the identification of potential chemical carcinogens. Some of these aspects will be covered in great detail in succeeding chapters.

ACKNOWLEDGMENTS

The authors wish to express their appreciation to Ms. M. A. Montgomery for her assistance in compiling information regarding federal agencies, and to Ms. D. Foer for her clerical assistance.

REFERENCES

1. **Lehmann, P.,** *Cancer and the Worker,* New York Academy of Sciences, New York, 1977.
2. **Poland, A., Glover, E., and Kende, A. S.,** Stereospecific, high affinity binding of 2,3,7,8-tetrachlorodibenzo-p-dioxin by hepatic cytosol. Evidence that the binding species is receptor for induction of aryl hydrocarbon hydroxylase, *J. Biol. Chem.,* 251, 2936, 1976.
3. **Wilding, G., Paigen, B., Vessel, E. S.,** Genetic control of interindividual variations in racemic warfarin binding to plasma and albumin of twins, *Clin. Pharmacol. Ther.,* 22, 831, 1977.
4. **Flamant, R.,** Epidemiological research on the relationship between tobacco, alcohol and cancer, *Prog. Biochem. Pharmacol.,* 14, 36, 1978.
5. World Health Organization, Prevention of Cancer, Tech. Rep. Ser. No. 276, World Health Organization, Geneva, 1964.
6. **Pott, P.,** Cancer scrotic, in *Chirurgical Observations,* Hawes, Clarke and Collins, London, 1775, 63.
7. **Muir, C. S.,** Geographical differences in cancer patterns, in *Host Environmental Interactions in the Etiology of Cancer in Man,* No. 7, Doll, R. and Vodopija, J., Eds., IARC Scientific Publications, Lyon, France, 1.
8. **Armstrong, B. and Doll, R.,** Environmental factors and cancer incidence and mortality in different countries, with special reference to dietary practices, *Br. J. Cancer,* 15, 617, 1975.
9. **Berg, J. W.,** World-wide variations in cancer incidence as clues to cancer origins, in *Origins of Human Cancer,* Book A, Hiatt, H. H., Watson, J. D., and Winsten, J. A., Eds., Cold Spring Harbor Laboratory, New York, 1977, 15.
10. **Blot, W. J., Mason, T. J., Hoover, R., and Fraumeni, J. F.,** Cancer by county: etiologic implications, in *Origins of Human Cancer,* Book A, Hiatt, H. H., Watson, J. D., and Winsten, J. A., Eds., Cold Spring Harbor Laboratory, New York, 1977, 21.
11. **Mason, T. J. and McKay, F. W.,** U.S. Cancer Mortality by County: 1950-1969, DHEW Publ. No. (NIH) 74-615, U. S. Government Printing Office, Washington, D.C., 1973.
12. **Mason, T. J., McKay, F. W., Hoover, R., Blot, W. J., and Fraumeni, J. F., Jr.,** Atlas of Cancer Mortality for U.S. Counties: 1950-1969, DHEW Publ. No. (NIH) 75-780, U.S. Government Printing Office, Washington, D.C., 1975.
13. **Clemmesen, J.,** Statistical studies in the aetiology of malignant neoplasms. V. Trends and risks, *Acta Pathol. Microbiol. Scand.,* Suppl., 261, 1977.
14. **Hammond, E. D.,** The epidemiological approach to the etiology of cancer, *Cancer,* 35, 652, 1975.
15. **Wagoner, J. K.,** Occupational carcinogenesis: the two hundred years since Percivall Pott, *Ann. N. Y. Acad. Sci.,* 271, 1, 1976.
16. **Doll, R.,** Introduction, in *Origins of Human Cancer,* Book A, Hiatt, H. H., Watson, J. D., and Winsten, J. A., Eds., Cold Spring Harbor Laboratory, New York, 1977, 1.
17. **Kouri, R. E., Rude, T. H., Curren, R. D., Brandt, K. C., Sosnowski, R. G., Schechtman, L. M., Benedict, W. M., and Henry, C. J.,** Biological activity of tobacco smoke and tobacco smoke-related chemicals, *Environ. Health Perspect.,* 29, 63, 1979.
18. **Reif, A. E.,** Public information on smoking: an urgent responsibility for cancer research workers, *J. Nat. Cancer Inst.,* 57, 1207, 1976.

19. **Bingham, E., Niemeier, R. W., and Reid, J. B.,** Multiple factors in carcinogenesis, *Ann. N. Y. Acad. Sci.,* 271, 14, 1976.

20. **Upton, A. C.,** Radiation effects, in *Origins of Human Cancer,* Book A, Hiatt, H. H., Watson, J. D., and Winsten, J. A., Eds., Cold Spring Harbor Laboratory, New York, 1977, 477.

21. **Hutchison, G. B.,** Carcinogenic effects of medical irradiation, in *Origins of Human Cancer,* Book A, Hiatt, H. H., Watson, J. D., and Winsten, J. A., Eds., Cold Spring Harbor Laboratory, New York, 1977, 501.

22. **Scott, E. L. and Stref, M. L.,** Ultraviolet radiation as a cause of cancer, in *Origins of Human Cancer,* Book A, Hiatt, H. H., Watson, J. D., and Winsten, J. A., Eds., Cold Spring Harbor Laboratory, New York, 1977, 529.

23. **Linsell, C. A. and Peers, F. G.,** Field studies on liver cell cancer, in *Origins of Human Cancer,* Book A, Hiatt, H. H., Watson, J. D., and Winsten, J. A., Eds., Cold Spring Harbor Laboratory, New York, 1977, 549.

24. **Armstrong, B. K.,** The role of diet in human carcinogenesis with special reference to endometrial cancer, in *Origins of Human n Cancer,* Book A, Hiatt, H. H., Watson, J. D., and Winsten, J. A., Eds., Cold Spring Harbor Laboratory, New York, 1977, 557.

25. **Weisburger, J. H., Cohen, L. A., and Wynder, E. L.,** On the etiology and metabolic epidemiology of the main human cancers, in *Origins of Human Cancer,* Book A, Hiatt, H. H., Watson, J. D., and Winsten, J. A., Eds., Cold Spring Harbor Laboratory, New York, 1977, 567.

26. **Wynder, E. L., Peters, J. A., Vivona, S.,** Nutrition in the causation of cancer, *Cancer Res.,* 35, 3238, 1975.

27. **McLean, A. E. M. and Magee, P. N.,** Increased renal carcinogenesis by dimethylnitrosamine in protein deficient rats, *Br. J. Exp. Pathol.,* 51, 587, 1970.

28. **McLean, A. E. M.,** Diet and the chemical environment as modifiers of carcinogenesis, in *Host-Environmental Interactions in the Etiology of Cancer in Man,* No. 7, Doll, R. and Vodopija, J., Eds., IARC Scientific Publications, Lyon, France, 223.

29. **Miller, J. A.,** Naturally occurring substances that can induce tumors, in *Toxicants Occurring Naturally in Foods,* Strong, F. M., Ed., National Academy of Sciences, Washington, D. C., 1973, 508.

30. **Miller, J. A. and Miller, E. C.,** Carcinogens occurring naturally in foods, *Fed. Proc.,* 35, 1316, 1976.

31. **Tazima, Y.,** Naturally occurring mutagens of biological origin, *Mutat. Res.,* 26, 225, 1974.

32. **Kraybill, H. F.,** Global distribution of carcinogenic pollutants in water, *Ann. N.Y. Acad. Sci.,* 298, 80, 1977.

33. **Kraybill, H. F.,** Distribution of chemical carcinogens in aquatic environments, *Prog. Exp. Tumor Res.,* 20, 3, 1976.

34. **Harris, R. H., Page, T., and Reiches, N. A.,** Carcinogenic hazards of organic chemicals in drinking water, in *Origins of Human Cancer,* Book A, Hiatt, H. H., Watson, J. D., and Winsten, J. A., Eds., Cold Spring Harbor Laboratory, New York, 1977, 309.

35. *Aquatic Pollutants and Biologic Effects with Emphasis on Neoplasia,* Kraybill, H. F,, Daive, C. J., Harshbarger, J. C., and Tardiff, R. G., Eds., New York Academy of Sciences, New York, 1977.

36. **Stich, H. F. and Acton, A. B.,** The possible use of fish tumors in monitoring for carcinogens in the marine environment, *Prog. Exp. Tumor Res.,* 20, 44, 1976.

37. **Dunn, B. P. and Stich, H. F.,** Release of the carcinogen benzo(a)pyrene from environmentally contaminated mussels, *Bull. Environ. Contam. Toxicol.,* 15, 398, 1976.

38. **Dunn, B. P. and Stich, H. F.,** The use of mussels in estimating benzo(a)pyrene contamination of the marine environment, *Proc. Soc. Exp. Biol. Med.,* 150, 49, 1975.

39. **Hoover, R.,** Effects of drugs — immunosuppression, in *Origins of Human Cancer,* Book A, Hiatt, H. H., Watson, J. D., and Winsten, J. A., Eds., Cold Spring Harbor Laboratory, New York, 1977, 369.

40. **Weiss, N. S.,** Exogenous estrogens and the incidence of neoplasms in tissues of müllerian origin, in *Origins of Human Cancer,* Book A, Hiatt, H. H., Watson, J. D., and Winsten, J. A., Eds., Cold Spring Harbor Laboratory, New York, 1977, 413.

41. **Pike, M. C., Edmondson, H. A., Benton, B., and Henderson, B. E.,** Liver adenomas and oral contraceptives, in *Origins of Human Cancer,* Book A, Hiatt, H. H., Watson, J. D., and Winsten, J. A., Eds., Cold Spring Harbor Laboratory, New York, 1977, 423.

42. **Adamson, R. H. and Sieber, S. M.,** Antineoplastic agents as potential carcinogens, in *Origins of Human Cancer,* Book A, Hiatt, H. H., Watson, J. D., and Winsten, J. A., Eds., Cold Spring Harbor Laboratory, New York, 1977, 429.

43. **Bueding, E. and Batzinger, R. P.,** Hycanthone and other antischistosomal drugs: lack of obligatory association between chemotherapeutic effects and mutagenic activity, in *Origins of Human Cancer,* Book A, Hiatt, H. H., Watson, J. D., Winsten, J. A., Eds., Cold Spring Harbor Laboratory, New York, 1977, 445.

44. **Goldman, P., Ingelfinger, J. A., and Friedman, P. A.,** Metronidazole, isoniazid, and the threat of human cancer, in *Origins of Human Cancer,* Book A, Hiatt, H. H., Watson, J. D., and Winsten, J. A., Eds., Cold Spring Harbor Laboratory, New York, 1977, 465.

45. **Herbst, A. L., Scully, R. E., Robboy, S. J., Welch, W. R., and Cole, P.,** Abnormal development of the human genital tract following prenatal exposure to diethystilbestrol, in *Origins of Human Cancer,* Book A, Hiatt, H. H., Watson, J. D., and Winsten, J. A., Eds., Cold Spring Harbor Laboratory, New York, 1977, 399.

46. **Jick, H. and Smith, P. G.,** Regularly used drugs and cancer, in *Origins of Human Cancer,* Book A, Hiatt, H. H., Watson, J. D., and Winsten, Eds., Cold Spring Harbor Laboratory, New York, 1977, 389.

47. **Hammond, E. C., Garfinkel, L., Seidman, H., and Lew, E. A.,** Some recent findings concerning cigarette smoking, in *Origins of Human Cancer,* Book A, Hiatt, H. H., Watson, J. D., and Winsten, J. A., Eds., Cold Spring Harbor Laboratory, New York, 1977, 101.

48. **Higginson, J. and Jensen, O. M.,** Epidemiological review of lung cancer in man, in *Air Pollution and Cancer in Man,* No. 16, Mohr, U., Schmähl, D., Tomatis, L., Eds., IARC Scientific Publications, Lyon, France, 1977, 169.

49. **Sawicki, E.,** Chemical composition and potential "genotoxic" aspects of polluted atmospheres, in *Air Pollution and Cancer in Man,* No. 16, Mohr, U., Schmähl, D., and Tomatis, L., Eds., IARC Scientific Publications, Lyon, France, 1977, 127.

50. **Mohr, U., Schmähl, D., and Tomatis, L., Eds.,** *Air Pollution and Cancer in Man,* No. 16, IARC Scientific Publications, Lyon, France, 1977.

51. **Bridbord, K., Finklea, J. F., Wagoner, J. K., Moran, J. B., and Caplan, P.,** Human exposure to polynuclear aromatic hydrocarbons, in *Carcinogenesis, Polynuclear Aromatic Hydrocarbons: Chemistry, Metabolism, and Carcinogenesis,* Vol. 1, Freudenthal, R. I. and Jones, P. W., Eds., Raven Press, New York, 1976, 319.

52. **Davies, I. W., Harrison, R. M., Perry, R., Ratnayaka, D., and Wellings, R. A.,** Municipal incinerator as a source of polynuclear aromatic hydrocarbons in the environment, *Environ. Sci. Technol.,* 10, 451, 1976.

53. **Hayatsu, R., Scott, R. G., Moore, L. P., and Studier, M. H.,** Aromatic units in coal, *Nature,* 257, 378, 1975.

54. **Gross, G. P.,** Gasoline Composition and Vehicle Exhaust Gas Polynuclear Aromatic Content, 2nd and 3rd Ann. Rep., CRC-APRAC, Proj. No. CAPE-6-68, Coordinating Research Council.

55. **Sawicki, E.,** Airborne carcinogens and allied compounds, *Arch. Environ. Health,* 14, 46, 1967.

56. **Grimmer, G.,** Analysis of automobile exhaust condensates, in *Air Pollution and Cancer in Man,* No. 16, Mohr, U., Schmähl, D., and Tomatis, L., Eds., IARC Scientific Publications, Lyon, France, 1977, 29.

57. **Preussmann, R.,** Chemical carcinogens in the human environment: problems and quantitative aspects, *Oncology,* 33, 51, 1976.

58. **Schmeltz, I. and Hoffman, D.,** Formation of polynuclear aromatic hydrocarbons from combustion of organic matter, in *Carcinogenesis, Polynuclear Aromatic Hydrocarbons: Chemistry, Metabolism, and Carcinogenesis,* Vol. 1, Freudenthal, R. I. and Jones, P. W., Eds., Raven Press, New York, 1976, 225.

59. **Waxweiler, R. J., Stringer, W., Wagoner, J. K., and Jones, J.,** Neoplastic risk among workers exposed to vinyl chloride, *Ann. N. Y. Acad. Sci.,* 271, 40, 1976.

60. **Infante, P. F.,** Oncogenic and mutagenic risks in communities with polyvinyl chloride production facilities, *Ann. N. Y. Acad. Sci.,* 271, 49, 1976.

61. **Maltoni, C.,** Vinyl chloride carcinogenicity: an experimental model for carcinogenesis studies, in *Origins of Human Cancer,* Book A, Hiatt, H. H., Watson, J. D., and Winsten, J. A., Eds., Cold Spring Harbor Laboatory, New York, 1977, 119.

62. **Nelson, N.,** The chloroethers — occupational carcinogens: a summary of laboratory and epidemiology studies, *Ann. N. Y. Acad. Sci.,* 271, 81, 1976.

63. **Lemen, R. A., Johnson, W. M., Wagoner, J. K., Archer, V. E., and Saccomanno, G.,** Cytologic observations and cancer incidence following exposure to BCME, *Ann. N. Y. Acad. Sci.,* 271, 71, 1976.

64. **Nelson, N.,** The carcinogenicity of chloro ethers and related compounds: a brief note, in *Origins of Human Cancer,* Book A, Hiatt, H. H., Watson, J. D., Winsten, J. A., Eds., Cold Spring Harbor Laboratory, New York, 1977, 115.

65. **Corbett, T. H.,** Cancer and congenital anomalies associated with anesthetics, *Ann. N. Y. Acad. Sci.,* 271, 58, 1976.

66. **Sakabe, H., Matsushita, H., and Koshi, S.,** Cancer among benzoyl chloride manufacturing workers, *Ann. N. Y. Acad. Sci.,* 271, 67, 1976.

67. **Lloyd, J. W.**, Cancer risks among workers exposed to chloroprene, *Ann. N. Y. Acad. Sci.*, 291, 91, 1976.
68. **Infante, P. F., Wagoner, J. K., and Young, R. J.**, Chloroprene: Observations of carcinogenesis and mutagenesis, in *Origins of Human Cancer*, Book A, Hiatt, H. H., Watson, J. D., and Winsten, J. A., Eds., Cold Spring Harbor Laboratory, New York, 1977, 205.
69. **McMichael, A. J., Andjelkovic, D. A., and Tyroler, H. A.**, Cancer mortality among rubber workers: an epidemiologic study, *Ann. N. Y. Acad. Sci.*, 271, 125, 1976.
70. **Redmond, C. K., Strobino, B. R., and Cypess, R. H.**, Cancer experience among coke by-product workers, *Ann. N. Y. Acad. Sci.*, 271, 102, 1976.
71. **Hammond, E. C., Selikoff, I. J., Lawther, P. L., and Seidman, H.**, Inhalation of benzpyrene and cancer in man, *Ann. N. Y. Acad. Sci.*, 271, 116, 1976.
72. **Vigliani, E. C.**, Leukemia associated with benzene exposure, *Ann. N. Y. Acad. Sci.*, 271, 143, 1976.
73. **Milham, S., Jr.**, Cancer mortality patterns associated with exposure to metals, *Ann. N. Y. Acad. Sci.*, 271, 243, 1976.
74. **Newman, J. A., Archer, V. E., Saccomanno, G., Kuschner, M., Auerbach, O., Brondahl, R. D., and Wilson, J. C.**, Histologic types of bronchogenic carcinomas among members of copper-mining and smelting communities, *Ann. N. Y. Acad. Sci.*, 271, 260, 1976.
75. **Doll, R.**, Cancer of the lung and nose in nickel workers, *Br. J. Ind. Med.*, 15, 217, 1958.
76. **Cooper, W. C.**, Cancer mortality patterns in the lead industry, *Ann. N. Y. Acad. Sci.*, 271, 250, 1976.
77. **Lemen, R. A., Lee, J. S., Wagoner, J. K., and Blejer, H. P.**, Cancer mortality among cadmium production workers, *Ann. N. Y. Acad. Sci.*, 271, 273, 1976.
78. **Archer, V. E., Gillam, J. D., and Wagoner, J. K.**, Respiratory disease mortality among uranium miners, *Ann. N. Y. Acad. Sci.*, 271, 280, 1976.
79. **Hernberg, S.**, Incidence of cancer in population with exceptional exposure to metals, in *Origins of Human Cancer*, Book A, Hiatt, H. H., Watson, J. D., and Winsten, J. A., Eds., Cold Spring Harbor Laboratory, New York, 1977, 147.
80. **Epstein, S. S.**, The carcinogenicity of organochlorine pesticides, in *Origins of Human Cancer*, Book A, Hiatt, H. H., Watson, J. D., and Winsten, J. A., Eds., Cold Spring Harbor Laboratory, New York, 1977, 243.
81. **Allen, J. R. and Norback, D. H.**, Carcinogenic potential of the polychlorinated biphenyls, in *Origins of Human Cancer*, Book A, Hiatt, H. H., Watson, J. D., and Winsten, J. A., Eds., Cold Spring Harbor Laboratory, New York, 1977, 173.
82. **Morgan, R. W. and Shettigara, P. T.**, Occupational asbestos exposure, smoking, and laryngeal carcinoma, *Ann. N. Y. Acad. Sci.*, 271, 308, 1976.
83. **Anderson, H. A., Lilis, R., Daum, S. M., Fischbein, A. S., and Selikoff, I. J.**, Household-contact asbestos neoplastic risk, *Ann. N. Y. Acad. Sci.*, 271, 311, 1976.
84. **Gillam, J. D., Dement, J. M., Lemen, R. A., Wagoner, J. K., Archer, V. E., and Blejer, H. P.**, Mortality patterns among hard rock gold miners exposed to an asbestiform mineral, *Ann.N. Y. Acad. 3Sci.*, 271, 336, 1976.
85. **Dement, J. M., Zumwalde, R. D., and Wallingford, K. M.**, Discussion paper: asbestos fiber exposures in a hard rock gold mine, *Ann. N. Y. Acad. Sci.*, 271, 345, 1976.
86. **Selikoff, I. J.**, Lung cancer and mesothelioma during prospective surveillance of 1249 asbestos insulation workers, 1963-1974, *Ann. N. Y. Acad, Sci.*, 271, 448, 1976.
87. **Bayliss, D. L., Dement, J. M., Wagoner, J. K., and Blejer, H. P.**, Mortality patterns among fibrous glass production workers, *Ann. N. Y. Acad. Sci.*, 271, 324, 1976.
88. **IARC**, Ann. Rep. 90-91, 1975, IARC, Monographs on the Evaluation of Carcinogenic Risk of Chemicals to Man, Vol. 1-14, 1972-1977.
89. **Tomatis, L.**, The IARC program on the evaluation of the carcinogenic risk of chemicals to man, *Ann. N. Y. Acad. Sci.*, 271, 396, 1976.
90. **Kolbye, A. C., Jr.**, Cancer in humans: exposures and responses in a real world, *Oncology*, 33, 90, 1976.
91. **Montesano, R. and Tomatis, L.**, Eds., *Chemical Carcinogenesis Essays*, No. 10, IARC Scientific Publications, Lyon, France, 1974.
92. **Montesano, R., Bartsch, H., and Tomatis, L.**, Eds., *Screening Tests in Chemical Carcinogenesis*, No. 12, IARC Scientific Publications, Lyon, France, 1976.
93. **Berky, J. and Sherrod, P. C.**, Eds., *Short-term In Vitro Testing for Carcinogenesis, Mutagenesis and Toxicity*, Franklin Institute Press, Philadelphia, 1978.
94. **Kilbey, B. J., Legator, M., Nichols, W., and Ramel, C.**, Eds., *Handbook of Mutagenicity Test Procedures*, Elsevier, New York, 1977.
95. **Hollaender, A.**, Ed., *Chemical Mutagens, Principles and Methods for their Detection*, Vol. 1-4, Plenum Press, New York, NY, 1971.

96. McCann, J., Choi, E., Yamasaki, E., and Ames, B. N., Detection of carcinogens as mutagens in the Salmonella/microsome test: assay of 300 chemicals, *Proc. Nat. Acad. Sci. U.S.A.*, 72, 5135, 1975.

97. Ames, B. N., McCann, J., and Yamasaki, E., Carcinogens are mutagens: a simple test system, *Mutat. Res.*, 33, 27, 1975.

98. McCann, J., Springarn, N. E., Kobori, J., and Ames, B. N., Detection of carcinogens as mutagens: bacterial tester strains with R factor plasmids, *Proc. Nat. Acad. Sci. U.S.A.*, 72, 979, 1975.

99. Ames, B. N., Durston, W. E., Yamasaki, E., and Lee, F. D., Carcinogens are mutagens: a simple test system combining liver homogenates for activation and bacteria for detection, *Proc. Nat. Acad. Sci. U.S.A.*, 70 2281, 1973.

100. Schechtman, L. M., State of the art: chemically induced mammalian cell mutagenesis and transformation, in *Proc. of the Workshop on Methodology for Assessing Reproductive Hazards in the Workplace*, National Institute for Occupational Health and Society for Occupational and Environmental Health, Submitted.

101. Heidelberger, C., Chemical carcinogenesis, *Ann. Rev. Biochem.*, 44, 79, 1975.

102. Heidelberger, C., Chemical oncogenesis in culture, *Adv. Cancer Res.*, 18, 317, 1973.

Chapter 2

METABOLISM OF CHEMICAL CARCINOGENS

Richard E. Kouri, Leonard M. Schechtman, and Daniel W. Nebert

TABLE OF CONTENTS

I. INTRODUCTION

The previous chapter has discussed at length some of the recent epidemiological data which have created a growing concern that environmental chemicals may be responsible for a considerable proportion of all human cancers. Most of these chemicals are so lipophilic that they would remain in the body indefinitely were it not for phase I and phase II enzyme systems.[1] During phase I metabolism, one or more polar groups (such as hydroxyl) are introduced ino the parent molecule thereby presenting the phase II conjugating systems (such as UDP glucuronosyltransferase) with a substrate. These conjugates are sufficiently polar to be excreted from the cell and from the body. Thus the raison d'etre for many of these enzyme systems is to make many of these lipophilic compounds water soluble so that they can be excreted from the body.

Recent work has shown that one particular group of enzymes known collectively as the cytochrome P-450 mediated monooxygenases[2,3] is very important in the metabolism of a great many exogenous and/or endogenous chemical compounds. These multicomponent membrane-bound enzyme systems metabolize exogenous compounds such as polycyclic aromatic hydrocarbons, halogenated hydrocarbons, insecticides, ingredients in soaps, and deodorants, strong mutagens such as N-methyl-N′-nitro-N-nitrosoguanidine, nitrosamines, aminoazo dyes and diazo compounds, N-acetyl-arylamines and nitrofurans, numerous aromatic amines such as those found in hair dyes, nitro aromatics and heterocyclics, wood terpenes, epoxides, carbonates, alkylhalides, safrole derivatives, certain fungal toxins and antibiotics, many chemotherapeutic agents used to treat human cancer, most drugs, and even such simple compounds such as vinyl chloride. Endogenous compounds, like steroids, biogenic amines, indoles, thyroxine and fatty acids all serve as substrates for this enzyme complex.[4-9] Many of these aforementioned substrates are, in fact, metabolized to more biologically active forms as the result of the activity of these enzyme systems. An example of such compounds are benzo(a)pyrene (BP), 3-methylcholanthrene, dimethylnitrosamine and vinyl chloride. On the other hand, compounds such as N-methyl-N′-nitro-N-nitrosoguanidine[10] or sodium dichromate, sodium azide, and captan[11] are in fact detoxified by the action of these enzyme systems. The active intermediates from many of these compounds are thought to be reactive species such as carbonium ions or alkylating agents.[12] Both species act as electrophiles and seem to be capable of random damage to critical cellular macromolecules thereby leading to such biological effects like cytotoxicity, mutation, and cancer.

Because of the complexity of these monooxygenases and the presence of phase II conjugating enzyme systems, it is very important to consider that the fate of a particular chemical resides in a delicate balance between those enzymes capable of potentiating the effects of these chemicals and those enzymes capable of detoxifying these chemicals to their reactive intermediates. Thus, within a given tissue or cell, a multitude of potential pathways exist for the metabolism of almost any of these chemical compounds. One recent approach has been suggested as a simple method to break down these rather complex series of reactions to a controllable number of individual steps. This approach takes advantage of the fact that there is very often a rate-limiting step in these complex series of reactions so that regardless of the length of the number of steps involved in a specific pathway, one individual step is usually much slower than all the rest and hence determines the average rate of the the whole process of steps. The questions then become:

1.   Can we identify which of these steps is rate-limiting?

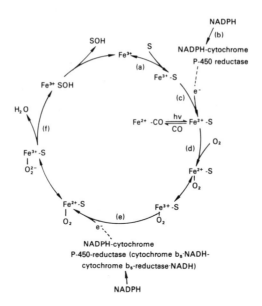

FIGURE 1. Mechanism of microsomal cytochrome P-450-dependent hydroxylations. (From Estabrook, R. W., Hildebrandt, A. G., Baron, J., Ritter, K. J., and Liebman, K., *Biochem., Biophys.
Res. Commun.*, 42, 132, 1971. With permission.)

2.   Are there naturally-occurring variations in the level of activity of this particular
      step?
3.   Is there a genetic basis for the regulation of these naturally-occurring differences?
4.   Can these differences result from the action of a single gene or multiple genes?
5.   Is there genetic linkage between the presence or absence of this locus and a bio-
      logical effect?

These rather basic approaches have been used very nicely not only to break down and
analyze the rate-limiting step in monooxygenase metabolism, but also to correlate the
levels of these enzymes to such biological endpoints as carcinogenesis, mutagenesis,
and cytotoxicity. In this chapter we would like to review the data which suggest that
there are naturally-occurring variations in the steady-state levels of these monooxygenases; that these naturally-occurring variations are under host-gene regulation by a small
number of genes; that there is a genetic correlation between levels of these enzymes
and such biological endpoints as mutagenicity, carcinogenicity, and cytotoxicity; and
that metabolism at specific positions of many of these chemicals carcinogens is associated with generation of mutagenic and/or carcinogenic intermediates. We will also
attempt to update the information regarding the existence of genetic regulation of
monooxygenase activity in man and its potential role in determining susceptibility of
man to chemical carcinogenesis.

II. THE MIXED FUNCTION OXIDASES

A. General Characteristics
   A postulated scheme for microsomal electron transport reactions associated with
cytochrome P-450 function and the monooxygenase activities is shown in Figure 1.

The following steps have been suggested (see Reference 13 for discussion of these steps):

1. Association of substrate to oxidized cytochrome P-450
2. One-electron reduction of NADPH-cytochrome P-450 reductase by NADPH
3. One-electron reduction of cytochrome P-450-substrate complex by reduced NADPH-cytochrome P-450 reductase
4. Addition of molecular oxygen to reduced cytochrome P-450-substrate complex
5. Reduction of oxygenated reduced NADPH-cytochrome P-450-substrate complex by the second electron, probably from reduced NADPH-cytochrome P-450 reductase
6. Decomposition of oxygenated reduced cytochrome P-450-substrate complex to yield hydroxylated substrate, oxidized cytochrome P-450, and water

The functional components of the mixed function oxidase system consist of at least two protein components: a hemoprotein called cytochrome P-450 and a flavoprotein called NADPH-cytochrome P-450 reductase. Cytochrome P-450 is the substrate and the oxygen binding site of the enzyme system, whereas the reductase serves as an electron carrier shuttling electrons from NADPH to cytochrome P-450. The enzyme system can be solubilized with detergent and resolved chromatographically into three components.[15] These three components are identified as cytochrome P-450, NADPH-cytochrome P-450 reductase, and a lipid Fraction which can be successfully replaced by phosphotidylcholine.[16,17] Both cytochrome P-450 and NADPH-cytochrome P-450 reductase have been purified.[18-24] All three components are necessary for the metabolism of a variety of drugs, steroids, alkanes, and polycyclic hydrocarbons.[21,25,26]

Of the three components involved in microsomal drug metabolism, cytochrome P-450 is undoubtedly the most important because of its vital role in oxygen activation and substrate binding.[25,27] There is now immunologic evidence in rat liver[28] for at least six different forms of P-450. One of these forms, cytochrome P_1-450 or P-448* is induced by polycyclic aromatic hydrocarbons in many mammalian cells both in vivo[8,9] and in culture.[33,34] This specific enzyme system utilizing P_1-450 and metabolizing a variety of polycyclic aromatic hydrocarbons is called aryl hydrocarbon hydroxylase (AHH). AHH activity results from a tri-molecular complex, the interaction of cytochrome P-450, the polycyclic aromatic hydrocarbon substrate and molecular oxygen. The incorporation of one atom of molecular oxygen into the aromatic substrate results in formation of arene oxides. These reactive arene oxides may rearrange spontaneously to form a phenol, be converted enzymatically to a *trans*-dihydrodiol or glutathione conjugate or become covalently bound to cellular nucleic acids and proteins. A scheme depicting these events is shown in Figure 2. The phenol can also be conjugated with UDP-glucuronic acids. These conjugated products are considerably more polar than the parent compound, arene oxide, phenol or dihydrodiol and therefore are more readily excreted. It has recently been shown[36] that the dihydrodiol and perhaps the phenol

---

* The nomenclature for the various forms of cytochrome P-450 is currently inadequate considering that four or more forms are distinguishable by electrophoretic[29] or immunochemical[28] techniques. The eventual better understanding of chemical and catalytic properties[29,30] should, in time, permit a more suitable nomenclature to be devised. In fact, two or more polycyclic aromatic hydrocarbon-inducible forms of P-450 have been separated electrophoretically,[31] and developmentally[32] in the mouse rat, and rabbit liver and in rabbit lung and kidney. The form having the higher molecular weight—about 56,000 or 57,000 daltons—is arbitrarily defined in this report as "cytochrome P_1-450" and has been shown[31,32] to rise and fall concomitant with AHH activity. Whether P_1-450 is exactly the same among these species and among liver and various nonhepatic tissues remains to be elucidated. Since this report deals principally with tumors of lung and skin the term "cytochrome P_1-450" is used throughout.

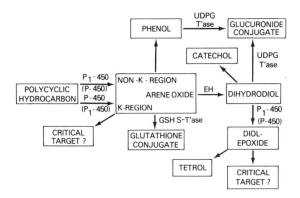

FIGURE 2. Scheme by which polycyclic aromatic hydrocarbons are metabolized in the liver and presumably in other mammalian tissues. (From Kouri, R. E., Rude, T. H., Joglekar, R., Dansette, P. M., Jerina, D. M., Atlas, S. A., Owens, I. S., and Nebert, D. W., *Cancer Res.*, 38, 2777, 1978. With permission.)

may be sufficiently nonpolar to be oxygenated a second time by the P-450 enzymes. The importance of this second monooxygenation will be discussed later.

B. Genetic Regulation

The level of AHH activity is increased dramatically by pretreatment with polycyclic aromatic hydrocarbons. This increase, or induction, is observed in the liver, lung, bowel, kidney, lymph nodes, skin, bone marrow, pigmented epithelium of the retina, brain, mammary gland, uterus, testes, and the ovary, of a variety of responsive mouse strains, but is absent or markedly decreased in these same tissues from other nonresponsive mouse strains.[8,9] This "responsiveness" to aromatic hydrocarbons was originally designated the *Ahh* locus,[37] and finally was designated the *Ah* locus;[38] the allele Ah^b denotes the allele carried by the C57 Bl/6 (B6) inbred strain and Ah^d denotes the allele carried by the DBA/2 (D2) inbred strain. Numerous studies indicate that an important product of the *Ah* locus in mice is a cytosolic receptor[7,39] capable of binding to certain polycyclic aromatic inducers (see Figure 3). Such a complex in some manner activates structural genes thereby leading to increases in enzymes which metabolize these inducers and other polycyclic aromatic noninducing compounds. In addition to innocuous products, reactive metabolites may also be generated. Induction of one or more forms of cytochrome P_1-450 is associated with the induction of the numerous monooxygenase activities listed in Figure 4. How so many substrates with very different chemical structures can be oxygenated by a single enzyme active site is not understood. The most likely possibility is that there are several or many forms of cytochrome P_1-450.

With BP as the substrate in vitro, AHH activity is equated with the rate of formation of 3-hydroxybenzo(a)pyrene (3-OH BP) and probably other phenols having similar wavelengths of fluorescent activation and emission (see Figure 5). These phenols may be formed either by a direct hydroxylation or in a two-step process via an arene oxide. Recent data suggest the latter mechanism to be more important.[42] During in vitro incubation, a substantial percentage (20 to 50%) of the total BP metabolites are not phenolic products and therefore are not detected by the standard fluorometric assay in alkali.[43] However, it has been observed that the proportional amounts of phenolic products from control, or 3-methylcholanthrene or phenobarbital-treated animals found by the standard fluorometric assay remain relatively constant,[44] thereby ensuring the continued use of this simple and very sensitive fluorometric assay.

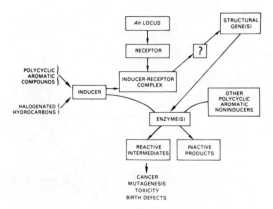

FIGURE 3.   Simplified scheme demonstrating the relationship of the *Ah* locus in the mouse to cancer, mutagenesis, toxicity, and birth defects. (From Kouri, R. E. and Nebert, D. W., *Origins of Human Cancer,* Book A, Hiatt, H. H., Watson, J. D., and Winsten, J. A., Eds., Cold Spring Harbor Laboratory, New York, 1978, 811. With permission.)

The level of AHH activity in liver, kidney, bowel, and lung tissue in B6, D2, and (B6D2) F1 mice in response to exposure to different concentrations of the polycyclic aromatic hydrocarbon β-naphthoflavone is shown in Figure 6. At every dose level, AHH activity is highest in the B6, less high in the (B6D2)F1 and much lower in the D2 strain. In fact, the D2 strain is virtually nonresponsive to β-naphthoflavone at any of these concentrations. The time-dependent increase in AHH activity in pulmonary and hepatic tissue after intratracheal inoculation of 3-methylcholanthrene is shown in Figure 7. The dose of 3-methylcholanthrene was 500 µg/mouse, which is a dose capable of transiently inducing hepatic AHH for about 3 days in the B6 and (B6D2)F1 mice. The D2 strain does show a slight but significant increase in pulmonary AHH activity by 2 days. However, the activity barely reaches levels of activity found in the noninduced B6 strain (see Reference 46 for discussion). Using AHH induction as an indicator of phenotype, several laboratories have found (see Table 1) that about half, or slightly more than half, of all inbred strains examined are responsive (as are wild mice, random bred mice, and about 20 inbred rat strains tested — unpublished data) and the remaining mouse strains are nonresponsive. Thus, during the past 60 or 70 years of developing these inbred strains, it would seem that there has developed a stable mutation whereby certain of these strains either quantitatively or qualitatively lack the gene product of the *Ah* locus, the cytosolic receptor molecule.[39]

Induction of AHH activity and cytochrome P_1-450 by 3-methylcholanthrene is expressed almost exclusively as an autosomal dominant trait among offspring of the appropriate crosses between the B6 and D2 inbred strains. The top two panels in Figure 8 show that the B6 mice are fully responsive to intraperitoneally administered 3-methylcholanthrene, whereas, the D2 strain is unresponsive. The (B6D2)F1's are responsive, but to a slightly lower level than the B6 strain. In the F_1 × B6 backcross, all progeny are responsive to 3-methylcholanthrene. In the F_1 × D2 backcross 50% of the offspring are nonresponsive and indistinguishable from the D2 parent. In the F2 population, approximately 75% of the progeny are responsive, 25% nonresponsive. The same distribution is also observed in pulmonary tissue after intratracheal administration of 3-methylcholanthrene (second panel, Figure 8). Thus, in this system, a single autosomal dominant gene seems to regulate AHH responsiveness in this cross. The last panel in

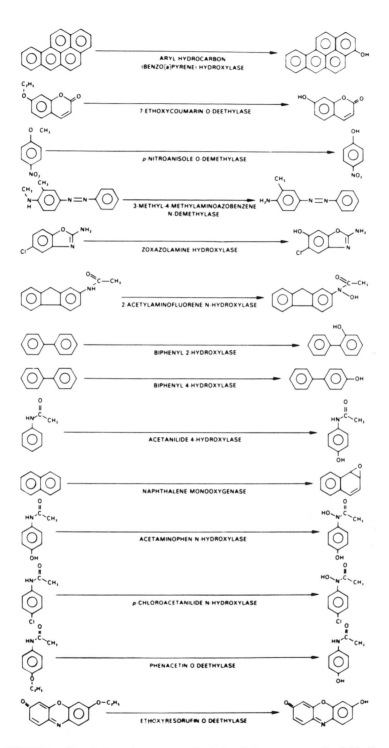

FIGURE 4. Chemical reactions representing induced monooxygenase "activities" associated with cytochrome(s) P$_1$-450 induction and the Ah^b allele in the mouse. Not shown in UDP glucuronosyl transferase activity with 4-methylumbelliferone as substrate, a membrane-bound, metabolically coordinated enzyme whose induction appears to be closely correlated with the Ah^b allele. Only the substrate and the major product are shown. (From Owens, I. S. and Nebert, D. W., *Pharmacologist*, 17, 217, 1975. With permission.)

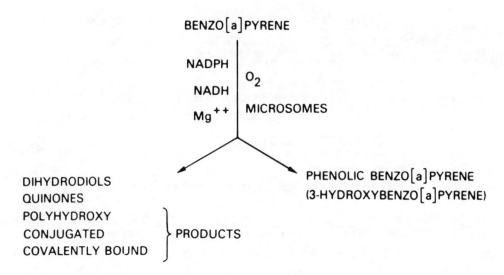

FIGURE 5.   Current concept of the AHH activity. The substrate BP is oxygenated to arene oxides which rearrange nonenzymically to phenols or are oxygenated to phenolic derivatives by direct oxygen insertion. Other oxygenated derivatives of BP, including dihydrodiols and quinones, are not measured by this assay. One unit of AHH activity is defined as that amount of enzyme catalyzing per min at 37°C the formation of hydroxylated product causing fluorescence equivalent to that of 1 pmole of 3-hydroxybenzo(a)pyrene. (Reprinted from Nebert, D. W. and Felton, J. S., *Fed. Proc.,* 31, 1315, 1976. With permission.)

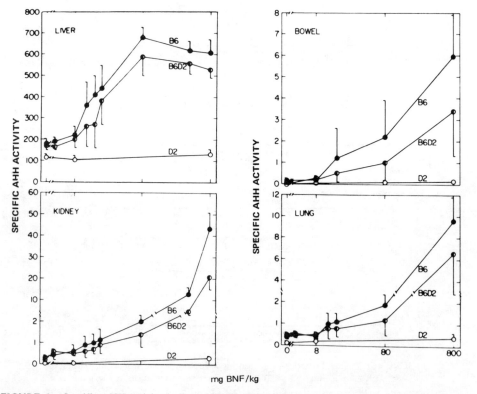

FIGURE 6.   Specific AHH activity in liver, kidney, bowel, and lung of B6, D2, or (B6D2)F₁ mice as a function of the dosage of β-naphthoflavone. Brackets denote standard deviation. Each symbol represents the mean of five or six individual determinations per group. All mice used were immature females of identical age. All determinations of enzyme activity in a given tissue were performed in the same assay on the same day. (From Niwa, A., Kumaki, K., Nebert, D. W., and Poland, A. P., *Arch. Biochem. Biophys.,* 166, 559, 1975. With permission.)

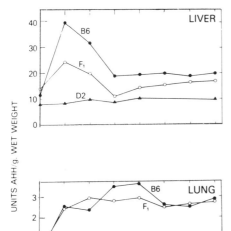

FIGURE 7. Kinetics of hepatic and pulmonary AHH induction following intratracheal administration of MC, 500 μg in 20 μl of 0.2% gelatin-0.85% NaCl, to B6, (B6D2)F₁, and D2 mice. The mice weighed between 15 and 20 g. Each symbol represents the mean of four animals determined individually. For further details, see Reference 46. (Reprinted from Kouri, R. E. and Nebert, D. W., *Origins of Human Cancer,* Book A, Hiatt, H. H., Watson, J. D., and Winsten, J. A., Eds., Cold Spring Harbor Laboratory, New York, 1977, 811. With permission.)

TABLE 1

Determination of Genetic Responsiveness or Nonresponsiveness at the *Ah* Locus in Various Strains and Substrains of the House Mouse *Mus musculus*

Responsive inbred strains	Nonresponsive strains	Ref.
C57BL/6N	DBA/2N	47,48
C57BL/6J	DBA/2J	37
C57L/J	DBA/1J	
C3H/HeJ	AKR/J	
DE/J	129/J	
BALB/cJ	RF/J	
CBA/J	LP/J	
A/J	ST/bJ	
A/HeJ	SJL/J	
SM/J	SWR/J	
PL/J	AU/SsJ	
SEC/1ReJ	NZW/BLN	49
	NZB/BLN	
C3H/HeN	AKR/N	50
BALB/cAnN	BRSUNT/N	
CBA/HN		
A/HeN		
STR/N		
NH/LwN		
P/JN		
AL/N		
C57BL/6Cum		51
C3H/fMai		
B10.BR/J		
C58/J		
BALB/cCR		
C57BL/10		
	DBA/2Cum	52
SEA/GnJ	NZB/BLNJ	53
C3HeB/FeJ		
C3H/fCum		54
AKXL—38A	AKXL—38	29,55

Figure 8 shows that in crosses involving the C3H/fCum (C3) and D2 strains, that responsiveness to intraperitoneally administered 3-methylcholanthrene segregates as a single autosomal co-dominant, or additive trait. That is, the (C3D2)F1 has intermediate AHH levels in response to 3-methylcholanthrene, the (C3D2)F1 × C3 has a 1:1 ratio of the intermediate to high. The (C3D2)F1 × D2 has a 1:1 ratio of intermediate to low, and the F2 has a 1:2:1 ratio of low to intermediate to high. For the sake of convenience, the data in Figure 8 are given both in terms of units AHH activity/mg microsomal protein and units AHH activity/gm wet weight tissue. The lack of induction of AHH activity and P₁-450 by 3-methylcholanthrene is expressed as an autosomal dominant trait among the offspring of the appropriate crosses between C57BL/6N and AKR/N parent strains.[54,55] The simplest genetic model to explain most (but still not all) of the data includes a minimum of 6 alleles at two different loci.[56] However, for all intents and purposes, we may regard genetic expression at the *Ah* locus among the offspring from the appropriate crosses between B6 and D2 strains and between C3 and D2 strains as dominant and additive, respectively. Because of the distinct phenotypes generated in progeny from the F1 × D2 backcross and the F2 generation, we can evaluate the possible importance of (steady-state levels of) reactive intermediates in the

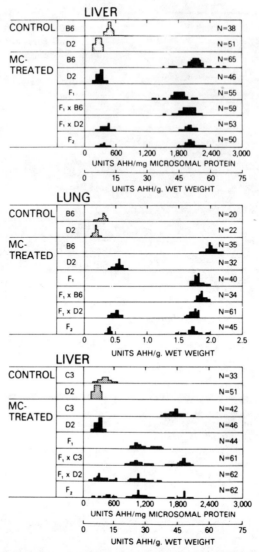

FIGURE 8.   Genetic variance in hepatic (top) and pulmonary (middle) AHH activity in control and MC-treated offspring from appropriate crosses between B6 and D2 inbred strains and hepatic AHH activity (bottom) in control and MC-treated offspring from appropriate crosses between C3 and D2 inbred strains, Histograms for liver samples represent specific AHH activity in control mice and in mice treated intraperitoneally 24 hr beforehand with MC (100 mg/kg body wt); controls received corn oil intraperitoneally. For lung samples, the mice received intratracheally, 24 hr beforehand, 500 μg MC, in 20 μl of 0.2% gelatin-0.85% NaCl; controls received the sterile vehicle alone. The mice weighed between 15 and 20 g. The number of mice examined individually is given at the right for each group. (From Kouri, R. E. and Nebert, D. W., *Origins of Human Cancer,* Book A, Hiatt, H. H., Watson, J. D., and Winsten, J. A., Cold Spring Harbor Laboratory, New York, 1977, 811. With permission.)

mechanism of chemically induced carcinogenesis, mutagenesis, or toxicity among siblings in the same litter or among individuals sharing the same uterus. This genetic probe is a particularly powerful experimental model system in the research areas of chemical carcinogenesis, pharmacology, toxicology, and teratology, because the test compounds studied often cause undesirable side effects such as sedation, malnutrition, hormone imbalance, etc., that are hard to distinguish from specific pharmacologic, toxicologic, or carcinogenic effects of the compound.

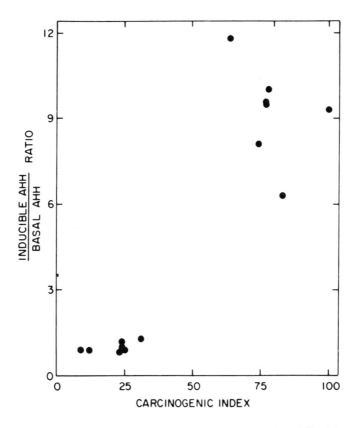

FIGURE 9.   Relationship between the carcinogenic index (defined by Iball 1939) for subcutaneous MC and the genetically mediated induction of AHH activity by MC for each of 14 inbred strains: the correlation coefficient r is 0.90 (P <0.001). Each closed circle represents the average result from a group of 30 inbred mice of a certain strain. The carcinogenic index was evaluated after a subcutaneous dose of 150 μg MC had been given to a minimum of 30 weanling mice of each strain. The inducible AHH/basal AHH ratio reflects the mean hepatic AHH activity in MC-treated mice divided by the mean hepatic enzyme activity in control mice (N >5 for each of the two groups). Whether the MC-inducible AHH activity in the nonhepatic tissues appears to segregate as a single gene with the inducible hepatic AHH activity has not been examined for many of these strains. (From Nebert, D. W., Benedict, W. F., and Kouri, R. E., *Chemical Carcinogenesis,* T'so, P. O. P. and DiPaolo, J. A., Eds., Marcel Dekker, New York, 1974, 271. With permission.)

III. ASSOCIATION BETWEEN THE *Ah* LOCUS AND SUSCEPTIBILITY TO CHEMICALLY INDUCED CANCERS

A. Polycyclic Aromatic Hydrocarbon Carcinogenesis
1. The Subcutaneous Model System

Fibrosarcomas initiated by subcutaneously administered 3-methylcholanthrene are associated with genetically mediated aromatic hydrocarbon responsiveness among 14 inbred strains of mice (Figure 9). Table 2 demonstrates that the carcinogenic index for subcutaneously administered 3-methylcholanthrene in offspring from crosses involving the B6 and D2 inbred parental strains is in fact associated or genetically linked with

TABLE 2

Relationship between Aromatic Hydrocarbon Responsiveness and Susceptibility to Subcutaneous 3-Methylcholanthrene (MC)-and BP-initiated Tumors among Offspring from Appropriate Crosses Involving the B6, C3, and D2 Strains of Mice

Strain or offspring	Expression at Ah locus[a]	Carcinogenic index for MC	Strain or offspring	Expression at Ah locus[a]	Carcinogenic index for MC	for BP
B6	+ +	61	C3	+ +	73	56
D2	0	11	D2	0	10	4
(B6D2)F₁	+ +	43	(C3D2)F₁	+	37	19
F₁ × B6	+ +	58	F₁ × C3	+ +	74	27
				+	60	24
F₁ × D2	+ +	54	F₁ × D2	+	46	1
	0	8		0	9	1
F₂	+ +	63				
	0	6	F₂	+ +	69	31
				+	61	7
				0	17	2

Note: Animals received as weanlngs 150 μg MC or BP in trioctanoin subcutaneously, and the carcinogenic index was determined over an 8 month period. (For further details, see References 52, 54.)

[a]   The phenotypic expression at the *Ah* locus is ranked as follows: + + = fully responsive, 0 = nonresponsive, + = intermediate responsive, as judged by the data illustrated in Figure 8.

the *Ah*[b] allele; the carcinogenic index is greater than 42 in all responsive phenotype groups and less than 12 in all nonresponsive phenotype groups.

With respect to the carcinogenic index for subcutaneous 3-methylcholanthrene in offspring from crosses involving the C3 and D2 lines, however, some unexpected values are obtained (see Table 2). Although the intermediate phenotype has intermediate carcinogenic index values among (C3D2)F1 individuals and among offspring from the (C3D2)F1 × D2 backcross (37 and 47, respectively), the values among progeny of the (C3D2)F1 × C3 backcross and the (C3D2)F2 generation are more susceptible to 3-methylcholanthrene initiated tumors than can be accounted for by their inducible AHH activity alone (carcinogenic indices of 60 and 61, respectively). There was also an increase (carcinogenic index of 17) in nonresponsive F2 individuals. We conclude that there probably exist other genes carried by the C3 mouse that make this strain particularly sensitive to 3-methylcholanthrene tumorigenesis.

With respect to BP tumorigenesis, the carcinogenic index for subcutaneous BP (Table 2) is disproportionately low among (C3D2)F1 progeny (value of 19) and among all offspring from both backcrosses and the F1 × F1 intercross. The intermediate phenotype of the (C3D2)F1 × D2 backcross is particularly resistant to BP carcinogenesis, having a carcinogenic index (value of 1) lower than that for the D2 parent. It seems likely that the D2 strain carries other genes that confer even a higher resistance to BP-induced tumors than would be expected from their AHH content alone. Nonetheless, the *Ah* locus still plays a major role in the susceptibility of these animals to BP tumorigenesis because both the (C3D2)F1 × C3 progeny and the (C3D2)F2 generation demonstrate a close association between tumor susceptibility caused by BP and inducible AHH activity. Thus, though some other genes may also influence susceptibility to BP-and/or 3-methylcholanthrene initiated tumors, the primary determinant for cancer susceptibility is the allele(s) regulating inducible AHH activity in various mouse tissues. Among recombinant inbred sublines having C57BL/6N and AKR/N as the progenitor strains, in which the lack of induction is expressed as an autosomal dominant trait,[56] susceptibility to 3-methylcholanthrene-initiated tumors remains linked with inducible

AHH activity.[54] Also, among recombinant inbred sublines having C57L/J and AKR/ J as the progenitor strains, the Ah^b-containing subline was highly susceptible to 3-methylcholanthrene subcutaneous sarcomas, whereas the Ah^d-containing subline was relatively resistant.[55]

2. The Lung Model System

The model system of tumorigenesis initiated by subcutaneous 3-methylcholanthrene or BP suffers from the shortcoming that AHH activity is determined in liver, whereas tumor formation occurs in subcutaneous connective tissue. The lung offers an alternate model system in which pulmonary AHH can be specifically and preferentially induced by intratracheal 3-methylcholanthrene.[46,54,58] AHH induction in the lung appears to be under genetic controls similar to that in the liver (Figure 8). Mouse lung is known to be susceptible to 3-methylcholanthrene induced bronchogenic squamous cell carcinomas,[59] and it is well known that carcinomas—not sarcomas—are the most frequently observed type of tumor in man. A statistically significant ($P < 0.01$) correlation between lung tumors produced by intratracheal 3-methylcholanthrene and the Ah^b allele is shown in Table 3. This correlation is most clearly seen in offspring from the (B6D2)F1 × D2 backcross, in which the responsive individuals were observed to be more than three times more susceptible to lung cancer than the nonresponsive individuals. Again, some contribution of genes other than the Ah locus seem to be responsible for the increased susceptibility to 3-methylcholanthrene-initiated pulmonary tumors found in the F1 and F2 offspring and the progeny from both backcrosses.

3. The Leukemia Model System

Two recent studies suggest genetic linkage between leukemia induction by percutaneous treatment with 3-methylcholanthrene,[61] or oral administration of BP,[62] and the Ah^d allele (the allele controlling for AHH nonresponsiveness). The results seem best explained on the basis of "first-pass elimination" kinetics. That is, the relative high degree of AHH activity (and induction) in the bowel (400 to 800 fold) and liver (2 to 8 fold) of Ah^b/Ah^b and Ah^b/Ah^d mice results in the much more rapid metabolism of BP and/or 3-methylcholanthrene to innocuous products which are then excreted in the feces and urine, when compared with the hydroxylase induction of less than 70-fold in the bowel and no induction in the liver of Ah^d/Ah^d mice.[63] Thus the nonresponsive animals actually seem to be exposed to higher concentrations of the carcinogens in the extra-hepatic tissue than are the responsive animals.

In summary, 3-methylcholanthrene and BP are either metabolized to higher steady-state levels of a proximal or ultimate carcinogenic intermediate(s) in the subcutaneous connective tissue or lung of responsive mice because of increased P_1-450 content in responsive mice, compared with nonresponsive mice, or are predominantly metabolized to a particular proximal or ultimate carcinogen(s) because of a marked change in the P_1-450/P-450 ratio. On the other hand, these high levels of AHH activity or P_1-450 content may also function in limiting the amount or type of metabolites available to other tissue (e.g., bone marrow) and actually protect these other tissues from chemically-induced cancers (e.g., leukemia).

B. Aromatic Amine Carcinogenesis

One other class of chemical carcinogens which has been studied in the genetic model described above is the aromatic amines. N-hydroxylation of 2-acetylaminofluorene is genetically linked to the Ah locus.[64] Thorgiersson et al.[8,65] have recently shown that this genetic difference in N-hydroxylation is genetically linked to 2-acetylaminofluorene and acetaminophen-produced hepatotoxicity, and also 2-acetylaminofluorene-induced mutagenicity in vitro. Preliminary studies have also suggested an association

TABLE 3

Tumorigenic Effect of Intratracheal Instillation of MCA Among Offspring From Appropriate Crosses Involving the B6 and D2 Strains of Mice

Strain or offspring	Expression at Ah locus[a]	Treatment	Number of mice	Type of lung tumor[b]						Incidence of lung tumors (%)[c]
				Normal	Alveolar adenoma	Broncho-alveolar lesion	Adeno-squamous carcinoma	Squamous neoplasm	Squamous cell carcinoma with metastasis	
B6	+ +	control	46	44 (96)	2 (4)	0	0	0	0	0
B6	+ +	MC	22	6 (27)	7 (32)	7 (32)	1 (5)	2 (9)	2 (9)	23
D2	0	MC	13	11 (85)	1 (8)	1 (8)	0	0	0	0
F₁	+ +	MC	30	4 (13)	22 (73)	6 (20)	8 (27)	2 (7)	1 (3)	37
F₁ × B6	+ +	MC	24	1 (4)	8 (33)	3 (13)	4 (17)	6 (25)	3 (13)	54
F₁ × D2	0	MC	12	5 (42)	4 (33)	1 (8)	1 (8)	0	1 (8)	17
	+ +	MC	11	1 (9)	4 (36)	2 (18)	1 (9)	3 (27)	55	55

Note: MCA, 500 µg in 20 µl of 0.2% gelatin-0.85% NaCl sterile solution, was given four times at weekly intervals to weanling mice of either sex, and the incidences and types of lung tumors were determined at autopsy 4 months later or at any earlier time in the case of premature death. For the sake of this presentation, data analysis was performed only on those conditions which were truly neoplastic, i.e., adenocarcinoma, squamous cell neoplasms, and bronchogenic squamous cell carcinomas. A complete pathological description of these lesions is presented elsewhere.[60]

a   Expression is the same as that outlined in Table 2.

b   Percent incidence is given in parentheses.

c   Percent of individuals with lung lesions are expressed relative to total number of survivors at 12 months when experiment was terminated. The incidences of pulmonary aberrancies include all pathologic lesions from adenosquamous carcinoma to frank squamous cell carcinoma with accompanying metastasis.

Reprinted from Kouri, R. E. and Nebert, D. W., *Origins of Human Cancer*, Book A, Hiatt, H. H., Watson, J. D., and Winsten, J. A., Eds., Cold Spring Harbor Laboratory, New York, 1977. With permission.

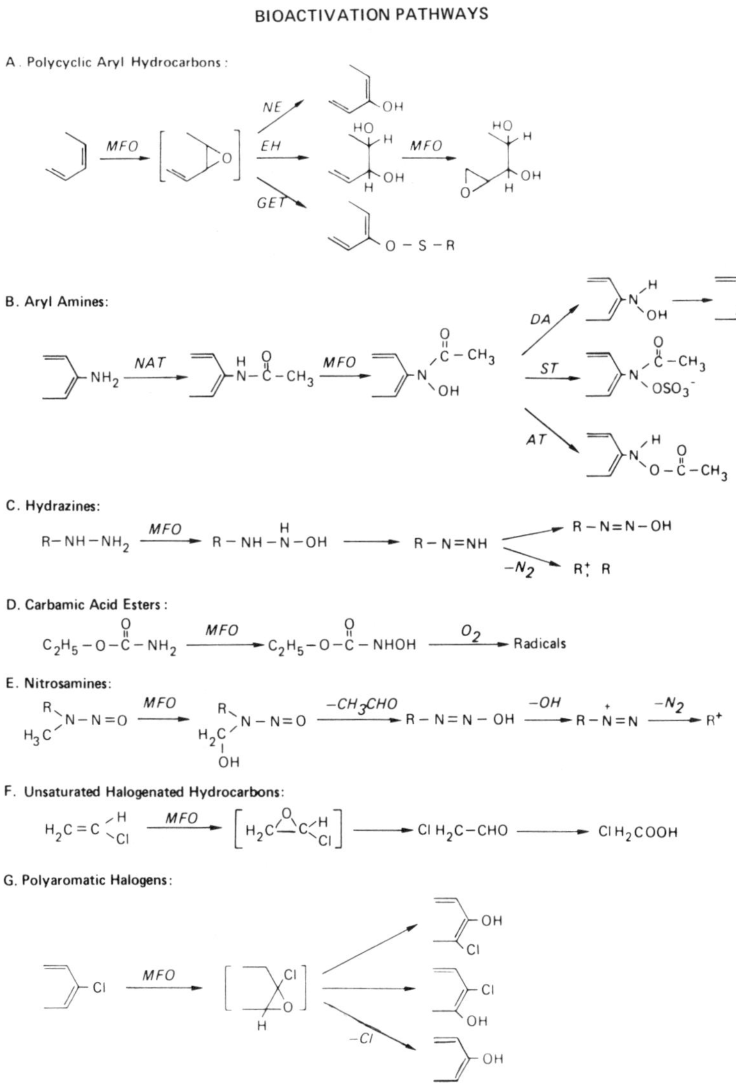

FIGURE 10.   Scheme for activation of 7 classes of chemical carcinogens. Abbreviations: MFO, mixed-function oxidases; NE, not enzymatic; EH, epoxide hydrase; GET, glutathione s-epoxide-transferase; NAT, N-acetyltransferase; DA, deacetylase; ST, sulfotransferase; AT, acyltransferase.

between 2-acetylaminofluorene-induced hepatic (and perhaps bladder) carcinogenesis and the *Ah* locus.[235] This latter observation is now in the process of being confirmed. Metabolism of the aromatic amine 6-aminochrysene to forms mutagenic to tester strains of *Salmonella typhimurium* has been recently shown to be genetically linked to the *Ah* locus.[66] Studies to determine the relationship between 6-aminochrysene induced carcinogenesis and the *Ah* locus are presently on test in our laboratory.

C. Other Chemical Classes of Carcinogens

As shown in Figure 4 the metabolism of many chemical carcinogens is genetically linked to the *Ah* locus and hypothetically this gene could control further metabolism of these chemicals to the forms that are carcinogenic in model test systems or carcinogenic to man. A proposed scheme for activation of seven different classes of chemical carcinogens is given in Figure 10. The site at which P-450-dependent mixed-function oxidases (MFO) are proposed to play a role in this bioactivation are depicted in this scheme. (See figure legend for definition of abbreviations.)

IV. NONGENETIC TESTS IMPLICATING AHH LEVELS IN CANCER SUSCEPTIBILITY

Five main classes of chemicals have been used as inhibitors of carcinogen metabolism and subsequently tested for their capacity to alter susceptibility to chemical carcinogenesis in vivo. These five chemical classes are (1) antioxidants, (2) isomers of the benzoflavones, (3) steroid hormones, (4) physiological biogenic amines, and (5) specific inducers of MFO activity.

Antioxidants such as butylated hydroxytoluene, butylated hydroxyanisol, vitamin A and disulfiram seem to alter either directly or indirectly the metabolism of a variety of known carcinogens[67-69] and also have been reported to inhibit carcinogenesis induced by such factors as 7,12-dimethylbenz(a)anthracene,[67,70] BP,[70] urethane,[70] uracil mustard,[70] 7,8-hydroxy-methyl-12-methylbenz(a)anthracene,[70] dibenz(a,h) anthracene,[70] dimethylhydrazine,[71] and 2-acetylaminofluorene.[72] This last paper points out one of the problems associated with this inhibitor plus carcinogen study. That is, these authors observed that butylated hydroxytoluene rather than inhibiting carcinogenesis seemed to enhance 2-acetylaminofluorene-induced hepatic tumors, Thus, depending on experimental design, one might observe inhibition or enhancement of susceptibility to chemical carcinogenesis.

The compound 7,8-benzoflavone (α-naphthoflavone) is a potent inhibitor and weak inducer of AHH activity while its isomer, 5,6-benzoflavone (β-naphthoflavone) is an inducer but a poor inhibitor of AHH activity.[73] 7,8-benzoflavone can inhibit 7,12-dimethylbenz(a)anthracene-induced mammary tumors[74] or skin tumors,[75-77] 3-methylcholanthrene-induced skin tumors[78] and cyclopentaphenanthrene-induced skin tumors.[79] 7,8-benzoflavone failed to inhibit BP induced tumors.[76] Moreover, in certain instances, the isomer 5,6-benzoflavone, which induces AHH activity is also active in inhibiting carcinogenicity in vivo.[73] Thus, as observed for the antioxidants, depending on the experimental design, inhibitors or inducers of AHH activity can enhance or inhibit chemical carcinogenesis.

Anti-inflammatory steroids, such as dexamethasone, can inhibit chemically induced AHH activity in vivo.[80] Not only do these steroids inhibit skin tissue mediated covalent binding of 3-methycholanthrene to DNA in vitro,[81] but also inhibit skin tumorigenesis in vivo.[80,81]

Recent studies[82] have shown that some thiols, unsaturated aliphatic acids, and biogenic amines can inhibit BP induced carcinogenesis in vivo, and many of these chemicals inhibit AHH activity in vivo. What is interesting in this latter study is the fact that many of these chemicals are physiological chemicals. That is, compounds such as: *cis*-aconitic acid, L-cysteine, dithiothreitol, and putrescine were shown to inhibit significantly the BP-induced carcinogenesis in vivo. Thus many of the observed differences in susceptibility among various species could result from variations in physiologic levels of these chemicals.

Phenobarbital is an example of an inducer of hepatic monooxygenase activity[3] which, when given simultaneously with the hepatocarcinogens, 4-(dimethylamino)-azobenzene or 2-acetylaminofluorene, decreases the carcinogenic effects of these chemicals.[83] When given subsequent to the carcinogen treatment however, phenobarbital enhances the carcinogenic effects of these chemicals.[83,84] Polychlorinated biphenyls, on the other hand, represent a class of environmental pollutants which induce hepatic

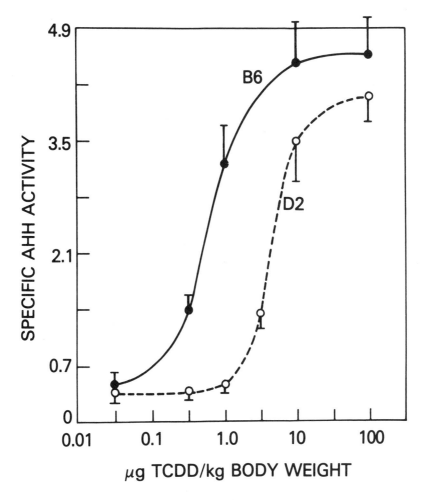

FIGURE 11. Semilog plot of dose-response curve for hepatic AHH induction by i.p. TCDD in B6 and D2 mice. The enzyme was assayed 3 days after TCDD had been administered at the indicated doses. Each point represents the mean AHH activity of 6 combined livers. Bar, S. D. (Reprinted from Kouri, R. E., Rude, T. H., Joglekar, R., Dansette, P. M., Jerina, D. M., Atlas, S. A., Owens, I. S., and Nebert, D. W., *Cancer Res.*, 38, 2777, 1978. With permission.)

monooxygenases[85] yet seem to inhibit hepatocarcinogenesis induced by 3'-methyl-4-dimethylaminoazobenzene, 2-acetylaminofluorene, and diethylnitrosamine.[86] A way to obviate these problems of enhancement vs. suppression is to use a chemical which is capable of inducing AHH activity, but is only a weak substrate for this activity. Moreover, the data would be more easily interpreted if conditions could be found whereby the chemical induces AHH activity but the test carcinogen cannot. One chemical with these desirable properties is 2,3,7,8-tetrachlorodibenzo(p)dioxin (TCDD). TCDD is a potent inducer of AHH activity and cytochrome P_1-450 in both responsive and nonresponsive strains of mice.[35,87] That is, TCDD can induce AHH activity in those strains genetically nonresponsive to 3-methylcholanthrene (e.g., the D2 strain). The AHH levels in response to various doses of TCDD is shown in Figure 11. A dose of approximately 10 μg of TCDD/kg body weight results

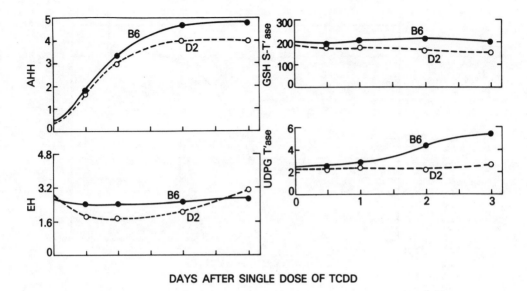

DAYS AFTER SINGLE DOSE OF TCDD

FIGURE 12.   Kinetics of hepatic AHH, epoxide hydrase (EH, GSH S-transferase (GSH S T'ase) and UDP glucuronsyltransferase (UDPG T'ase) activities in B6 and D2 mice following a single i.p. dose of TCDD. Specific activities of each enzyme activity, are given on the ordinates and are as described in Reference 35. Ten B6 and 10 D2 mice were given injections for each time point, so that each point represents at the time of assay a minimum of 4 livers combined. (From Kouri, R. E., Rude, T. H., Joglekar, R., Dansette, P. M., Jerina, D. M., Atlas, S. A., Owens, I. S., and Nebert, D. W., *Cancer Res.*, 38, 2777, 1978. With permission.)

in almost complete induction of AHH activity in both the D2 and B6 strains of mice. As discussed earlier, the balance between metabolic formation of an ultimate carcinogen and its detoxification depends upon the relative concentrations of several enzymes involved in the pathway of the polycyclic hydrocarbon metabolism. The effect of TCDD on four of these enzymes is shown in Figure 12. AHH activity is induced to a similar level in both B6 and D2 mice. Epoxide hydrase activity remains unaltered in B6 mice during the first 48 hr of TCDD treatment and in D2 mice there is a slight but significant ($p < 0.05$) decrease in hepatic epoxide hydrase levels during the first 48 hr following treatment with TCDD. This decrease is transitory and disappears by 3 days after TCDD treatment. Glutathione S-epoxide transferase activity in both strains remains unchanged. The induced UDPG-transferase activity begins to appear by 24 hr after the B6 mice received a high dose of TCDD. The induction is not even twofold in B6 during the first 48 hr after TCDD treatment. In D2 mice no significant increases in the UDPG-transferase are observed even 72 hr after the dose of TCDD. Therefore, we conclude that the magnitude of genetically regulated AHH induction by TCDD is by far the largest in comparison with any change in any of the other three enzymes.

The effect of intraperitoneal TCDD, given 2 days to or simultaneously with subcutaneous 3-methylcholanthrene, on subsequent tumor formation in B6 and D2 mice is shown in Table 4. Neither vehicle (*p*-dioxane or trioctanion) nor TCDD (at 100 μg/kg body weight) causes any tumors. The carcinogenic index of 3-methylcholanthrene alone is 65 in B6, compared with 1 in D2 mice. This result is within experimental variation of previous carcinogenic indexes of 61 and 11 in B6 and D2 mice, respec-

TABLE 4

Effects of i.p. TCDD on MCA-initiated s.c. Tumors

Inbred strain	Treatment −2 days	Treatment 0 days	Number of mice dying because of treatment[a]	Number of mice at risk for tumors[b]	Number of mice with tumors[c]	% of mice with tumors	Av. latency (days)	Carcinogenic index[d]
B6	i.p. p-dioxane	s.c. trioctanoin	1	39	0	0		
	ip. TCDD (100 µg/kg)	s.c. trioctanoin	20	27	0	0		
	None	s.c. MCA	1	36	29	81	125	65
	None	i.p. TCDD (100 µg/kg)	20	30	0	0		
	None	i.p. TCDD (100 µg/kg) + s.c. MCA	30	43	33	71	123	63
	None	i.p. TCDD (1 µg/kg)	4	46	0	0		
	None	i.p. TCDD (1 µg/kg) + s.c. MCA	6	27	27	100	132	76
D2	i.p. TCDD (100 µg/kg)	s.c. MCA	20	25	21	84	129	65
	i.p. TCDD (1 µg/kg)	s.c. MCA	6	23	16	70	140	50
	i.p. p-dioxane	s.c. trioctanoin	6	22	0	0		
	i.p. TCDD (100 µg/kg)	s.c. trioctanoin	24	25	0	0		
	None	s.c. MCA	3	34	1	3	217	1
	None	i.p. TCDD (100µg/kg)	30	38	0	0		
	None	i.p. TCDD (100 µg/kg) + s.c. MCA	43	43	10	23	178	13[e]
	None	i.p. TCDD (1 µg/kg)	5	48	0	0		
	None	i.p. TCDD (1 µg/kg) + s.c. MCA	5	34	5	15	199	7
	i.p. TCDD (100 µg/kg)	s.c. MCA	20	28	0	0		
	i.p. TCDD (1 µg/kg)	s.c. MCA	6	31	0	0		

Note: See Reference 35 for details relating to this table.

a   During the first 28 days following treatment.

b   Defined as the number of mice surviving the 36-week observation period.

c   At the end of the 36-week experiment.

d   Percentage of incidence of tumors, divided by the average latency in days, multiplied by 100.

e   This carcinogenic index value lies outside (greater than) the 99% confidence interval (i.e., $<p$ 0.01) constructed from 7 different studies over the past 5 years during which 150 µg of MCA were given s.c. to D2 mice. These studies included 295 D2 mice; the mean ± S.D. for all 7 studies was a carcinogenic index of 5.43 ± 2.70.

tively.[54] In B6 mice, neither the high nor the low dose of intraperitoneal TCDD, given 2 days prior to or simultaneously with subcutaneous 3-methylcholanthrene affects significantly the carcinogenic index. In D2 mice, intraperitoneal TCDD given 2 days prior to 3-methylcholanthrene does not affect the carcinogenic index; yet, the intraperitoneal TCDD given concomitantly with 3-methylcholanthrene increases the carcinogenic index in this experiment approximately five to tenfold.

With the responsive B6 strain, we conclude that any further induction of AHH activity and its associated P_1-450 by TCDD has little effect on further enhancing the metabolism of 3-methycholanthrene to the ultimate carcinogen. A carcinogenic index between 50 and 76 is apparently the maximal limit for 3-methylcholanthrene initiated tumors in this mouse strain under these experimental conditions. In the nonresponsive D2 strain, it was decided to examine further 3-methylcholanthrene tumor formation when the TCDD is given subcutaneously, rather than intraperitoneally, with subcutaneous 3-methycholanthrene (Table 5). In this second experiment, 3-methylcholanthrene alone gives a carcinogenic index of 6; *p*-dioxane administered intraperitoneally 2 days before the 3-methylcholanthrene does not affect the carcinogenic index, and 100 μg TCDD/kg body weight, injected intraperitoneally 2 days prior to the 3-methylcholanthrene produces a carcinogenic index of 10. The simultaneous intraperitoneally administration of *p*-dioxane, the low intraperitoneal TCDD dose, or subcutaneously administered *p*-dioxane with3-methylcholanthrene does not enhance the carcinogenic index. However, the high intraperitoneal TCDD dose or the low subcutaneous TCDD dose given concomitantly with 3-methylcholanthrene approximately triples the carcinogenic index (from 5 to 14 or 15), and the high subcutaneous TCDD dose given together with 3-methylcholanthrene raises the carcinogenic index to 38. TCDD, at a dose causing death in 30 to 70% of each group of mice treated, is not at all carcinogenic in the survivors examined 36 weeks later. Moreover, the toxicity of TCDD at this high dose does not appear to be associated with the aromatic hydrocarbon "responsiveness" regulated by the *Ah* locus, as has been shown[88] to be the cause for large doses of intraperitoneal BP, 7,12-dimethylbenz(a)anthracene, 3-methylcholanthrene or β-naphthoflavone. The high subcutaneous TCDD dose (Table 5) is much less lethal than the high intraperitoneal dose and enhances the 3-methylcholanthrene carcinogenic index in D2 mice from about 5 to 38, approximately halfway between the carcinogenic index for B6 mice and the carcinogenic index for D2 mice. Therefore, it was concluded that although TCDD is not carcinogenic, it is a cocarcinogen.

A possible mechanism of action for the subcutaneous TCDD would be that AHH activity and its associated cytochrome P_1-450 is induced locally at the site of inoculation. Thus, when TCDD is given together with subcutaneous 3-methylcholanthrene in the genetically nonresponsive mouse, 3-methylcholanthrene is now metabolized much more effectively to the ultimate carcinogen in the nonresponsive mouse.

Why does the carcinogenic index in D2 mice rise only to 38 rather than 60 or 70, as is found in B6 mice? Unexpected susceptibility or resistance to 3-methylcholanthrene or BP initiated tumors among progeny from appropriate genetic crosses between the C3 and D2 strains has been reported (see Table 2, References 9, 54). These data suggest that other gene(s) carried by the D2 strains may cause this strain to be more resistant to polycyclic hydrocarbon-initiated cancers than could be accounted for by regulation of AHH activity by the *Ah* locus alone. Conversely, other gene(s) carried by the C3 strain may cause this strain to be more sensitive to such chemically induced tumors than expected solely on the basis of the hydroxylase inducibility. The nature of some of these other genes will be the subject of other chapters in this book.

TABLE 5

Effect of i.p. or s.c. TCDD given 2 Days Prior to or Simultaneously with s.c. MCA on Tumorigenesis in D2 Mice Experimental Protocols Are Identical to Those Described in Table 5

Treatment		Number of mice dying because of treatment	Number of mice at risk for tumors	Number of mice with tumors	% of mice with tumors	Av. latency (days)	Carcinogenic index
−2 days	0 days						
None	s.c. MCA	0	30	3	10	177	6
i.p. p-dioxane	s.c. MCA	10	40	4	10	194	5
i.p. TCDD (100 µg/kg)	s.c. MCA	35	65	9	14	145	10
None	i.p. p-dioxane × s.c. MCA	5	45	5	11	176	6
None	i.p. TCDD (100 µg/kg) + s.c. MCA	38	62	17	27	183	15[a]
None	i.p. TCDD (1 µg/kg) + s.c. MCA	22	78	8	10	162	6
None	s.c. p-dioxane + s.c. MCA	2	68	8	12	180	6
None	s.c. TCDD (100 µg/kg)	8	42	0	0		
None	s.c. TCDD (100 µg/kg) + s.c. MCA	18	82	46	56	146	38[a]
None	s.c. TCDD (1 µg/kg)	2	48	0	0		
None	s.c. TCDD (1 µg/kg) + s.c. MCA	2	98	21	21	154	14[a]

Note: See Reference 35 for details pertaining to this table.

[a] These carcinogenic index values lie outside the 99% confidence interval, as described in Table 4, footnote e.

V. AHH AND ITS ROLE IN OTHER IN VIVO CONDITIONS

A. Chemically Induced Cytotoxicity

Massive intraperitoneal doses of BP, 7,12-dimethylbenz(a)anthracene, 3-methyl-cholanthrene or 5,6-benzoflavone, polychlorinated biphenyls and lindane (the insecticide hexachlorocyclohexane)[88] result in toxicity which is genetically linked to the Ah^b allele. The actual reason or explanation for the cause of this earlier death of responsive mice is not understood. The route of inoculation plays a major role in this toxicity. When the dosage and the route of administration of BP are changed, that is, a lower dose is given orally,[88] the survival time of nonresponsive mice is less than 4 weeks whereas no significant early death is seen in genetically responsive mice even after 6 months of continuous feeding of BP daily. The apparent cause of early death in the nonresponsive mice ingesting BP is pancytopenia resulting from toxic chemical depression of the bone marrow.[88] Other toxic responses in vivo that have been associated with the Ah^b allele include (1) increased susceptibility to 7,12-dimethylbenz(a)anthracene-induced skin inflammation,[89] (2) shortened zoxazolamine-induced paralysis time,[90] (3) increased susceptibility to stillborns, fetal resorptions, and malformations caused by 3-methylcholanthrene or 7,12-dimethylbenz(a)anthracene given to pregnant mothers,[91] (4) increased susceptibility to acetaminophen-produced hepatic necrosis,[64] and (5) increased susceptibility to cataract formation caused by intraperitoneal acetaminophen.[92] Two other toxins which have recently been shown to be influenced by the monooxygenase enzyme system (though not necessarily the Ah locus) are vinyl chloride[93] and the lung toxin 4-ipomeanol.[94] Both these studies suggest that hepatic injury and pulmonary injury induced by vinyl chloride or 4-ipomeanol, respectively, is the specific result of monooxygenase systems metabolizing these compounds to cytotoxic forms *in situ*.

B. AHH Responsiveness as a Marker for Environmental Pollution

1. Cigarette Smoke

Exposure to whole cigarette smoke results in a prompt rapid increase in pulmonary AHH activity, in rats,[95] and in mice.[58,95-97] Even placental tissue from women who smoke during pregnancy contains enhanced AHH levels.[98,99] Thus cigarette smoke contains chemicals that are capable of inducing AHH activity in vivo. Kinetics of cigarette smoke-induced AHH activity in mouse pulmonary tissue are shown in Figure 13. Pulmonary AHH activity rapidly increases following exposure to cigarette smoke and reaches peak activity by 6 hr after exposure. In rats this relative increase occurs as early as 4 hr after exposure.[95] This increase is followed by a plateau of enzyme activity where the half life of the induced enzyme is at least 24 hr. This increase in AHH activity is quite different from that induced by 3-methylcholanthrene (see Figure 13), in that the cigarette smoke-induced enzyme activity increases much more rapidly and the halflife of the induced enzyme is considerably shorter when compared with the 3-methylcholanthrene-induced pulmonary monooxygenases. Recent information in our laboratory suggests that this smoke-associated increase in enzyme activity is the result of specific induction of the P_1-450 cytochrome because enhanced 0-deethylation of ethoxyresorufin is observed following exposure to whole cigarette smoke.[96] This substrate has been shown to be a specific substrate for the P_1-450 enzyme system.[100] The pulmonary enzyme increases following exposure to whole cigarette smoke when measured using either BP or ethoxyresorufin as substrates for these enzymes is shown in

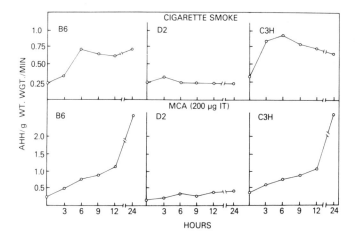

FIGURE 13. Mice were treated with 200 μg MCA/0.2% gelatin-saline solution intratracheally (IT) and sacrificed at the time periods specified. Mice were exposed to four cigarettes from a Walton smoking machine employing a 2-sec puff, 10% smoke, 30-sec exposure, and 30-sec purge. Mice were given a 2-min rest period before exposure to the next cigarette. The times for sacrifice were determined after the fourth cigarette. Lungs were excised and frozen at −70°C until assayed. AHH units are expressed as nmoles 3-OH BP formed/min/g wet weight tissue. Average activity of three animals is given. (From Kouri, R. E., Rude, T. H., Curren, R., Brandt, K. R., Sosnowski, R. G., Schechtman, L. M., Benedict, W. F., and Henry, C. J., *Environ. Health Perspect.*, 29, 63, 1979. With permission.)

Table 6. When BP is the substrate, induced AHH activity can be detected only when the mouse has been exposed to smoke from a single cigarette, and this induction is dependent on new RNA and protein synthesis (see Table 6). Use of ethoxyresorufin as a substrate confirms that some new RNA and protein synthesis is a necessary requirement for smoke-induced monooxygenase activity. Because no basal enzyme activity can be detected, enhanced 0-deethylase activity in pulmonary tissue can therefore be observed after as little as one puff of a reference cigarette (data not shown). Particular fractions of cigarette smoke condensate materials can induce AHH activity in vivo.[58] and can competitively inhibit BP metabolism in vitro.[58] However, neither whole cigarette smoke nor specific fractions of the cigarette smoke condensate induces pulmonary AHH activities in accordance with regulation by the Ah^b allele.[95-97] We believe that the level of induction is too small and irreproducible for genetic analysis.

2. Other Environmental Chemicals

A variety of other environmental factors can alter the monooxygenase capacity of mammals.[101,102] These factors include general nutrition,[103] level of water pollution,[104,105] level of air pollution,[106,107] and environmental contaminants that enter the food chain.[101,108,109] The level of AHH activity in hepatic tissues from salmon[105] and salamanders[104] seems to be directed related to the level of organic pollutants in the water, and AHH activity in rats and mice is altered by such factors as type of cage bedding,[110] insecticides and pesticides,[108,111] and room deodorizers.[107] A myriad of chemicals seem responsible for these effects including polychlorinated biphenyls,[109] methylated benzenes and methylated napthalenes,[108] chlorinated dibenzo(p)dioxins

TABLE 6

Effect of Cycloheximide and Actinomycin D on Smoke Induced Lung AHH
and ETR O-deethylase Activity in BC3F₁ Mice[a]

Treatment	AHH activity[b]	O-deethylase activity[c]
Machine controls	0.35	0.04
Smoke	0.70	0.61
Smoke + saline (0.02 ml)	0.67	0.83
Smoke + propylene glycol (0.02 ml)	0.53	0.83
Smoke + cycloheximide (500 μg/g body wt.)	0.32	0.14
Smoke + actinomycin D (1 μg/g body wt.)	0.42	0.15

[a]   Cycloheximide and actinomycin D were injected intraperitoneally in saline
or propylene glycol immediately before exposure to one 2A1 cigarette on a
Walton smoking machine. Mice were sacrificed 6 hr after end of smoke
exposure. Procedures were as described by Van Cantfort and Gielen.[95]

[b]   AHH units are expressed as nmol 3-OH BP formed/min/g wt. wgt. tissue.
Average activity of 3 animals.

[c]   O-deethylase units are expressed as nmoles resorufin formed min/g wt.
wgt. tissue according to the procedures of Burke and Mayer.[101]

and dibenzofurans,[111] and dieldrin-based insecticides such as, P, P′ -DDT, and lindane[91,112] With certain of these chemicals, such as the dibenzo(p) *d* ioxins, the level of
induction of AHH is being used as a tool to show direction as to future chemical
analysis for these classes of chemicals suspected to be contaminating a given food
stuff.[236]

C. AHH and Promotion

In certain model systems, two specific stages of carcinogenesis can be identified.
The first stage involves the actual initiation of the transformed event and the second
stage involves the nonspecific proliferation of this transformed cell into a palpable
tumor[113,114] (see also Chapter 5, this book). It has been suggested that many chemical
carcinogens such as 3-methylcholanthrene possess both initiation and promotion activity; however, it is not known whether the metabolites responsible for initiation are the
same as those responsible for promotion of carcinogenesis. Various BP-metabolites
have been tested for initiation and/or promotion activity in the mouse skin assay.[115-122] Results indicate that the metabolites having the highest initiating activity
(e.g., the BP-7,8 dihydro-7,8-dihydroxy), also are capable of being a complete carcinogen (that is, possess both initiating and promoting activity). The only BP-metabolite
actually tested for its ability to promote skin carcinogenesis, 3-OH BP, was found to
have no promoting capacity.[118] Thus, although promotion could play an important
role in determining the carcinogenic potential of a given chemical, the roles of metabolic activation or inactivation in this promotion process have in fact not been well
defined.

VI. AHH AND ITS ROLE IN IN VITRO TEST SYSTEMS

A. Cytotoxicity

Since the early work of Haddow,[123] it has been known that many of the polycyclic aromatic hydrocarbons are both growth inhibiting and cytotoxic. Most tumor cells and established cell lines, in contrast to freshly explanted cells or tissues, are relatively resistant to the toxic effects of these aromatic hydrocarbons.[124,125] Resistance does not result from the inability of these cells to incorporate these hydrocarbons.[124] Their disparate response seems to result from the fact that neoplastic cells show considerably less hydrocarbon metabolizing activities than do normal cells. In fact, there seems to be a direct correlation between hydrocarbon induced cytotoxicity and AHH enzyme levels in a variety of cell lines.[125,126] The phenols, dihydrodiols, and arene oxides are all more cytotoxic than the parent compounds.[127]

B. Mutagenesis

With the use of bacterial tester strains recently developed by Ames and his colleagues,[128] it has been shown that in vitro metabolic activation of 3-methylcholanthrene,[66] 6-aminochrysene,[66] 2-acetylaminofluorene,[66] and BP[129] is closely associated with the *Ah* locus. This result is especially interesting in view of the recent studies suggesting that specific BP metabolites are in fact much more mutagenic in vitro to both bacterial[127,130,131] and mammalian cells[127,132] than is the parent compound BP. The incorporation of the in vitro metabolic activation system with these bacterial mutagenesis systems has resulted in the characterization of at least some of the metabolically active forms of benz(a)anthracene[133] and 3-methylcholanthrene.[134] Moreover, use of the purified components of the monooxygenase enzyme system has been able to show very nicely the two step activation of BP to one of its mutagenic metabolites. The first step employs the cytochrome P-450-dependent monooxygenase and the second step requires purified epoxide hydrase.[131] Characterization of the active metabolites of BP will be discussed later in this chapter.

The versatility of these partially purified enzyme preparations is exemplified by recent studies on the metabolic activation of cigarette smoke condensate material to their mutagenic forms in vitro. Although S-9 (9000 × g supernatant) preparations from rat or mouse hepatic tissue can activate cigarette smoke condensate material to mutagenic forms in vitro,[96,135-137] S-9 preparations from mouse pulmonary tissue seem to lack this ability.[96,136,137] For reasons as yet unknown, the tissue hypothetically at risk to the action of cigarette smoke related materials (i.e., the mouse lung) does not seem capable of activating these chemicals to their biologically active form, even though the lung tissue is capable of activating other chemical carcinogens such as aflatoxin B_1, 2-aminofluorene, or 7,8-dihydro-7,8-dihydroxy BP to their mutagenic forms.[96,137]

The mammalian mutagenesis systems that have utilized an exogenous in vitro metabolic activation system include V-79 Chinese hamster cells,[138-140] L5178Y mouse lymphoma cells,[141] and the BALB 3T3 C1. A31-1 cells.[142,143] Both whole cell activation systems[138] and partially purified enzyme preparations[139-142] have been used in many of these model systems and a comparison of the advantages and disadvantages of these activation systems is presented in Table 7. it seems the mammalian mutagenesis bioassays are amenable to the sort of studies that the bacterial systems have used with such great success. The major advantage of being able to carry out in vitro metabolic activation of chemicals with mammalian cells is that, in addition to mutagenesis, the endpoint of neoplastic transformation can also be quantitated.

TABLE 7

Comparison of S-9 and Cell-Mediated Systems for Bioactivation of Chemical Carcinogens

ADVANTAGES

S-9	SHE Cells	Hepatocytes
1. Relatively easy to prepare and stable at −70°C	1. Relatively easy to prepare	1. High MFO activity
2. Level of MFO activity can be controlled by varying species or strain of animals, tissue of origin, or kind of inducer	2. High MFO activity which is unaffected by lethal (5000 R) X-irradiation	2. Cells attach to dishes and are mitotically arrested without the need for X-irradiation
3. Reaction time can be stricly controlled	3. Both cells and MFO activity are stable at −120°C for indefinite periods	3. Cells and MFO activity are stable at −120°C
4. Permits some degree of control in amounts and kinds of metabolites generated	4. Metabolites are continually generated for long periods of time ($\sim$ 24 hr) so that long-term exposures are possible	4. Used as a source of metabolic activity in mutagenicity tests and is presently being used for transformation assays
5. Can be made sterile by filtration through 0.45 μ filters	5. Has been used in mammalian mutagenesis tests with high success, but in transformation tests with only limited success	5. Metabolic profile of whole cells may be more analogous to in vivo condition
6. Has been used in conjunction with bacterial and mammalian mutagenesis systems with great success		
7. Versatile: i.e., can be used with bacterial and mammalian cell mutagenesis and mammalian cell transformation assay systems		

DISADVANTAGES

S-9	SHE Cells	Hepatocytes
1. High inherent toxicity to test cells; therefore, level of MFO added is determined by this toxicity	1. Inability to strictly control level of MFO activity	1. Time-consuming and relatively difficult preparation
2. MFO activity is not linear with time and only relatively short incubation times (< 4 hr) are feasible	2. Limited control over time of co-incubation	2. Inability to strictly control level of MFO activity
3. Requires an exogenous NADPH-generating system; cost of assay is relatively high	3. Metabolism is mostly that of fibroblasts, and these cells do not activate certain carcinogens (e.g., 2-AAF)	3. MFO activity very labile (half-life of only $\sim$ 4 hr)
	4. Level of MFO is limited by number of SHE cells per culture vessel	4. Some enhanced stability to these enzymes if other cells are present, but the mechanism of this action is not understood
		5. Level of MFO is limited by the number of hepatocytes attaching to the culture flask

TABLE 8

BP-Metabolizing Activity of Various Rodent Cells in Vitro

Cell line[a]	Nanomoles BP metabolized[b]	Relative activity[c]
FU 5-5	25.0	1
BALB/3T3 C1. A31-714	6.4	0.26
BALB/3T3 C1. A31-1	19.8	0.79
C3H 10T½ C1.8	20.5	0.82
V-79 C1.8	< 1.4	<0.06
SHE—12f	67.1	2.68

[a] FU 5-5 is an established rat hapatoma line that has maintained its monooxygenase activity after repeated subculture in vitro. V-79 C1.8 is an established Chinese hamster line that has virtually lost its monooxygenase activity. The 3T3, 10T½ and SHE lines are described in Reference 142.

[b] Nanomoles converted to water-soluble forms/mg protein/ 24 hr.

[c] Relative BP metabolizing activity.

C. Neoplastic Transformation

A common problem associated with almost every target cell system employed in in vitro carcinogenesis (and mutagenesis) studies is the inherent lack of, low level of, or rapidly dissipating level of carcinogen/mutagen metabolizing activity. The problem is further compounded by the fact that most chemical carcinogens and mutagens require metabolic activation in order to exhibit biological activity.[142] Table 8 shows the relative inherent enzyme activities of several rodent cell lines used in transformation and mutation studies, in terms of their hydrocarbon metabolizing capacities (total amount of organic soluble BP converted to water-soluble forms/min/mg protein). It is obvious that the cell lines differ widely in their mono-oxygenase activities and that these differences could account, in part, for the differences in their sensitivity to different chemical carcinogens (and mutagens). In order to render such target cells more universally sensitive to a wide variety of chemicals, to low concentrations of chemicals, and/or to chemicals of weak biological activity, exogenous supplementary metabolizing activity has been supplied either in the form of intact "feeder" cells or subcellular enzyme fractions (e.g., S-9 or miscrosomal fractions, usually derived from hepatic tissues). Each of these approaches offers its own advantages and disadvantages (see Table 7).

One of the main considerations that needs to be recognized when dealing with exogenous metabolic activation systems is that there is no likely single ideal source of metabolizing activity which is capable of metabolically activating all pro-mutagens and pro-carcinogens to their bioactive forms. Thus the choice of the appropriate activation system is necessarily a function of the specific problem being addressed. It may be that in order to identify the myriad of potentially biohazardous agents and to limit the poosibility of false negative results attributed to a lack of target cell sensitivity to a given particular chemical, a whole battery of activation systems will be required.

The inclusion of exogenous mammalian enzyme fractions for supplying metabolic activity in vitro has been useful with mammalian cell transformation tests.[143-145] Using this approach, an assay has been developed employing a single target cell system for the simultaneous assessment of the mutagenic and carcinogenic potential of chemicals requiring metabolic activation.[145] The assay employs a subclone of the BALB/3T3 C1. A31 line.[146] The 3T3 cells are treated with the test chemical in either of two ways:

STANDARD SUSPENSION ASSAY FOR CHEMICALLY-INDUCED MUTATION AND TRANSFORMATION

OF BALB/3T3 A CLONE A31 CELLS *In Vitro*

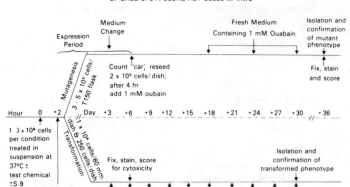

FIGURE 14.   Scheme for the simultaneous in vitro assessment of the cytotoxic, mutagenic, and carcinogenic potential of chemical agents employing a 2 hr treatment of target 3T3 cells in suspension. Cells can be treated either in the presence or absence of an exogenously supplied S-9 preparation and an NADPH-generating system.

1.   In suspension for 2 hr at 3°C in the presence of a reaction mixture containing an Aroclor-1254-induced rat hepatic S-9 and an NADPH-generating system, in accordance with methods previously described for bacterial systems[147] and mammalian cells in culture,[148] and modified for use with BALB/3T3 cells[143,145]

2.   For 24 hr at 37°C under conditions in which cells are attached to the petri dish surface in the presence of the same reaction mixture

Flow charts depicting each of these approaches are presented in Figures 14 and 15, respectively. This assay has successfully detected the mutagenic and phenotypic transforming effects of different classes of chemicals including polycyclic aromatic hydrocarbons, aromatic amines, alkylating agents, and various complex biological mixtures such as pesticides, dyes, and environmental pollutants. Furthermore, the assay technique permits the examination of the molecular realtionship between carcinogenesis and mutagenesis.

D. Covalent Binding of AHH Metabolites to DNA

Although RNA or protein might be the critical intracellular target at which chemical carcinogenesis is initiated, considerable interest has centered on DNA and chemicals which bind covalently to DNA as important early events in the initiation of tumors.[149] When polycyclic aromatic hydrocarbon carcinogens are topically applied to mouse skin, covalent binding of the compounds to cellular macromolecules results.[150] Subsequently the incubation of BP was shown[151,152] to produce covalent binding of unknown metabolites to DNA. Since the initial products of double-bond oxidation was thought to be epoxides,[153] it was assumed that these particular metabolites were probably formed by the microsomal cytochrome P-450-mediated monooxygenase systems and that these intermediates then interacted with a variety of cellular macromolecules including DNA, rearranged nonenzymatically to form phenols, were hydrated to form trans-dihydrodiols, and were then conjugated with glutathione (see Figure 2).

STANDARD PLATE ASSAY FOR CHEMICALLY-INDUCED MUTATION AND TRANSFORMATION
OF BALB/3T3 CLONE A31 CELLS *In Vitro*

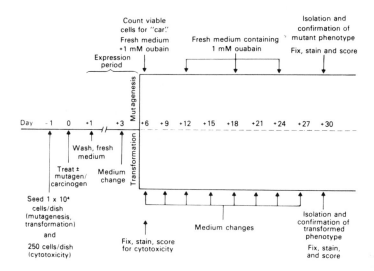

FIGURE 15.   Scheme for the simultaneous in vitro assessment of the cytotoxic, mutagenic and carcinogenic potential of chemical agents employing a
24 hr treatment of target 3T3 cells which have previously been allowed to
adhere to the growing surface of petri dishes. Cells can be treated either in
the presence or absence of an exogenously supplied S-9 preparation and an
NADPH-generating system.

1. Measurements of DNA Binding

Techniques have now been developed so that the nature of the carcinogen bound to
nucleic acid can be studied.[154] This method has shown great promise in that distinct
peaks eluted from the Sephadex LH20 column can be demonstrated to change in elution profile, depending on the carcinogen incubated with the microsomes and cofactors, whether rat liver microsomes or cells in culture are used, and on the use of microsomal enzyme inhibitors in vitro.[155-159] Use of this technique has shown that: (1) there
are at least nine distinct carcinogen-metabolite-DNA peaks following in vitro DNA
binding of BP metabolites generated with liver[129,160-163] or skin microsomes,[129] (2) eight
peaks are associated with increased P_1-450 content and are greater with liver microsomes from genetically responsive inbred strains (e.g., C3, B6) than from genetically
nonresponsive strains (e.g., D2),[160,161,163] (3) all nine peaks are greater wit skin nicro-
somes in vitro from C3 and B6 than from D2 mice,[129] and (4) using various synthetic
metabolites of BP[162] and various inducers in vivo and inhibitors in vitro,[163] the major
reactive intermediate compromising each of the nine chromatographic peaks was tentatively identified (Table 9). The capacity of a given microsomal preparation to metabolize BP to forms that bind to DNA parallel its capacity to metabolize BP to forms
mutagenic to the TA1538 and TA98 tester strains of *Salmonella typhimurium*.[129] No
specific BP metabolite-nucleoside peak is linked to this mutagenic event. The comparison of the profile of the nine BP metabolite-nucleoside complex(es) generated in vitro
with susceptibility to BP carcinogenesis for the AHH responsive B6 and C3 strains
and the nonresponsive D2 strain, demonstrates the following; a good correlation between total DNA-binding and susceptibility to BP carcinogenesis for the B6 and C3
when compared to the D2 strain; a lack of correlation between either total bound BP-
metabolites, or any particular BP-metabolite-nucleoside, complex(es) and susceptibil-

TABLE 9

Postulated Identification of BP Metabolites Produced In Vitro by Mouse Liver Microsomes That Bind to DNA

Peak	Fraction number at which peaks occur	Precursor	Ultimate active form of BP metabolite which is the major contributor to the peak[a]
A	62	Dihydrodiol(s)	Unknown dihydrodiol oxide(s)
B	71	Quinone(s)	Quinone-oxide(s) (or quinone-derived free radicals)
C	86	Dihydrodiol(s)	Unknown dihydrodiol oxide(s)
D	98	Quinone(s)	Quinone-oxide(s) (or quinone-derived free radicals)
E	105	7,8-Dihydrodiol	7,8-Diol-9,10-epoxides (both cis and trans)
F	122	Quinone(s)	Quinone-oxide(s) (or quinone-derived free radicals)
F'	115	BP	7,8-Oxide
G	134	BP	4,5-Oxide
H	155	Phenol(s)	Unknown penol oxide(s)
I	171	Quinone(s)	Quinone-oxide(s) (or quinone-derived free radicals)

[a] See Reference 129.

ity to BP carcinogenesis for the B6 and C3 strains. Thus, as mentioned previously in this chapter, although the capacity of the inbred strains to metabolize a chemical carcinogen plays a major role in the susceptibility of that strain to cancers induced by that chemical, there are other factors which influence the ultimate susceptibility to chemical carcinogenesis. Some of the factors will be discussed at length in other chapters of this book.

2. Measure of DNA Damage

As a result of the binding of chemical carcinogens or their metabolites to DNA, perturbations or distortions of the DNA helicies are observed. These distortions serve as stimuli for the DNA repair enzymes. As a direct result of the chemical-DNA interacti or as a result of DNA-repair enzymes attempting to restore this distortion, strand breakage often occurs. This strand breakage can be detected and quantified by measuring the elution rate of DNA under alkaline conditions.[164] This technique has been used to measure the amount of DNA damage induced by a number of chemical carcinogens using both in vitro[165] and in vivo[166,167] model systems. In vitro activation of chemicals that require metabolic activation can also be studied by this technique.[165] Recent studies in our laboratory suggest that the level of AHH activity in a given tissue preparation parallels the extent of BP metabolized to forms that cause damage to DNA.[237] The nature of the chemical or its metabolite that causes this damage has not been as yet defined.

3. DNA Repair

Monofunctional alkylating agents (such as methylmethane sulfonate, which do not require metabolic activation), polycyclic aromatic hydrocarbons (which do require metabolic activation), and multifunctional agents (such as mitomycin C which can cross-link DNA strands[168]—all can bind to DNA and stimulate DNA repair. These processes, which include pre and post replication repair, also express some selectivity or priority related to the type of DNA damage that is repaired. The concept that the DNA repair capacity of an individual may be genetically regulated and can play a major role in determining the alternate susceptibility to chemically-induced cancer will be discussed at length in Chapter 3.

E. Identification of Active Forms of Chemical Carcinogens; the "Bay-Region" Theory of Polycyclic Aromatic Hydrocarbon Induced Cancers

Numerous theories have attempted to correlate structure with carcinogenic activity. The most successful of the early theories was the "K-region" hypothesis of Pullman and Pullman.[169] In this theory, the hydrocarbon must possess a "K-region" with high electron density in order to be carcinogenic. If the molecule also has an "L-region", this region must be rather inactive in order for the hydrocarbon to remain carcinogenic. Prototypes for the "K-region" and "L-region" are the 9,10-position in phenanthrene and the 9,10-position in anthracene, respectively. This theory provides a fairly good ranking of the carcinogenic potential of a given set of polycyclic aromatic hydrocarbons; however, certain "K-region" oxides of these chemicals are observed to possess very weak carcinogenic activity in vivo.[170-175] Certain in vitro model systems, such as bacterial mutagenesis,[176] mammalian mutagenesis,[177] or mammalian transformation[178] yield data which tend to support the "K-region" theory; that is, the "K-region" arene oxides of BP, the 4,5-oxide and 11,12-oxide are the most active primary oxidative metabolite in the bacterial mutagenesis and mammalian mutagenesis bioassays.[179-180]

However, the ultimate carcinogenic metabolites need not be primary oxidative metabolites. Borgen et al.[181] showed that the 7,8-dihydro-7,8-dihydroxy BP is the substrate which is metabolized most extensively to DNA bound products. The realization that a 7,8-dihydro-7,8-dihydroxy BP-9,10-epoxide is responsible for the binding to DNA[36] suggested that secondary metabolites may be very important in the bioactivation of polycyclic aromatic hydrocarbons. Studies of DNA adducts formed when BP is applied to mouse skin,[182] of RNA adducts formed when cultured bovine bronchial mucosa are exposed to BP,[183] of DNA adducts formed when primary cultures of Syrian hamster embryo cells[36] are exposed to BP, of DNA adducts formed when yeast RNA or certain polyribonucleotides are exposed to BP,[184] and of DNA adducts formed when deproteinized DNA is exposed to BP plus known microsomal enzyme preparations,[129] indicate that BP 7,8-diol-9,10-epoxides rather than the "K-region" 4,5-oxides are responsible for most of the covalent binding to DNA.

A comparison of the biological activity of BP and thirteen BP derivatives in three in vivo carcinogenesis assays and two in vitro mutagenesis assays is shown in Table 10 (see Reference 185 for details). Sensitivity of the subcutaneous model system to the seven arene oxides of BP compare very favorably with the results with the other in vivo systems of skin carcinogenesis of leukemia/lymphomas and lung carcinogenesis following arene-oxide treatment of newborn mice. That is, the diol-epoxide 2, the H_4-9, 10-epoxide, and the 7,8-oxide are the only arene oxides showing significant carcinogenic activity in vivo. The lower carcinogenic activity of the diol-epoxide 2 in the subcutaneous assay compared with the skin or newborn assay may be the result of instability of this chemical in the vehicles employed. Slaga et al.[118] suggest that the vehicle plays a major role in allowing for the biological activity of this diol-epoxide. Therefore, use of another vehicle such as tetrahydrofuran could very well enhance the activity of diol-epoxide 2, just as it enhanced the activity of this BP-metabolite in the skin model system. It seems likely that the high chemical reactivity and relatively high instability of these epoxides masks their potential biological effects in vivo (see discussion, Reference 192). On the other hand, the in vitro assays of bacterial mutagenesis using the *S. typhimurium* tester strains, and mammalian mutagenesis using the V-79 C1 8 Chinese hamster cell line are much more sensitive to these arene oxides. In fact,

TABLE 10

Comparison of Biological Activity of BP and BP-derivative in Various In Vitro and In Vivo Model Systems[a]

	Tumorigenesis			Mutagenesis	
Chemical	Skin (Ref. 115,119,120) SQ[b] (CI)	Skin (Ref. 115,119,120)	Newborn (Ref. 186—188)	Bacterial (Ref. 127—131,189,190)	V-79 (Ref. 127,122,189—191)
BP	+++ (55)	+++	++	+++	++
7,8-diol	++ (13)[c]	+++	+++	+++	++
	+ (0.3)				
7,8-diacetate	++ (8.5)	NT[d]	NT	NT	NT
H4-7,8-transdiol	±[e]	—	NT	—	—
9,10-H2	+ (1.3)	NT	NT	+++	NT
7,8-H2	+++ (63)	NT	NT	+++	NT
Diol epoxide-1	—	+++[f]	—	+++	+++
Diol epoxide-2	+ (1.9)	+	+++	+++	+++
H4-9,10-epoxide	+ (3.3)	—	NT	+++	+++
4,5-oxide	—	++	+	—	—
7,8-oxide	+ (3.0)	++	—	—	—
9,10-oxide	—	—	—	—	+++
11,12-oxide	—	—	—	—	—
2-OH BP	++ (6.9)	+++	+++	+	+

[a]   Relative activity of the compounds are presented.

[b]   From Reference 185, carcinogenic index given in parentheses.

[c]   Results when given in DMSO.

[d]   NT = not tested.

[e]   Tumors only found when simultaneously treated with TCDD.

[f]   Results when given in tetrahydrofuran.[118]

the highly mutagenic diol-epoxide 1, H_4-9,10-epoxide, 4,5-oxide, and the 11,12-oxide (only in the V-79 cells) have little or no capacity to cause tumors in the three in vivo systems. These in vitro assays may also arrive at a false negative conclusion. The 7,8-oxide causes no mutagenesis to either bacterial or mammalian cells in vitro; however, it has detectable carcinogenic activity in all three in vivo assays. These results exemplify the limitations of using these in vitro systems as sole criteria for determination of the potential biological activity of a chemical.

The BP-derivative, 2-OH BP, is active in all five model systems. The importance of this observation is difficult to assess at this time because 2-OH BP is not a known metabolite of BP (see discussion in Reference 119). Nonetheless, its relatively strong carcinogenic and mutagenic capacity suggests a need for additional work to determine whether 2-OH BP is formed from BP in any mammalian tissue and whether 2-OH BP contributes to the carcinogenic action of BP.

The carcinogenesis bioassay using the subcutaneous route of evauation shows very nicely the importance of the double bond at the 9,10 position to the carcinogenicity of BP. The 7,8-H_2 derivative, which lacks a double bond at the 7,8 position but still can be metabolized at the 9,10 position, is as carcinogenic as BP. The 9,10-H_2 derivative, which lacks a double bond at the 9,10 position and cannot be metabolized at this position, has very low carcinogenic potential. The activity of these chemicals in vivo parallels their mutagenic activity in bacteria. That is, the products of 7,8-H_2 BP metabolism are considerably more mutagenic than the products of 9,10-H_2 BP metabolism.[130]

The major problem with this subcutaneous assay is the inability to detect reproducibly the carcinogenic effects of the 7,8-dihydro-7,8-dihydroxy BP. When given in trioctanoin, only 2 of 99 animals developed tumors. BP-treated animals resulted in 65 of 76 animals with tumors. The 7,8-dihydro-7,8-dihydroxy BP given in DMSO resulted in a fairly high CI of 13 and in fact the 7,8-dihydro-7,8-dihydroxy BP in DMSO is more tumorigenic than any of the BP-metabolites tested and is as carcinogenic as BP given in DMSO. The 7,8-dihydro-7,8-dihydroxy BP is more polar than BP, however this polarity does not influence its uptake into cells.[191] The use of a chemical that is more nonpolar than the 7,8-dihydro-7,8-dihydroxy BP, the 7,8-diacetate (given in trioctanoin), is 10 times more carcinogenic than the 7,8-dihydro-7,8-dihydroxy BP. The reasons for this enhanced tumorigenicity are not known at this time. The second problem is that the 7,8-dihydro-7,8-dihydroxy BP is not an inducer for AHH activity in vivo[237] or in cell culture[191] and the subcutaneous connective tissue may not possess enough AHH activity to metabolize this chemical efficiently. Induction of AHH activity in the subcutaneous tissue by simultaneous administration with TCDD slightly enhances the tumorigenicity of both the 7,8-dihydro-7,8-dihydroxy BP and the 7,8-diacetate.[179]

Simultaneous treatment with TCDD and BP in this AHH-inducible strain of mouse has no effect on BP-induced tumorigenesis. This latter observation confirms a similar result using TCDD, 3-methylcholanthrene, and the AHH-inducible C57BL/6 mouse.[35] Recent studies in our laboratory[238] suggest that the 7,8-dihydro-7,8-dihydroxy BP possesses much higher carcinogenic potential than BP when administered intratracheally to C3 mice. A variety of tumors, including bronchogenic squamous cell carcinomas, alveologenic adenocarcinomas, and even mammary adenocarcinomas are observed after intratracheal inoculation of this diol. Thus the 7,8-dihydro-7,8-dihydroxy BP can be a very active carcinogen in C3 mice and the lower activity observed in this subcutaneous assay probably results from a combination of these problems discussed above.

Two BP-derivatives express very low carcinogenic activity per se. These are the H_4-7,8-transdiol and the 9,10-H_2-BP. Both of these compounds are saturated at the 9,10 positions and therefore neither can be metabolized directly to an arene oxide at this position. The H_4-7,8-transdiol also does not exert any biological effect even if given in a DMSO vehicle. However, simultaneous treatment with TCDD did allow for some carcinogenic activity of this chemical.[185] The low carcinogenic potential of the 9,10-H_2-BP and the H_4-7,8-transdiol (with TCDD) are consistent with the hypothesis that most of the tumorigenic activity of BP can be accounted for by metabolism at the 9,10 position of this chemical carcinogen; at the so-called "bay region."[192] The fact that some carcinogenic potential was observed with the H_4-7,8-transdiol and the 9,10-H_2-BP suggests that either there are enzymatic mechanisms in vivo that can reconstitute the double bond at the 9,10 position, or that metabolism elsewhere on the BP molecule may also contribute to the overall carcinogenicity of BP. The data, especially with the 7,8-H_2-BP derivative, suggests that in these in vivo tumor systems probably less than 10% of the overall carcinogenicity of BP can be attributed to metabolism at other than this "bay region."

The "bay-region" of an aromatic hydrocarbon refers to the hindered region between the 4- and 5- positions in the phenanthrene molecule. The regions between the 1- and 12- positions of benz(a)anthracene are "bay-regions." It should be pointed out that all hydrocarbons that have a "bay-region" also have "K-regions." The aforementioned example of BP showed that the 7,8-diol-9,10-epoxy-7,8,9,10-tetrahydro derivative is at least one of the ultimate biologically-active metabolites of this carcinogen. Nucleophilic attack on this diol-epoxide occurs at the C-10 position suggesting the involvement of carbonium ions.[194] Assessment of the relative ease of formation of cardonium ion formation from diol epoxides has been attempted.[192,195] Results suggest that using a perturbational molecular orbital procedure described by Dewar,[196] a parameter Δ_{deloc}, can be calculated which reflects the stability of formation of carbonium ions at that position, and imply the existence of more reactive diol epoxides.[192,195] For a given polycyclic aromatic hydrocarbon, diol-epoxides in which the oxiran (e.g., epoxide) oxygen forms part of a "bay-region" were calculated to be more reactive than diol-epoxides in which the oxiran oxygen was remote from the "bay-region."[195] Moreover, the diol-epoxides of highly carcinogenic hydrocarbons should be more reactive than those "bay-region" diol epoxides of weak or noncarcinogenic aromatic hydrocarbons.[195,197] Measurements of the biological activity of the "bay-region" derivative of BP,[192] benz(a)anthracene,[192] 7,12-dimethylbenz(a)anthracene,[198] 3-methylcholanthrene,[199] dibenz(a,h)anthracene,[200] and chrysene.[201] All are consistent with the idea that the formation of diol epoxides of the "bay-region" results in the generation of at least one of the carcinogenic and mutagenic metabolites of polycyclic aromatic hydrocarbons.

VII. EVIDENCE FOR *Ah* LOCUS IN MAN

In 1973 two published reports[202,203] aroused the hopes of clinical geneticists and oncologists that a test for the detection of AHH levels in the human population was possible. The extent of AHH induction by 3-methylcholanthrene in cultured mitogen-activated lymphocytes was examined in 353 healthy subjects, ranging in age from 2 to 89 and including 67 families with 165 children.[202] The distribution of inducibilities in the patients tested in the Houston area was trimodal, the groups being designated as having "low", "intermediate", and "high" inducibility. The data were consistent with a hypothesis of two alleles at a single locus and gave an excellent fit to the Hardy-Weinberg equilibrium, with a frequency of 0.717 for the low-inducibility allele and 0.283 for the high-inducibility allele (although the sample is biased by including parents and siblings). Fifty patients with bronchogenic carcinoma were then compared with

46 patients having other types of tumors and with 85 healthy control.[203] The authors concluded that a person having the intermediate-inducibility phenotype has a 16 times increased risk and a person having the high-inducibility phenotype has a 46 times increased risk, of developing bronchogenic carcinoma, compared with persons having the low-inducibility phenotype. Laryngeal carcinoma was also reported[204] to be associated with the high-inducibility phenotype. However, this report suffered from a major shortcoming: the values for patients free of cancer were not obtained under the same conditions as those for patients with cancer. In fact, control, cancer-free patients in Lund, Sweden were not studied at all, but rather the incidence of AHH-inducibility phenotypes was taken directly from the studies of Kellerman and co-workers[203] in Houston, Texas. Three other laboratories have suggested that lung cancer patients have higher AHH capacities when compared to noncancerous individuals.[205-209] In one study,[205] the lung cancer patients were observed to have higher levels of hydrocarbon metabolizing capacity than control patients, and in the other,[206] the total AHH capacity was similar among the two groups, but rather, the noninduced or control lymphocytes expressed lower AHH levels in the lung cancer patients; therefore, the inducibility ratio (induced activity per noninduced activity) was significantly elevated in these lung cancer patients. AHH activity can be detected in pulmonary alveolar macrophages,[210] this activity is correlated with AHH levels in mitogen-activated lymphocytes in noncancer patients,[207-209] but there is a disassociation in lung cancer patients.[207-209] Lung cancer susceptibility seems correlated with high AHH activity in either the lymphocytes or the pulmonay alveolar macrophages, but not both.[208,209]

There are reports that suggest that lung cancer patients possess similar or even lower AHH capacities as noncancer patients,[211-213] even patients whose lung tumors have been removed and have been clinically free of the disease for a period of time express no high levels of AHH activity when compared to noncancer controls.[212] However, this latter observation is difficult to evaluate because only the AHH inducibility ratios are presented, no actual AHH data are given. Even using very similar assay conditions,[205,213] two different laboratories have come to opposite conclusions as to the role of AHH in lunr cancer susceptibility in man. Opposite conclusions as to the relationship between high lymphocyte AHH levels and such parameters as in vivo drug half-life,[214-216] high monocyte AHH levels,[217-219] or yearly seasonal variations,[220-222] have also been reported.

The easiest explanation of these seemingly disparate observations resides in the mitogen activation step itself. Culture conditions such as lot and type of serum supplement,[214,222-224] type and lot of mitogens,[223-225] initial concentrations of lymphocytes,[222] type and concentration of AHH inducer,[222] length of incubation time,[222] presence of heparin in culture medium,[226] and even such in vivo conditions as age of donor, percentage of T- or B-cells, day of menstrual cycle, nutrition or disease state and use of drugs, all can influence the mitogen activation of lymphocytes and their associated AHH activities.[227] Since these laboratories employed different mitogen-activation conditions, and since only a few studies have simultaneously measured for mitogen activation,[211,213,222,228,229] it seems quite likely that many of these observed differences in AHH levels simply reflect variations in mitogen responsiveness, rather than specific differences in the capacity to metabolize chemical carcinogens. Recent studies have shown that when the degree of mitogen responsiveness is held relatively constant, real differences in AHH levels exist among individuals.[214,222,228-230] Moreover, a significant heritable component regulating AHH levels exists.[214,230,231] Thus, people seem to possess naturally occurring variations in their capacity to metabolize some chemical carcinogens,[214,222,228-234] but whether these differences are regulated by an *Ah* locus, or are related to cancer susceptibility requires much additional work.

ACKNOWLEDGMENT

The authors extend their appreciation to many collaborators including Drs. S. Thorgiersson, D. Felton, W. F. Benedict, and A. Boobis whose efforts made this chapter possible. The authors also wish to thank The Council for Tobacco Research, New York, for their continued support of many of these studies.

REFERENCES

1. **Williams, R. T.**, *Detoxification Mechanisms. The Metabolism and Detoxification of Drugs, Toxic Substances, and Other Organic Compounds,* 2nd ed., John Wiley & Sons, New York, 1959.
2. **Mason, H. S.**, Mechanisms of oxygen metabolism, *Adv. Enzymol.,* 19, 79, 1957.
3. **Conney, A. H. and Burns, J. J.**, Metabolic interactions among environmental chemicals and drugs, *Sciences,* 178, 576, 1972.
4. **Jerina, D. M. and Daly, J. W.**, Arene oxides: a new aspect of drug metabolism, *Science,* 185, 573, 1974.
5. **Sims, P. and Grover, P. L.**, Epoxides in polycyclic aromatic hydrocarbon metabolism and carcinogenesis, *Adv. Cancer Res.,* 20, 165, 1974.
6. **Heidelberger, C.**, Chemical carcinogenesis, *Ann. Rev. Biochem.,* 44, 79, 1975.
7. **Nebert, D. W., Robinson, J. R., Niwa, A., Kumaki, K., and Poland, A. P.**, Genetic expression of aryl hydrocarbon hydroxylase activity in the mouse, *J. Cell Physiol.,* 83, 393, 1975.
8. **Thorgeirsson, S. S. and Nebert, D. W.**, The *Ah* locus and the metabolism of chemical carcinogens and other foreign compounds, *Adv. Cancer Res.,* 25, 149, 1977.
9. **Kouri, R. E. and Nebert, D. W.**, Genetic regulation of susceptibility to polycyclic-hydrocarbon-induced tumors in the mouse, in, *Origins of Human Cancer,* Book A, Hiatt, H. H., Watson, J. D., and Winsten, J. A., Eds., Cold Spring Harbor Laboratory, New York, 1977, 811.
10. **Czygan, P., Greim, H., Garro, A., Schaffner, F., and Popper, H.**, The effect of dietary protein deficiency on the ability of isolated hepatic microsomes to alter the mutagenicity of a primary and a secondary carcinogen, *Cancer Res.,* 34, 119, 1974.
11. **DeFlora, S.**, Metabolic deactivation of mutagens in the Salmonella-microsome test, *Nature,* 271, 455, 1978.
12. **Miller, J. A. and Miller, E. C.**, Chemical carcinogenesis, mechanisms and approaches to its control, *J. Nat. Cancer Inst.,* 47, 5, 1971.
13. **Bjorkhem, I.**, Rate limiting step in microsomal cytochrome P-450 catalyzed hydroxylations, *Pharm. Ther.,* 1, 327, 1977.
14. **Estabrook, R. W., Hildebrandt, A. G., Baron, J., Ritter, K. J., and Leibman, K.**, A new spectral intermediate associated with cytochrome P-450 function in liver microsomes, *Biochem. Biophys. Res. Commun.,* 42, 132, 1971.
15. **Lu, A. Y. H. and Coon, M. J.**, Role of hemoprotein P-450 in fatty acid ω-hydroxylation in a soluble enzyme system from liver microsomes, *J. Biol. Chem.,* 243, 1331, 1968.
16. **Lu, A. Y. H., Junk, K. W., and Coon, M. J.**, Resolution of the cytochrome P-450—containing ω-hydroxylation system of liver microsomes into three components, *J. Biol. Chem.,* 244, 3714, 1968.
17. **Strobel, H. W., Lu, A. Y. H., Heidema, J., and Coon, M. J.**, Phosphatidylcholine requirement in the enzymatic reduction of hemoprotein P-450 and in fatty acid, hydrocarbon, and drug hydroxylation, *J. Biol. Chem.,* 245, 4851, 1970.
18. **Dignam, J. D. and Strobel, H. W.**, Preparation of homogenous NADPH-cytochrome P-450 reductase from rat liver, *Biochem. Biophys. Res. Commun.,* 63, 845, 1975.
19. **Imai, Y. and Sato, R.**, Gel-electrophoretically homogeneous preparation of cytochrome P-450 from liver microsomes of phenobarbital—pretreated rabbits, *Biochem. Biophys. Res. Commun.,* 60, 8, 1974.
20. **Iyanagi, T. and Mason, H. S.**, Some properties of hepatic reduced nicotinamide adenine dinucleotide phosphate—cytochrome *c* reductase, *Biochemistry,* 12, 2297, 1973.
21. **Levin, W., Ryan, D., West, S., and Lu, A. Y. H.**, Preparation of partially purified lipid-depleted cytochrome P-400 and reduced nicotinamide adenine dinucleotide phosphate—cytochrome *c* reductase from rat liver microsomes, *J. Biol. Chem.,* 249, 1747, 1974.

22. Kadlubar, F. F. and Ziegler, D. M., Properties of a NADH-dependent n-hydroxy amine reductase isolated from pig liver microsomes, *Arch. Biochem. Biophys.*, 162, 83, 1974.

23. van der Hoeven, T. A., Haugen, D. A., and Coon, M. J., Cytochrome P-450 purified to apparent homogeneity from phenobarbital-induced rabbit liver microsomes: catalytic activity and other properties, *Biochem. Biophys. Res. Commun.*, 60, 569, 1974.

24. Vermillion, J. L. and Coon, M. J., Highly purified detergent solubilized NADPH-cytochrome P-450 reductase from phenobarbital-induced rat liver microsomes, *Biochem. Biophys. Res. Commun.*, 60, 1315, 1974.

25. Lu, A. Y. H. and Levin, W., The resolution and reconstitution of the liver microsomal hydroxylation system, *Biochem. Biophys. Acta*, 344, 205, 1974.

26. van der Hoeven, T. A. and Coon, M. J., Preparation and properties of partially purified cytochrome P-450 and reduced nicotinamide adenine dinucleotide phosphate-cytochrome P-450 reductase from rabbit liver microsomes, *Biol. Chem.*, 249, 6302, 1974.

27. Lu, A. Y. H., Liver microsomal drug-metabolizing enzyme system: functional components and their properties, *Fed. Proc.*, 35, 2460, 1976.

28. Thomas, P. E., Lu, A. Y. H., Ryan, D., West, S. B., Kawalek, J., and Levin, W., Immunochemical evidence for six forms of rat liver cytochrome P-450 obtained using antibodies against purified rat liver cytochromes P-450 and P-448, *Mol. Pharmacol.*, 12, 746, 1976.

29. Haugen, D. A., Coon, M. J., and Nebert, D. W., Induction of multiple forms of mouse liver cytochrome P-450 evidence for genetically controlled *de novo* protein synthesis in response to treatment with β-naphthoflavone or phenobarbital, *J. Biol. Chem.*, 251, 1817, 1976.

30. Ryan, D., Lu, A. Y. H. West, S., and Levin, W., Multiple forms of cytochrome P-450 in phenobarbital- and 3-methylcholanthrene-treated rats. Separation and spectral properties, *J. Biol. Chem.*, 250, 2157, 1975.

31. Guenthner, T. M. and Nebert, D. W., Evidence in rat for temporal gene control of two inducible monooxygenase activities and two distinct forms of cytochrome P-450 regulated by the *Ah* locus, *Fed. Proc.*, 37, 858, 1978.

32. Atlas, S. A., Boobis, A. R., Felton, J. S., and Nebert, D. W., Ontogenetic expression of polycyclic aromatic compound inducible monooxygenase activities and forms of cytochrome P-450 in rabbit. Evidence for temporal control and organ specificity of two genetic regulatory systems, *J. Biol. Chem.*, 252, 4712, 1977.

33. Owens, I. A. and Nebert, D. W., Aryl hydrocarbon hydroxylase induction in mammalian liver-derived cell cultures. Stimulation of "cytochrome P_1-450-associated" enzyme activity by many inducing compounds, *Mol. Pharamacol.*, 11, 94, 1975.

34. Gielen, J. E. and Nebert, D. W., Aryl hydrocarbon hydroxylase induction in mammalian liver cell culture. III. Effects of various sera, hormones, biogenic amines, and other endogenous compounds on the enzyme activity, *J. Biol. Chem.*, 247, 7591, 1972.

35. Kouri, R. E., Rude, T. H., Joglekar, R., Dansette, P. M., Jerina, D. M., Atlas, S. A., Owens, I. S., and Nedert, D. W., 2,3,7,8-Tetrachlorodibenzo(p)dioxin acts as a cocarcinogen in causing 3-methylcholanthrene-initiated subcutaneous tumors in mice genetically "nonresponsive" at the *Ah* locus, *Cancer Res.*, 38, 2777, 1978.

36. Sims, P., Grover, P. L., Swaisland, A., Pal, K., and Hewer, A., Metabolic activation of benzo(a)pyrene proceeds by a diol-epoxide, *Nature*, 252, 326, 1974.

37. Thomas, P. E., Kouri, R. E., and Hutton, J. J., The genetics of aryl hydrocarbon hydroxylase induction in mice: a single gene difference between C5BL/6J and DBA/2J, *Biochem. Genet.*, 6, 157, 1972.

38. Green, M. C., Guideline for genetically determined biochemical variants in the house mouse, *Mus musculus*, *Biochem. Genet.*, 9, 369, 1973.

39. Poland, A. P. and Glover, E., Genetic expression of aryl hydrocarbon hydroxylase by 2,3,7,8-tetrachlorodibenzo-p-dioxin by hepatic cytosol: evidence for a receptor mutation in genetically nonresponsive mice, *Mol. Pharmacol.*, 11, 389, 1975.

40. Owens, I. S. and Nebert, D. W., Genetically-medicated UDPG transferase induction by polycyclic aromatic compounds associated with the "*Ah* locus" in the mouse, *Pharmacologist*, 17, 217, 1975.

41. Nebert, D. W. and Felton, J. S., The importance of genetic factors influencing the metabolism of foreign compounds, *Fed. Proc.*, 31, 1315, 1976.

42. Yang, S. K., Roller, P. P., Fu, P. P., Harvey, R. G. and Gelboin, N. V., Evidence of a 2,3-epoxide as an intermediate in the microsomal metabolism of benzo(a)pyrene to 3-hydroxybenzo(a)pyrene, *Biochem. Biophys. Res. Commun.*, 77, 1176, 1977.

43. Nebert, D. W. and Gelboin, H. V., Substrate-inducible microsomal aryl hydrocarbon hydroxylase in mammalian cell culture. I. Assay and properties of induced enzyme, *J. Biol. Chem.*, 243, 6242, 1968.

44. **Lu, A. Y. H., Levin, W., Vore, M., Conney, A. H., Thakker, D., Holder, G., and Jerina, D. M.,** Metabolism of benzo(a)pyrene by purified liver microsomal cytochrome P-448 and epoxide hydrase, in *Polynuclear Aromatic Hydrocarbons: Chemistry, Metabolism and Carcinogenesis,* Freudenthal, R. I. and Jones, P. W., Eds., Raven Press, New York, 1976, 115.

45. **Niwa, A., Kumaki, K., Nebert, D. W., and Poland, A. P.,** Genetic expression of aryl hydrocarbon hydroxylase activity in the mouse. Distinction between the "responsive" homozygote and heterozygote at the *Ah* locus, *Arch. Biochem. Biophys.,* 166, 559, 1975.

46. **Kouri, R. E., Rude, T., Thomas, P. E., and Whitmire, C. E.,** Studies on pulmonary aryl hydrocarbon hydroxylase activity in inbred strains of mice, *Chem. Biol. Interact.,* 13, 317, 1976.

47. **Nebert, D. W. and Gielen, J. E.,** Genetic regulation of aryl hydrocarbon hydroxylase induction in the mouse, *Fed. Proc.,* 31, 1315, 1972.

48. **Nebert, D. W., Goujon, F. M., and Gielen, J. E.,** Aryl hydrocarbon hydroxylase induction by polycyclic hydrocarbons: simple autosomal cominant trait in the mouse, *Nature London New Biol.,* 236, 107, 1972.

49. **Gielen, J. E., Goujon, F. M., and Nebert, D. W.,** Genetic regulation of aryl hydrocarbon hydroxylase induction. iI. Simple mendelian expression in mouse tissues *in vivo, J. Biol. Chem.,* 247, 1125, 1972.

50. **Nebert, D. W., Considine, N., and Owens, I. S.,** Genetic expression of aryl hydrocarbon hyoroxylase induction. VI. Control of other aromatic hydrocarbon-inducible monooxygenase activities at or near the same genetic locus, *Arch. Biochem. Biophys.,* 157, 148, 1973.

51. **Kouri, R. E., Salerno, R. A., and Whitmire, C. E.,** Relationships between aryl hydrocarbon hydroxylase inducibility and sensitivity to chemically induced subcutaneous sarcomas in various strains of mice, *J. Nat. Cancer Inst.,* 50, 363, 173.

52. **Kouri, R. E., Ratrie, H., III, and Whitmire, C. E.,** Evidence of a genetic relationship between susceptibility to 3-methycholanthrene-induced subcutaneous tumors and inducibility of aryl hydrocarbon hydroxylase, *J. Nat. Cancer Inst.,* 51, 197, 1973.

53. **Poland, A. P. and Glover, E.,** Genetic expression of aryl hydrocarbon hydroxylase by 2,3,7,8-tetrachlorodibenzo-*p*-dioxin: evidence for a receptor mutation in genetically non-responsive mice, *Mol. Pharmacol.,* 11, 389, 1975.

54. **Kouri, R. E.,** Relationship between levels of aryl hydrocarbon hydroxylase activity and susceptibility to 3-methylcholanthrene and benzo(a)pyrene-induced cancers in inbred strains of mice, in *Polynuclear Aromatic Hydrocarbons: Chemistry, Metabolism and Carcinogenesis,* Freudenthal, R. E. and Jones, P. W., Eds., Raven Press, New York, 1976, 139.

55. **Atlas, S. A., Taylor, B. A., Diwan, B. A., and Nebert, D. W.,** Inducible monooxygenase activities and 3-methylcholanthrene-initiated tumorigenesis in mouse recombinant inbred sublines, *Genetics,* 83, 537, 1976.

56. **Robinson, J. R., Considine, N., and Nebert, D. W.,** Genetic expression of aryl hydrocarbon hydroxylase induction. Evidence for the involvement of other genetic loci, *J. Biol. Chem.,* 249, 5851, 1974.

57. **Nebert, D. W., Benedict, W. F., and Kouri, R. E.,** Aromatic hydrocarbon-produced tumorigenesis and the genetic differences in aryl hydrocarbon hydroxylase induction, in *Chemical Carcinogenesis,* T'so, P.O.P. and DiPaolo, J. A., Eds., Marcel Dekker, New York, 1974, 271.

58. **Kouri, R. E., Demoise, C., and Whitmire, C. E.,** The significance of aryl hydrocarbon hydroxylase enzyme systems in the selection of model systems for respiratory carcinogenesis, in *Experimental Lung Cancer: Carcinogenesis and Bioassays,* Karbe, E. and Park, J. F., Eds., Springer-Verlag, New York, 1974, 48.

59. **Nettesheim, P. and Hammons, A. S.,** Induction of squamous cell carcinoma in the respiratory tract of mice, *J. Nat. Cancer Inst.,* 47, 69, 1971.

60. **Kouri, R. E., Rude, T., Billups, L., Whitmire, C. E., Sass, B., and Henry, C. J.,** Correlation of inducibility of aryl hydrocarbon hydroxylase with susceptibility to 3-methylcholanthrene-induced lung cancer, submitted, 1979.

61. **Duran-Reynols, M. L., Lilly, F., Bosch, A., and Blank, K. J.,** The genetic basis of susceptibility to leukemia induction in mice by 3-methylcholanthrene applied percutaneously, *J. Exp. Med.,* 147, 459, 1978.

62. **Nebert, D. W. and Jensen, N. M.,** Benzo(a)pyrene-initiated leukemia in mice. Association with allelic differences at the *Ah-locus, Biochem. Pharmacol.,* 27, 149, 1979.

63. **Nebert, D. W., Levitt, R. C., Jensen, N. M., Lambert, G. H., and Felton, J. S.,** Birth defects and aplastic anemia: differences in polycyclic hydrocarbon toxicity associated with the *Ah* locus, *Arch. Toxicol.,* 39, 109, 1977.

64. **Thorgeirsson, S. S., Felton, J. S., and Nebert, D. W.,** Genetic differences in the aromatic hydrocarbon-inducible *n* -hydroxylation of 2-acetylaminofluorene and acetaminophen-produced hepatotoxicity in mice, *Mol. Pharmacol.,* 11, 159, 1975.

65. Thorgeirsson, S. S., Wirth, P. J., Nelson, W. L., and Lambert, G. H., Genetic regulation of metabolism and mutagenicity of 2-acetylaminofluorene and related compounds in mice, in *Origins of Human Cancer,* Book B, Hiatt, H. H., Watson, J. D., and Winsten, J. A., Cold Spring Harbor Laboratory, New York, 1977, 869.

66. Felton, J. S. and Nebert, D. W., Mutagenesis of certain activated carcinogens *in vitro* associated with genetically mediated increases in monooxygenase activity and cytochrome P_1-450, *J. Biol. Chem.,* 250, 6769, 1975.

67. Slaga, R. J. and Bracken, W. M., The effects of antioxidants on skin tumor initiation and aryl hydrocarbon hydroxylase, *Cancer Res.,* 37, 1631, 1977.

68. Speier, J. and Wattenberg, L. S., Alterations in microsomal metabolism of benzo(a)pyrene in mice fed butylated hydroxyanisole, *J. Nat. Cancer Inst.,* 55, 469, 1975.

69. Hill, D. L. and Shih, T. W., Vitamin A compounds and analogs as inhibitors of mixed-function oxidases that metabolize carcinogenic polycyclic hydrocarbons and other compounds, *Cancer Res.,* 34, 564, 1974.

70. Wattenberg, L. W., Inhibition of chemical carcinogen-induced pulmonary neoplasia by butylated hydroxyanisole, *J. Nat. Cancer Inst.,* 50, 1541, 1973.

71. Wattenberg, L. W., Inhibition of dimethylhydrazine-induced neoplasia of the large intestine by disulfiram, *J. Nat. Cancer Inst.,* 54, 1005, 1975.

72. Peraino, C., Fry, R. J. M., Stafferat, E., and Christopher, J. P., Enhancing effects of phenobarbitone and butylated hydroxytoluene on 2-acetylamino fluorene induced hepatic tumorigenesis in the rat, *Food Cosmet. Toxicol.,* 15, 93, 1977.

73. Diamond, L., McFall, R., Miller, J., and Gelboin, H. V., The effects of two isomeric benzoflavones on aryl hydrocarbon hydroxylase and the toxicity and carcinogenicity of polycyclic hydrocarbons, *Cancer Res.,* 32, 731, 1972.

74. Dao, T. L., Inhibition of tumor induction in chemical carcinogenesis in the mammary gland, *Prog. Exp. Tumor Res.,* 14, 59, 1972.

75. Gelboin, H. V., Weibel, F. and Diamond, L., Dimethylbenz(a)anthracene tumorigenesis and aryl hydrocarbon hydroxylase in mouse skin: inhibition by 7,8-benzoflavone, *Science,* 170, 169, 1970.

76. Kinoshita, N. and Gelboin, H. V., Aryl hydrocarbon hydroxylase and polycyclic aromatic hydrocarbon tumorigenesis: effect of the enzyme inhibitors 7,8-benzoflavone on tumorigenesis and macromolecular binding, *Proc. Nat. Acad. Sci. U.S.A.,* 69, 824, 1972.

77. Kinoshita, N. and Gelboin, H. V., The role of aryl hydrocarbon hydroxylase in 7,12-dimethylbenz(a)anthracene skin tumorigenesis: or the mechanism of 7,8-benzoflavone inhibition of tumorigenesis, *Cancer Res.,* 32, 1329, 1972.

78. Slaga, T. J., Thompson, S., Berry, D. L., Digiovanni, J., Juchau, M., and Viaje, A., The effects of benzoflavone on polycyclic hydrocarbon metabolism and skin tumor initiation, *Chem. Biol. Interact.,* 17, 297, 1977.

79. Coombs, M. M., Bhott, T. S., and Vose, C. W., The relationship between metabolism, DNA binding, and carcinogenicity of 15,16-dihydro-11-methylcyclopenta(a)phenanthrene-17-one in the presence of a microsomal enzyme inhibitor, *Cancer Res.,* 35, 305, 1975.

80. Thompson, S. and Slaga, T. J., The effects of dexamethasone on mouse skin initiation and aryl hydrocarbon hydroxylase, *Eur. J. Cancer,* 12, 363, 1976.

81. Slaga, T. J., Viage, A., and Bracken, W., The effects of anti-inflammatory agents on skin tumor initiation and aryl hydrocarbon hydroxylase, *Res. Commun. Chem. Pathol. Pharmacol.,* 16, 337, 1977.

82. Kallistratos, G. and Kallistratos, U., The influence of some thiols, unsaturated aliphatic acids and biogenic amines on the inhibition of 3,4-benzpyrene carcinogenesis, *Chimika Chronika,* 5, 115, 1976.

83. Peraino, C., Fry, M. R., and Staffeldt, D., Reduction and enhancement by phenobarbital of hepatocarcinogenesis induced in the rat by 2-acetylaminofluorene, *Cancer Res.,* 31, 1506, 1971.

84. Kitagawa, T. and Sugano, H., Enhancement of azo-dye hepatocarcinogenesis with dietary phenobarbital in rats, *Gann,* 8, 255, 1977.

85. Alvares, A. and Kappas, A., The inducing properties of polychlorinated biphenyls on hepatic monooxygenases, *Clin. Pharmacol. Ther.,* 22, 809, 1977.

86. Makiura, S., Aoe, H., Sugihara, S., Hirao, K., Arai, M., and Sate, N., Inhibitory effect of polychlorinated biphenyls on liver tumorigenesis in rats treated with 3'-methyl-4-dimethyl-aminoazobenzene, N-2-fluorenylacetamide, and diethylnitrosamine, *J. Nat. Cancer Inst.,* 53, 1253, 1974.

87. Poland, A. P., Glover, F., Robinson, J. R., and Nebert, D. W., Genetic expression of aryl hydrocarbon hydroxylase activity. Induction of monooxygenase activities and cytochrome P_1-450 formation by 2,3,7,8-tetrachlorodibenzo-*p*-dioxin in mice genetically "nonresponsive" to other aromatic hydrocarbons, *J. Biol. Chem.,* 249, 5599, 1974.

88. **Robinson, J. R., Felton, J. S., Levitt, R. C., Thorgiersson, S. S., and Nebert, D. W.,** Relationship between "aromatic hydrocarbon responsiveness" and the survival times in mice treated with various drugs and environmental compounds, *Mol. Pharmacol.*, 11, 850, 1975.

89. **Thomas, P. E., Hutton, J. J., and Taylor, B. A.,** Genetic relationship between aryl hydrocarbon hydroxylase inducibility and chemical carcinogen induced skin ulceration in mice, *Genetics*, 74, 655, 1973.

90. **Robinson, J. R. and Nebert, D. W.,** Genetic expression of aryl hydrocarbon hydroxylase induction. Presence or absence of association with zoxazolamine, diphenylhydantoin, and hexobarbital metabolism, *Mol. Pharmacol.*, 10, 484, 1974.

91. **Nebert, D. W., Thorgeirsson, S. S., and Lambert, G. H.,** Genetic aspects of toxicity during development, *Environ. Health Perspect.*, 18, 35, 1976.

92. **Shichi, H., Gaasterland, D. E., Jensen, N. M., and Nebert, D. W.,** *Ah* locus: genetic differences in susceptibility to cataracts induced by acetaminophen, *Science*, 200, (4341), 539, 1978.

93. **Reynolds, E. S., Masler, M. T., Szabo, S., Jaeger, R. J., and Murphy, S. D.,** Hepatotoxicity of vinyl chloride and 1, 1-dichloroethane, *Am. J. Path.*, 81, 219, 1975.

94. **Boyd, M. R.,** Role of metabolic activation in the pathogenesis of chemically induced pulmonary disease. Mechanism of action of the lung toxic furan, 4-ipomeanol., *Environ. Health Perspect.*, 16, 127, 1976.

95. **van Cantfort, J. and Gielen, J.,** Induction by cigarette smoke of aryl hydrocarbon hydroxylase activity in the rat kidney and lung, *Int. J. Cancer*, 19, 538, 1977.

96. **Kouri, R. E., Rude, T. H., Curren, R., Brandt, K. R., Sosnowski, R. G., Schechtman, L. M., Benedict, W. F., and Henry, C. J.,** Biological activity of tobacco smoke, smoke condensate and condensate fractions, *Environ. Health Perspect.*, 29, 63, 1979.

97. **Abramson, R. K., Taylor, B. A., Tomlin, D., and Hutton, J. J.,** Genetics of aryl hydrocarbon hydroxylase induction in mice: response of the lung to cigarette smoke and 3-methylcholanthrene, *Biochem. Genet.*, 15, 723, 1977.

98. **Welch, R. M., Harrison, Y. E., Gommi, B. W., Poppers, P. J., Finster, M., and Conney, A. H.,** Stimulatory effect of cigarette smoking on the hydroxylation of 3,4-benzopyrene and the N-demethylation of 3-methyl-γ-monomethyl-aminoazobenzene by enzymes in human placentas, *Clin. Pharmacol. Ther.*, 10, 100, 1969.

99. **Nebert, D. W., Winkler, J., and Gelboin, H. V.,** Aryl hydrocarbon hydroxylase activity in human placenta from cigarette smoking and non-smoking women, *Cancer Res.*, 29, 1763, 1969.

100. **Burke, M. D. and Mayar, R. T.,** Ethoxyresorufin: direct fluorometric assay of a microsomal O-dealkylation which is preferentially inducible by 3-methylcholanthrene, *Drug Metab. Dispos.*, 2, 583, 1974.

101. **Fouts, J. R.,** Overview of the field: environmental factors affecting chemical or drug effects in animals, *Fed. Proc.*, 35, 1162, 1976.

102. **Gillette, J. R.,** Environmental factors in drug metabolism, *Fed. Proc.*, 35, 1142, 1976.

103. **Campbell, T. C. and Hages, J. R.,** Role of nutrition in the drug-metabolizing enzyme system, *Pharmacol. Rev.*, 26, 171, 1974.

104. **Busbee, D. L., Guyden, J., Kingston, R., Rose, R. L., and Cantrell, E. T.,** Metabolism of benzo(a)pyrene in animals with high aryl hydrocarbon hydroxylase levels and rates of spontaneous cancer, *Cancer Lett.*, 4, 61, 1978.

105. **Gruger, E. H., Wehell, M. M., Numoto, P. T., and Craddock, D. T.,** Induction of hepatic aryl hydrocarbon hydroxylase or salmon exposed to petroleum dissolved in seawater and to petroleum and polychlorinated biphenyls, separate, and together, in food, *Environ. Contam. Toxicol.*, 17, 512, 1977.

106. **Palmer, M. S., Exley, R. W., and Coffin, D. L.,** Influence of pollutant gases on benzpyrene hydroxylase activity, *Arch. Environ. Health*, 25, 439, 1972.

107. **Cinti, D. L., Lemelin, M. A., and Christian, J.,** Induction of liver microsomal mixed-function oxidases by volatile hydrocarbons, *Biochem. Pharmacol.*, 25, 100, 1976.

108. **Fabacher, D. L. and Hodgson, E.,** Hepatic mixed-function oxidase activity in mice treated with methylated benzenes and methylated napthalenes, *J. Toxicol. Environ. Health*, 2, 1143, 1977.

109. **Burckner, J. V., Jiang, W. D., Brown, J. M., Putcha, L., Chu, C. K., and Stella, V. J.,** The influence of ingestion of environmentally encountered levels of a commercial polychlorinated biphenyl mixture (aroclor 1254) on drug metabolism in the rat, *J. Pharmacol. Exp. Ther.*, 202, 22, 1977.

110. **Vesell, E. S., Lang, C. M., White, W. J., Passonanti, G. J., Hill, R. N., Clemens, T. L., Liu, D. K., and Johnson, W. D.,** Environmental and genetic factors affecting the response of laboratory animals to drugs, *Fed. Proc.*, 35, 1125, 1976.

111. **Poland, A. and Kende, A.,** 2,3,7,8-tetrachlorodibenzo-*p*-dioxin: environmental contaminant and molecular probe, *Fed. Proc.*, 35, 2404, 1976.

112. Conaway, C. C., Mudhukar, B. V., and Matsumura, F., P_1P^1-DDT: studies on induction mechanisms of microsomal enzymes in rat liver systems, *Environ. Res.,* 14, 305, 1977.

113. Boutwell, R. K., Some biological aspects of skin carcinogenesis, *Prog. Exp. Tumor Res.,* 4, 207, 1964.

114. Berenblum, I., Historical perspective, in *Mechanisms of Tumor Promotion and Co-carcinogenesis,* Slaga, T. J., Sivak, A., and Boutwell, R. K., Eds., Raven Press, New York, 1978, 1.

115. Levin, W., Wood, A. W., Yagi, H., Dansette, P. M., Jerina, D. M., and Conney, A. H., Carcinogenicity of benzo(a)pyrene 4,5- 7,8-, and 9,10-oxides on mouse skin, *Proc. Nat. Acad. Sci. U.S.A.,* 73, 243, 1976.

116. Chouroulinkov, I., Gentel, A., Grover, P., and Sims, P., Tumour-initiating activities on mouse skin of dihydrodiols derived from benzo(a)pyrene, *Br. J. Cancer,* 34, 523, 1976.

117. Levin, W., Wood, A. W., Yagi, H., Jerina, D. M., and Conney, A. H., (±) -trans-7,8-dihydroxy-7,8-dihydrobenzo(a)pyrene: a potent skin carcinogen when applied topically to mice, *Proc. Nat. Acad. Sci. U.S.A.,* 73, 3867, 1976.

118. Slaga, T. J., Viage, A., Bracken, W. M., Berry, D. L., Fischer, S. M., Miller, D. R., and Leclerc, S. M., Skin-tumor-initiating ability of benzo(a)pyrene-7,8-diol-epoxide (anti) when applied topically in tetrahydrofuran, *Cancer Lett.,* 3, 23, 1977.

119. Wislocki, P. G., Chang, R. L., Wood, A. W., Levin, W., Yagi, N., Hernandez, O., Mah, H. D., Dansette, P. M., Jerina, D. M., and Conney, A. H., High carcinogenicity of 2-hydroxybenzo(a)pyrene arene oxides and diol-epoxides, *Cancer Res.,* 37, 3356, 1977.

120. Levin, W., Wood, A. W., Wislocki, P. G., Kapitulnik, J., Yagi, H., Jerina, D. M., and Conney, A. H., Carcinogenicity of benzo-ring derivatives of benzo(a)pyrene on mouse skin, *Cancer Res.,* 37, 3356, 1977.

121. Slaga, T. J., Bracken, W. M., Viage, A., Levin, W., Yagi, H., Jerina, D. M., and Conney, A. H., Comparison of the tumor-initiating activities of benzo(a)pyrene arene oxides and diol-epoxides, *Cancer Res.,* 37, 4130, 1977.

122. Slaga, T. J., Bracken, W. M., Dresner, S., Levin, W., Yagi, H., Jerina, D. M., and Conney, A. H., Skin tumor-initiating activities of the twelve isomeric phenols of benzo(a)pyrene, *Cancer Res.,* 38, 678, 1978.

123. Haddow, A., The influence of carcinogenic substances on sarcomata induced by the same other compounds, *J. Pathol. Bacteriol.,* 47, 581, 1938.

124. Diamond, L., Metabolism of polycyclic hydrocarbons in mammalian cell cultures, *Int. J. Cancer,* 8, 451, 1971.

125. Gelboin, H. V., Huberman, E., and Sachs, L., Enzymatic hydroxylation of benzopyrene and its relationship to cytotoxicity, *Proc. Nat. Acad. Sci. U.S.A.,* 64, 1188, 1969.

126. Lubet, R. A., Brown, D. Q., and Kouri, R. E., The role of 3-OH benzo(a)pyrene in mediating benzo(a)pyrene induced toxicity and transformation in cell culture, *Res. Commun. Chem. Pathol. Pharmacol.,* 6, 929, 1973.

127. Wislocki, P. G., Wood, A. W., Chang, R. L., Levin, W., Yagi, H., Hernandes, O., Jerina, D. M., and Conney, A. H., Mutagenicity and cytotoxicity of benzo(a)pyrene arene oxides, phenols, quinones, and dihydrodiols in bacterial and mammalian cells, *Cancer Res.,* 36, 3350, 1976.

128. Ames, B. N., McCann, J., and Yamasaki, E., Methods for detecting carcinogens and mutagens with the *Salmonella*/mammalian microsome mutagenicity test, *Mutat. Res.,* 31, 347, 1975.

129. Pelkonen, O., Boobis, A. R., Levitt, R. C., Kouri, R. E., and Nebert, D. W., Genetic differences in metabolic activation of benzo(a)pyrene in mice. Attempts to correlate tumorigenesis with binding reactives intermediates to DNA and with mutagenesis *in vitro, Pharmacology,* 18, 281, 1979.

130. Wood, A. W., Levin, W., Lu, A. Y. H., Ryan, D., West, S. B., Yagi, H., Mah, H. D., Jerina, D. M., and Conney, A. H., Structural requirement for the metabolic activation of benzo(a)pyrene to mutagenic products: effects of modifications in the 4,5-, 7,8- and 9,10- positions, *Mol. Pharamacol.,* 13, 1116, 1977.

131. Wood, A. W., Levin, W., Yagi, H., Hernandez, O., Jerina, D. M., and Conney, A. H., Mutagenicity and cytotoxicity of benzo(a)pyrene derivatives to mutagenic products by highly purified hepatic microsomal enzymes, *J. Biol. Chem.,* 251, 4482, 1976.

132. Huberman, E., Yang, S. K., McCourt, D. W., and Gelboin, H. V., Mutagenicity to mammalian cells in culture by (+) and (−) trans-7,8-dihydroxy-7,8-dihydro-benzo(a)pyrene and the hydrolysis and reduction products of two stereoisomeric benzo(a)pyrene 7,8-diol-9,10-epoxides, *Cancer Lett.,* 4, 35, 1977.

133. Wood, A. W., Chang, R. L., Levin, W., Lehr, R. E., Schaeffer-Ridder, M., Karle, J. M., Jerina, D. M., and Conney, A. H., Mutagenicity and cytotoxicity of benz(a)anthracene diol epoxides and tetrahydro-epoxides: exceptional activity of the bay region 1,2-epoxides, *Proc. Nat. Acad. Sci. U.S.A.,* 74, 2746, 1977.

134. **Thakker, O., Levin, W., Wood, A., Conney, A., Storming, T., and Jerina, D.**, Metabolic formation of 1,9,10- trihydroxy- 9,10-dihydro-3-methylcholanthrene—a potential ultimate carcinogen from 3-methylcholanthrene, *J. Am. Chem. Soc.*, 100, 645, 1978.

135. **Kier, L. D., Yamasaki, E., and Ames, B. N.**, Detection of mutagenic activity in cigarette smoke condensate, *Proc. Nat. Acad. Sci. U.S.A.*, 71, 4159, 1974.

136. **Hutton, J. J. and Hackney, C.**, Metabolim of cigarette smoke condensates by human and rat homogenates to form mutagens detectable by *Salmonella typhimurium* TA 1538, *Cancer Res.*, 35, 2461, 1975.

137. **Kouri, R. E., Brandt, K., Sosnowsk, R. G., Schechtman, L. M., and Benedict, W. F.**, *In vitro* activation of cigarette smoke condensate materials to their mutagenic forms, in *Proceedings Conference on Application of Short Term Bioassays in Fractionation and Analysis of Complex Environmental Mixtures*, Waters, M. D., Nesnow, S., Huisingh, J. L., Sandhu, S. S., Claxton, L., Eds., Environmental Research Information Center, Cincinnati, 1978, 495.

138. **Huberman, E. and Sachs, L.**, Cell-mediated mutagenesis of mammalian cells with chemical carcinogens, *Int. J. Cancer*, 13, 326, 1974.

139. **Krahn, D. F. and Heidelberger, C.**, Liver homogenate-mediated mutagenesis in Chinese hamster V-79 cells by polycyclic aromatic hydrocarbons and aflatoxins, *Mutat. Res.*, 4, 27, 1977.

140. **Kuroki, T., Drevon, C., and Montesano, R.**, Microsome-mediated mutagenesis in V-79 Chinese hamster cells by various nitrosamines, *Cancer Res.*, 37, 1044, 1977.

141. **Clive, D.**, A linear relationship between tumorigenic potency *in vivo* and mutagenic potency at the heterozygous thymidine kinase (TK$^{+/-}$) locus of L5178Y mouse lymphoma cells coupled with mammalian metabolism, in *Progress in Genetic Toxicology*, Scott, D., Bridges, B. A., and Sobels, F. H., Eds., Elsevier/North-Holland Biomedical Press, Amsterdam, 1977, 241.

142. **Kouri, R. E. and Schechtman, L. M.**, State of the art: *in vitro* activation systems, in *Short Term in Vitro Testing for Carcinogenesis, Mutagenesis and Toxicity*, Berky, J. and Sherrod, P. C., Eds., Franklin Institute Press, Philadelphia, 1978, 423.

143. **Schechtman, L. M. and Kouri, R. E.**, Control of benzo(a)pyrene-induced mammalian cell cytotoxicity, mutagenesis and transformation by exogenous enzyme fractions, in *Progress in Genetic Toxicology*, Scott, D., Bridges, B. A., and Sobels, F. H., Eds., Elsevier/North-Holland Biomedical Press, Amsterdam, 1977, 307.

144. **Pienta, R. J., Lebhert, W. B, and Poiley, J. A.**, Further evaluation of a hamster cell carcinogenesis bioassay, in *Proc. of 3rd Int. Symp. on the Detection and Prevention of Cancer*, Nieburgs, H. E., Ed., Marcel Dekker, New York, 1976, 21.

145. **Schechtman, L. M., Beard, S., Dively, C., Joglekar, R., and Slomiany, D.**, Simultaneous determination of the cytotoxic, mutagenic and transforming activities of benzo(a)pyrene (BP) metabolically activated *in vitro*, *Proc. Am. Assoc. Cancer Res.*, 19, 142, 1978.

146. **Aaronson, S. A. and Todaro, G. J.**, Development of 3T3-like lines from BALB/C mouse embryo cultures. Transformation susceptibility to SV 40, *J. Cell Physiol.*, 72, 141, 1968.

147. **Malling, H. V.**, Dimethylnitrosamine formation of mutagenic compounds by interaction with mouse liver microsomes, *Mutat. Res.*, 13, 425, 971.

148. **Umeda, M. and Saito, M.**, Mutagenicity of dimethylnitrosamine to mammalian cells as determined by the use of mouse liver microsomes, *Mutat. Res.*, 30, 249, 1975.

149. **Miller, E. C. and Miller, J. A.**, Biochemical mechanisms of chemical carcinogenesis, in *The Molecular Biology of Cancer*, Busch, H., Ed., Academic Press, New York, 1974, 337.

150. **Brookes, P. and Lawley, P. D.**, Evidence for the binding of polynuclear aromatic hydrocarbons to the nucleic acids of mouse skin: relation between carcinogenic power of hydrocarbons and their binding to deoxyribonucleic acid, *Nature*, 202, 781, 1964.

151. **Grover, P. L. and Sims, P.**, Enzyme-catalyzed reactions of polycyclic hydrocarbons with deoxyribonucleic acid and protein *in vitro*, *Biochem. J.*, 110, 159, 1968.

152. **Gelboin, H. V.**, A microsome-dependent binding of benzo(a)pyrene to DNA, *Cancer Res.*, 29, 1272, 1969.

153. **Boyland, E.**, The biological significance of metabolism of polycyclic compounds, *Biochem. Soc. Symp.*, 5, 40, 1950.

154. **Baird, W. M. and Brookes, P.**, Isolation of the hydrocarbon-deoxyribonucleoside products from the DNA of mouse embryo cells treated *in vitro* with 7-methylbenz(a)anthracene-^{3}H, *Cancer Res.*, 33, 2378, 1973.

155. **Sims, P. and Grover, P. L.**, Epoxides in polycyclic aromatic hydrocarbon metabolism and carcinogenesis, *Adv. Cancer Res.*, 20, 165, 1974.

156. **Baird, W. M., Dipple, A., Grover, P. L., Sims, P., and Brookes, P.**, Studies on the formation of hydrocarbon-deoxyribonucleoside products by the binding of derivatives of 7-methylbenz(a)anthracene to DNA in aqueous solution and in mouse embryo cells in culture, *Cancer Res.*, 33, 2386, 1973.

157. **Booth, J. and Sims, P.**, 8,9-dihydro-8,9-dihydroxybenz(a)anthracene 1,11-oxide: a new type of polycyclic aromatic hydrocarbon metabolite, *FEBS Lett.*, 47, 30, 1974.

158. **Swaisland, A. J., Hewer, H., Pal, K., Keysell, G. R., Booth, J., Grover, P. L., and Sims, P.**, Polycyclic hydrocarbon epoxides: the involvement of 8,9-dihydro-8,9-dihydroxybenz(a)anthracene 10,11-oxide in reactions with the DNA of benz(a)anthracene-treated hamster embryo cells, *FEBS Lett.*, 47, 34, 1974.

159. **King, H. W. S., Thompson, M. H., and Brookes, P.**, The benzo(a)pyrene deoxyribonucleoside products isolated from DNA after metabolism of benzo(a)pyrene by rat liver microsomes in the presence of DNA, *Cancer Res.*, 34, 1263, 1975.

160. **Nebert, D. W., Boobis, A. R., Yagi, H., Jerina, D. M., and Kouri, R. E.**, Genetic differences in mouse cytochrome P_1-450-mediated metabolism of benzo(a)pyrene *in vitro* and carcinogenic index *in vivo*, in *Biological Reactive Intermediates*, Jollow, D. F., Kocsis, J. J., Snyder, R., and Vainio, H., Eds., Plenum Press, New York, 1977, 125.

161. **Boobis, A. R., Nebert, D. W.**, Genetic differences in the metabolism of carcinogens and in the binding of benzo(a)pyrene metabolites to DNA, in *Advances in Enzyme Regulations*, Weber, G., Eds., Pergamon Press, New York, 1977, 339.

162. **Pelkonen, O., Boobis, A. F., Yagi, H., Jerina, D., Nebert, D. W.**, Tentative identification of benzo(a)pyrene metabolites-nucleoside complexes produced *in vitro* by mouse liver microsomes, *Mol. Pharmacol.*, 14, 306, 1978.

163. **Boobis, A. R., Nebert, D. W., and Pelkonen, O.**, Effects of microsomal enzyme inducers *in vivo* and inhibitors *in vitro* on the covalent binding of benzo(a)pyrene metabolites to DNA catalyzed by liver microsomes from genetically responsive and non-responsive mice, *Biochem. Pharmacol.*, 28, 111, 1979.

164. **Kohn, K. W., Erickson, L. C., Regina, A. G., and Freidman, C. A.**, Fractionation of DNA from mammalian cells by alkaline elution, *Biochemistry*, 15, 4629, 1976.

165. **Swenberg, J. A., Petzold, G. L., and Harback, P. R.**, *In vitro* DNA damage/alkaline elution assay for predicting carcinogenic potential, *Biochem. Biophys. Res. Commun.*, 72, 732, 1976.

166. **Petzold, G. L. and Swenberg, J. A.**, Detection of DNA damage induced *in vivo* following exposure of rats to carcinogens, *Cancer Res.*, 38, 1589, 1978.

167. **Brambilla, G., Cavanna, M., Parodi, S., Sciaba, L., Pina, A., and Robbiano, L.**, DNA damage in liver, colon, stomach, lung, and kidney of BALB/c mice treated with 1,2-dimethylhydrazine, *Int. J. Cancer*, 22, 174, 1978.

168. **Tyer, V. N. and Szybaski, W.**, A molecular mechanism of mitomycin action: linking of complementary DNA strands, *Proc. Nat. Acad. Sci. U.S.A.*, 50, 355, 1963.

169. **Pullman, A. and Pullman, B.**, Electronic structure and carcinogenic activity of aromatic molecules, *Adv. Cancer Res.*, 3, 117, 1955.

170. **Miller, E. C. and Miller, J. A.**, Low carcinogenicity of the K-region epoxides of 7-methylbenz(a)anthracene and benz(a)anthracene in the mouse and rat, *Proc. Soc. Exp. Biol. Med.*, 124, 915, 1967.

171. **Boyland, E. and Sims, P.**, The carcinogenic activities in mice of compounds related to benz(a)anthracene, *Int. J. Cancer*, 2, 500, 1967.

172. **Sims, P.**, The carcinogenic activities in mice of compounds related to 3-methylcholanthrene, *Int. J. Cancer*, 2, 505, 1976.

173. **Burki, K., Wheeler, J. E., Akamatsu, Y., Scribner, J. E., Candelas, G., and Bresnick, E.**, Early differential effects of 3-methycholanthrene and its K-region epoxide on mouse skin. Possible implication in the two stage mechanism of tumorigenesis, *J. Nat. Cancer Inst.*, 53, 976, 1974.

174. **Grover, P. L., Sims, P., Mitchley, B. C. V., and Roe, F. J. C.**, The carcinogenicity of polycyclic hydrocarbon epoxides in newborn mice, *Br. J. Cancer*, 31, 182, 1975.

175. **Slaga, T. J., Berry, D. L., Juchau, M. R., Thompson, S., Buty, S. G., and Viaje, A.**, Effects of benzoflavones and trichloropropane oxide on polynuclear aromatic hydrocarbon metabolism and initiation of skin tumors, in *Polynuclear Aromatic Hydrocarbons: Chemistry, Metabolism and Carcinogenesis*, Freudenthal, R. and Jones, P. W., Eds., Raven Press, New York, 1976, 127.

176. **Ames, B. N., Sims, P., and Grover, P. L.**, Epoxides of carcinogenic polycyclic hydrocarbons are frameshift mutagens, *Science*, 176, 47, 1972.

177. **Huberman, E., Aspires, L., Heidelberger, C., Grover, P. L., and Sims, P.**, Mutagenicity to mammalian cells of epoxides and other derivatives of polycyclic hydrocarbons, *Proc. Nat. Acad. Sci. U.S.A.*, 68, 3195, 1971.

178. **Heidelberger, C.**, Chemical carcinogenesis in culture, *Adv. Cancer Res.*, 18, 317, 1973.

179. Jerina, D. M., Lehr, R. E., Yagi, H., Hernandez, O., Dansette, P. M., Wislocki, P. G., Wood, A. W., Chang, R. L., Levin, W., and Conney, A. H., Mutagenicity of benzo(a)pyrene derivatives and the description of a quantum mechanical model which predicts the ease of carbonium ion formation from diol epoxides, in *In Vitro Metabolic Activation in Mutagenesis Testing*, de Serres, F. J., Bend, J. R., and Philpot, R. M., Eds., Elsevier/North-Holland Biomedical Press, Amsterdam, 1976, 159.

180. Conney, A. H., Wood, A. W., Levin, W., Lu, A. Y. H., Chang, R. L., Wislocki, P. G., Goode, R. L., Holder, G. M., Dansette, P. M., Yagi, H., and Jerina, D. M., Metabolism and biological activity of benzo(a)pyrene and its metabolic products, in *Reactive Biological Intermediates*, Jollow, D., Kocsis, J., Snyder, R., and Vainio, H., Eds., Plenum Press, New York, 1977, 335.

181. Borgen, A., Darvey, H., Castagnoli, N., Crocker, T. T., Rasmussen, R. E., and Wang, I. Y., Metabolic conversion of benzo(a)pyrene by Syrian hamster liver microsomes and binding of metabolites to deoxyribonucleic acid, *J. Med. Chem.*, 16, 502, 1973.

182. Daudel, P., Duquesne, M., Vigny, P., Grover, P. L., and Sims, P., Fluorescence spectral evidence that benzo(a)pyrene-DNA products in mouse skin arise from diol-epoxides, *FEBS Lett.*, 57, 250, 1975.

183. Weinstein, I. B., Jeffrey, A. M., Jennette, K. W., Blobstein, S. H., Harvey, R. G., Harris, C., Autrup, H., Kasai, H., and Nakanishi, K., Benzo(a)pyrene diol epoxides as intermediates in nucleic acid binding *in vitro* and *in vivo*, *Science*, 193, 592, 1976.

184. Phillips, D. H., Grover, P. L., and Sims, P., Some properties of vicinal diol-epoxides derived from benz(a)anthracene and benzo(a)pyrene, *Chem. Biol. Interact.*, 20, 63, 1978.

185. Kouri, R. E., Rude, T. H., Levin, W., Wood, A., Yagi, H., and Jerina, D., Analysis of the subcutaneous carcinogenicity of benzo(a)pyrene (BP) and thirteen BP-derivatives in C3H/f Cum mice, *J. Natl. Cancer Inst.* March, 1980.

186. Kapitulnik, J., Levin, W., Conney, A. H., Yagi, H., and Jerina, D. M., Benzo(a)pyrene 7,8-dihydrodiol is more carcinogenic than benzo(a)pyrene in newborn mice, *Nature*, 266, 378, 1977.

187. Kapitulnik, J., Wislocki, P. G., Levin, W., Yagi, H., Jerina, D. M., and Conney, A. H., Tumorigenicity studies with diol-epoxides of benzo(a)pyrene which indicate that (±) trans-7β,8α-dihydroxy-9α,10α-epoxy-7,8,9,10-tetrahydrobenzo(a)pyrene is an ultimate carcinogen in newborn mice, *Cancer Res.*, 38, 354, 1978.

188. Levin, W., personal communication.

189. Wood, A. W., Goode, R. L., Chang, R. L., Levin, W., Conney, A. H., Yagi, H., Dansette, P. M., and Jerina, D. M., Mutagenic and cytotoxic activity of benzo(a)pyrene 4,5-, 7,8- and 9,10-oxides and the six corresponding phenols, *Proc. Nat. Acad. Sci. U.S.A.*, 72, 3176, 1975.

190. Wood, A. W., Wislocki, P. G., Chang, R. L., Levin, W., Lu, A. Y. H., Yagi, H., Hernandez, O., Jerina, D. M., and Conney, A. H., Mutagenicity and cytotoxicity of benzo(a)pyrene benzo-ring epoxides, *Cancer Res.*, 36, 3358, 1976.

191. Wislocki, P. G., Wood, A. W., Chang, R. L., Levin, W., Yagi, H., Hernandez, O., Jerina, D. M., and Conney, A. H., High mutagenicity and toxicity of a diol epoxide derived from benzo(a)pyrene, *Biochem. Biophys. Res. Commun.*, 68, 1006, 1976.

192. Jerina, D. M., Lehr, R., Schaefer-Ridder, M., Yagi, H., Karle, J. M., Thakker, D. R., Wood, A. W., Lu, A. Y. H., Ryan, D., West, W., Levin, W., and Conney, A. H., Bay-region epoxides of dihydrodiols: a concept which explains the mutagenic and carcinogenic activity of benzo(a)pyrene and benz(a)anthracene, in *Origins of Human Cancer*, Book B, Hiatt, H., Watson, J. D., Winsten, I., Eds., Cold Spring Harbor Laboratory, New York, 1977, 639.

193. Kano, I., Gielen, J. E., Yagi, H., Jerina, D. M., and Nebert, D. W., Subcellular events occurring during aryl hydrocarbon hydroxylase induction: no requirement for metabolism of polycyclic hydrocarbon inducer, *Mol. Pharm.*, 13, 1181, 1977.

194. Yagi, H., Thakker, D. R., Hernandez, O., Koruda, M., and Jerina, D. M., Synthesis and reactions of the highly mutagenic 7,8-diol-9,10-epoxides of the carcinogen benzo(a)pyrene, *J. Am. Chem. Soc.*, 99, 1604, 1977.

195. Lehr, R. E. and Jerina, D. M., Metabolic activations of polycyclic hydrocarbons: structure — activity relationships, *Arch. Toxicol.*, 39, 1, 1977.

196. Dewar, M. J. S., Ed., *The Molecular Orbital Theory of Organic Chemistry*, McGraw-Hill, New York, 1969, 214—217, 304—306.

197. Jerina, D. M. and Lehr, R. E., The bay-region theory: a quantum mechanical approach to aromatic hydrocarbon-induced carcinogenicity, in *Microsomes in Drug Oxidation*, Ullrich, V., Roots, I., Hildebrandt, A. J., Estabrook, R. W., and Conney, A. H., Eds., Pergamon Press, Oxford, 1977, 709.

198. Dipple, A. and Nebzydoski, J. A., Evidence for the involvement of a diol epoxide in the binding of 7,12-dimethylbenzo(a)anthracene to DNA in cells in culture, *Chem. Biol. Interact.*, 20, 17, 1978.

199. Wood, A. W., Chang, R. K., Levin, W., Thomas, P. E., Ryan, D., Storming, T. A., Thakker, D. R., Jerina, D. M., and Conney, A. H., Metabolic activation of 3-methylcholanthrene and its metabolites to products mutagenic to bacterial and mammalian cells, *Cancer Res.*, 38, 3398, 1978.

200. Wood, H. W., Levin, W., Thomas, P. E., Ryan, D., Karle, J. M., Yagi, H., Jerina, D. M., and Conney, A. H., Metabolic activation of dibenz(a,h) anthracene and its dihydrodiol to bacterial mutagens, Cancer Res., 38, 1967, 1978.

201. Wood, A. W., Levin, W., Ryan, D., Thomas, P. E., Yagi, H., Mah, H. D., Thakker, D. R., Jerina, D. M., and Conney, A. H., High mutagenicity of metabolically activated chrysene 1,2-dihydrodiol: evidence for bay-region activation of chrysene, Biochem. Biophys. Res. Commun., 78, 847, 1977.

202. Kellermann, G., Luyten-Kellermann, M., and Shaw, C. R., Genetic variation of aryl hydrocarbon hydroxylase in human lymphocytes, Am. J. Hum. Genet., 25, 327, 1973.

203. Kellermann, G., Shaw, C. R., and Luyten-Kellermann, M., Aryl hydrocarbon hydroxylase inducibility and bronchogenic carcinoma, N. Engl. J. Med., 289, 934, 1973.

204. Trell, E., Korsgaard, R., Hood, B., Kitzing, P., Norden, G., and Simonsson, B. G., Aryl hydrocarbon hydroxylase inducibility and laryngeal carcinomas, Lancet., 2, 140, 1976.

205. Guirgis, H. A., Lynch, H. T., Mate, T., Harris, R. E., Wells, I., and Caha, L., Aryl hydrocarbon hydroxylase activity in lymphocytes from lung cancer and normal controls, Oncology, 33, 105, 1976.

206. Arnott, M. S., Yamauchi, T., and Johnston, D. A., Aryl hydrocarbon hydroxylase in normal and cancer populations, in Carcinogens: Identification and Mechanisms of Action, Griffin, A. C. and Shaw, C. R., Eds., Raven Press, New York, 1979, 145.

207. McLemore, T. L., Martin, R. R., Busbee, D. L., Richie, R. C., Springer, R. R., Toppell, K. L., and Cantrell, E. T., Aryl hydrocarbon hydroxylase activity in pulmonary macrophages and lymphocytes from lung cancer and non-cancer patients, Cancer Res., 37, 1175, 1977.

208. McLemore, T. L., Martin, R. R., Pickard, L. R., Springer, R. R., Wray, N. P., Toppell, K. L., Mattox, K. L., Guinn, G. A., Cantrell, E. T., and Busbee, D. L., Analysis of aryl hydrocarbon hydroxylase activity in human lung tissue, pulmonary macrophages, and blood lymphocytes, Cancer, 41, 2292, 1978.

209. McLemore, T. L., Martin, R. R., Wray, N. P., Cantrell, E. T., and Busbee, D. L., Disassociation between aryl hydrocarbon hydroxylase activity in cultured pulmonary macrophages in blood lymphocytes from lung cancer patients, Cancer Res:, 38, 3805, 1978.

210. Cantrell, E. T., Warr, G. A., Busbee, D. L., and Martin, R. R., Induction of aryl hydrocarbon hydroxylase in human pulmonary alveolar macrophages by cigarette smoking, J. Clin. Invest., 52, 1881, 1973.

211. Paigen, B., Gurtoo, H. L., Minowada, J., Houten, L., Vincent, R., Paigen, K., Parker, N. B., Ward, E., and Hayner, N. T., Questionable relation of aryl hydrocarbon hydroxylase to lung-cancer risk, N. Engl. J. Med., 297, 346, 1977.

212. Ward, E., Paigen, B., Steenland, K., Vincent, R., Minowada, J., Gurtoo, H. L., Sartori, P., and Havens, M. B., Aryl hydrocarbon hydroxylase in persons with lung or laryngeal cancer, Int. J. Cancer, 22, 384, 1978.

213. Vaught, J. B., Gurtoo, H. L., Paigen, B., Minowada, J., and Sartori, P., Comparison of benzo(a)pyrene metabolism by human peripheral blood lymphocytes and monocytes, Cancer Lett., 5, 261, 1978.

214. Jett, J. R., Moses, H. L., Branum, E. L., Taylor, W. F., and Fontana, R. S., Benzo(a)pyrene metabolism and blast transformation in peripheral blood mononuclear cells from smoking and non-smoking populations and lung cancer patients, Cancer, 41, 192, 1978.

215. Atlas, S. A., Vesell, E. S., and Nebert, D. W., Genetic control of interindividual variations in the inducibility of aryl hydrocarbon hydroxylase in cultured human lymphocytes, Cancer Res., 36, 4619, 1976.

216. Kellermann, G., Luyten-Kellermann, M., Horning, M. G., and Stafford, M., Correlation of aryl hydrocarbon hydroxylase activity of human lymphocyte cultures and plasma elimination rates for antipyrene and phenylbutazone, Am. Soc. Pharmacol. Exp. Ther., 3, 47, 1975.

217. Kellerman, G., Luyten-Kellermann, M., Horning, M. G., and Stafford, M., Elimination of antipyrene and benzo(a)pyrene metabolism in cultured human lymphocytes, Clin. Pharmacol. Therap., 20, 72, 1976.

218. Lake, R., Pezzutti, M. R., Kropho, M. L., Freeman, A. E., and Igel, H. J., Measurement of benzo(a)pyrene metabolism in human monocytes, Cancer Res., 37, 2530, 1977.

219. Bast, R., Whitlock, J., Miller, H., Rapp, H., and Gelboin, H., Aryl hydrocarbon (Benzo(a)pyrene) hydroxylase in human peripheral blood monocytes, Nature, 250, 664, 1974.

220. Paigen, B., Minowada, J., Gurtoo, H. L., Paigen, K., Parker, N. B., Ward, E., Hayner, N. T., Bross, I. D. J., Bock, F., and Vincent, R., Distribution of aryl hydrocarbon hydroxylase inducibility in cultured human lymphocytes, Cancer Res., 37, 1829, 1977.

221. Richter, A., Kadar, D., Liszka-Hagmajer, E., and Kallow, W., Seasonal variation of aryl hydrocarbon hydroxylase inducibility in human lymphocytes in culture, Res. Commun. Chem. Pathol. Pharmacol., 19, 453, 1978.

222. **Kouri, R. E., Ratrie, H., III, Atlas, S. A., Niwa, A., and Nebert, D. W.**, Aryl hydrocarbon hydroxylase induction in human lymphocyte cultures by 2,3,7,8-tetrachlorodibenzo-*p*-dioxin, *Life Sci.,* 15, 1585, 1974.

223. **Kouri, R. E., Imblum, R. L., Sosnowski, R. G., Slomiany, D. J., and McKinney, C. H.**, Parameters influencing the quantitation of 3-methylcholanthrene induced aryl hydrocarbon hydroxylase activity in cultured human lymphocytes, *J. Toxicol. Environ. Health,* 2, 1079, 1979.

224. **Gurtoo, H. L., Bejba, N., and Minowada, J.**, Properties, inducibility, and an improved method of analysis of aryl hydrocarbon hydroxylase in cultured human lymphocytes, *Cancer Res.,* 35, 1235, 1975.

225. **Hart, P., Cooksley, W. G. E., Farrell, G. C., and Powell, L. W.**, 3-methylcholanthrene inducibility of aryl hydrocarbon hydroxylase in cultured human lymphocytes depends upon the extent of blast transformation, *Biochem. Pharmacol.,* 26, 1831, 1977.

226. **Kouri, R. E., Cantrell, E., and Tyrer, H.**, *Cancer Risk in Man and Carcinogen Metabolism,* Marcel Dekker, New York, 1980, in press.

227. **Arnott, M. S.**, personal communication.

228. **Burke, M. D., Mayer, R., and Kouri, R. E.**, 3-methylcholanthrene-induced monooxygenase (O-deethylation) activity of human lymphocytes, *Cancer Res.,* 37, 460, 1977.

229. **Kouri, R. E., Imblum, R. L., and Prough, R. A.**, Measurement of aryl hydrocarbon hydroxylase and NADH-dependent cytochrome *c* reductase activities in mitogen-activated human lymphocytes, in *Proc. of 3rd Int. Symp. of the Detection and Prevention of Cancer,* Nieburgs, H. E., Ed., Marcel Dekker, New York, 1977, 1659.

230. **Okuda, T., Vesell, E. S., Plotkin, E., Farone, R., Bast, R. C., and Gelboin, H. V.**, Interindividual and intraindividual variations in aryl hydrocarbon hydroxylase in monocytes from monozygotic and dizygotic twins, *Cancer Res.,* 37, 3904, 1977.

231. **Paigen, B., Gurtoo, H. L., Minowada, J., Ward, E., Houten, L., Paigen, K., Reilly, A., and Vincent, R.**, Genetics of aryl hydrocarbon hydroxylase in the human population and its relationship to lung cancer, in *Polycyclic Hydrocarbons and Cancer,* Ts'o, P. O. P. and Gelboin, H. V., Eds., Academic Press, New York, 1978, 391.

232. **Pelkonen, O., Sotaniemi, E., and Mokka, R.**, The *in vitro* metabolism of benzo(a)pyrene in human liver measured by different assays, *Chem. Biol. Interact.,* 16, 13, 1977.

233. **Harris, C. C., Autrup, H., Connor, R., Barrett, L. A., McDowell, E. M., and Trump, B. F.**, Interindividual variation in binding of benzo(a)pyrene to DNA in cultured human brochi, *Science,* 194, 1067, 1976.

234. **Yamasaki, H., Huberman, E., and Sachs, L.**, Metabolism of the carcinogenic hydrocarbon benzo(a)pyrene in human fibroblast and epithelial cells. II. Differences in metabolism to water-soluble products and aryl hydrocarbon hydroxylase activity, *Int. J. Cancer,* 19, 378, 1977.

235. **Thorgiersson, S. S.**, personal communication.

236. **Bradlaw, J.**, personal communication.

237. **Kouri, R. E.**, unpublished observation.

238. **Kouri, R. E.**, in preparation.

Chapter 3

REPAIR OF CHEMICAL CARCINOGEN-INDUCED LESIONS

Ronald E. Rasmussen

TABLE OF CONTENTS

I. INTRODUCTION

The first association of carcinogenesis in humans with an environmental chemical agent is most often attributed to Pott[1] who concluded that scrotal cancer in London chimney sweeps was the result of chronic skin contact with soot. It was early in the present century, however, before the most active principles in soot and other coal tar derivatives were shown to be the polynuclear aromatic hydrocarbons (PAH).[2] Also during this period demonstrations that cancer could be caused by physical agents such as X-rays[3] and viruses[4] began a revolution in the way that investigators thought about this collection of diseases. From being spontaneously occurring diseases of doubtful etiology, cancer in man and animals is now thought in most cases to be the result of specific interactions between environmental agents and living cells. On the basis of continuing epidemiological studies, some investigators have attributed up to 90% of human cancer to environmental causes.[5]

Two major hypotheses have been advanced to account for carcinogenesis: one postulates that the carcinogenic agent calls forth or stimulates preexisting cancer cells to proliferate;[6] the other proposes that normal cells are *transformed* either through chemical interaction leading to an alteration in cellular physiology (somatic mutation),[7] or possibly through infection by or induction of a virus which results from the chemical interaction of the carcinogen with cellular molecules.

Voluminous experimental data are available in support of both positions, and it may well be that one or the other is appropriate in any given case. Nonetheless, evidence continues to accumulate in favor of the hypothesis that a substantial fraction of carcinogenesis is the result of somatic mutation. Central to this hypothesis, in the case of chemical carcinogens, is the contention that they interact with the DNA molecule in such a way that a change in base sequence is produced which persists in DNA for sufficient time to perturb the normal evolution of the cell in which the event occurs. Since all normal mammals, and most other living organisms so far examined, have DNA repair systems capable of dealing with many different kinds of damage, including DNA-bound carcinogens,[8,9] it follows that DNA repair deficiencies or the inhibition of DNA repair should lead to increased susceptibility to chemical carcinogenesis. With similar reasoning, cocarcinogens might sometimes act through interference with DNA repair. Intellectually, this concept is satisfying, but, as with many other beautiful schemes, unequivocal supporting data are difficult to obtain. In this chapter the assumption is made that covalent binding or other interactions of carcinogenic chemicals with DNA which stimulate repair are relevant to the initiation of carcinogenesis. That is, at least some carcinogen-DNA interactions are the initiating events in carcinogenesis, and of these, a fraction is subject to repair by endogenous DNA repair mechanisms.

Whether DNA alterations produced by chemical binding or radiation persist long enough for their effects to be expressed as neoplasia or somatic mutation depends on several factors, among which are the efficiencies of the DNA repair mechanisms, which are of course dependent upon the genetic makeup of the organism concerned. This has been graphically shown in studies of radiation sensitive and resistant mutants in bacteria, where in several cases enzymes with specific repair functions have been isolated. This field has been reviewed recently by Grossman.[10] Bacterial studies of DNA repair have served as guides for studies in mammalian cells, and in fact suggested the experimental protocols which led to the discovery of DNA excision repair in mammalian cells.[11,12] As in bacteria, several DNA repair activities have been shown in mammalian cells, including rejoining of strand breaks,[13,14] excision of ultraviolet light-induced photoproducts,[15-17] and chemical adducts,[18,19] replacement of lost bases in

DNA,[20] and photoreactivation.[21,22] Evidence has also been presented that improper bases may be specifically removed without breakage of the deoxyribose-phosphate backbone of DNA.[23]

The above repair activities have all been associated with DNA repair which is initiated immediately following damage, and presumably before replication of the molecule. This repair is thought to be relatively error free.[24,25] That is, the fidelity of the repair is such that few mistakes are made which subsequently are seen as mutations or transformational events. DNA repair may take place following semiconservative replication of the damaged DNA in both bacteria and mammalian cells.[26] The latter repair, details of which are not entirely ilear, has been called "error prone" because of evidence that it is subject to perturbation by exogenous agents, in particular methylated xanthines.[27] Postreplication repair may have an especially important role in mutagenesis and carcinogenesis in mammalian cells, as discussed below.

II. RELATIONSHIPS BETWEEN DNA REPAIR AND CARCINOGENESIS

A. Background
1. Bacterial Studies

Recent developments in bacterial DNA repair mechanisms have been reviewed elsewhere[10,24] and only a summary will be given here to establish the relationship between mammalian and bacterial DNA repair systems. Although the first indications of repair of ultraviolet light (UV)-induced damage to bacteria were reported in the 1930s,[28] it was not until 1964 that biochemical evidence for the mechanisms involved was published. Setlow and Carrier[16] and Boyce and Howard-Flanders[15] showed the loss of UV-induced photoproducts (thymine dimers) from bacterial DNA, and suggested that an excision process was responsible. It was soon found that the ability to remove dimers from DNA was genetically controlled by several loci, and the loss of this ability was associated with increased sensitivity to the lethal effects of radiation[29,30] or chemicals which damage DNA.[31] Further evidence for the molecular mechanism of excision repair was presented by Pettijohn and Hanawalt[11] who showed that, following UV-irradiation, there occurred a partial breakdown of cellular DNA followed by resynthesis. Using the thymine analog, bromouracil (BrU) as a buoyant density label for newly synthesized DNA they showed that the DNA synthesized following UV-irradiation was intermediate in density between normal and the density expected if the thymine in new daughter strands had entirely been replaced by BrU. Further analysis indicated that the intermediate density DNA contained relatively short regions where BrU was substituted for thymine, suggesting a "repair patch." This interpretation was confirmed using other buoyant density labels, and the overall process is usually called excision-type repair or cut-and-patch repair. It is initiated by the binding of chemical agents to DNA as well as by UV.[18,19]

Other repair mechanisms found in bacteria are recombinational repair[32] in which exchange of nucleotide strands occurs between DNA molecules and S.O.S. repair where repair activity is induced by exposure of cells to UV or other mutagenic agents.[33]

One DNA repair mechanism that has proved especially accessible to study is photoreactivation.[21,34] In yeast and *Escherichia coli* a single enzyme combines with UV-induced pyrimidine dimers in DNA giving rise to a photoreceptor complex which absorbs near-UV light, the energy of which is used to split the dimer *in situ*.[34] However, the nature of the enzyme-dimer complex is not clear. The enzyme is not destroyed in the reaction. A most interesting finding is that caffeine at high concentration ($10^{-2} - 10^{-3}$M) apparently competes with the enzyme for its substrate in *E. coli*.[35] Again the molecular details are not known.

In addition to being able to repair their own DNA, most bacterial repair enzymes are free to interact with DNA of exogenous origins that may be ingested or injected by bacteriophage.[36] This implies that the enzymes are soluble, rather than being membrane bound, perhaps as a part of the DNA replication complex. In vitro studies have shown that many of the repair enzymes are not species-specific, but are specific for certain kinds of DNA lesions such as pyrimidine dimers,[37] single strand breaks,[38] and apurinic sites,[20] and regions of the double helix that may be distorted as the result of alkylation of bases.[39]

2. Mammalian DNA Repair Mechanisms
a. Unscheduled DNA Synthesis (UDS)

The term derives from the fact that the growth cycle of mammalian cells has a "scheduled" period of DNA synthesis; synthesis or incorporation of exogenous nucleotides into DNA at other times is thus "unscheduled." During studies of the effects of ionizing and UV radiation on cultured cells, and the influence of the presence of BU in place of thymine in DNA, autoradiographic (ARG) studies were undertaken to measure the fraction of cells progressing through DNA synthesis after various treatment. It was noticed that after exposure of monolayers of cells to moderate fluxes of UV, ³H-thymidine (³H-TdR) was incorporated into all cells in the culture, not only into that fraction in S phase and the presence of BrU in DNA in place of thymine enhanced this effect.[40] This finding suggested the presence of a repair process, and subsequent experiments confirmed this interpretation.[12] The presence of unscheduled DNA synthesis (UDS) was soon demonstrated in UV-irradiated human lymphocytes,[41] and other cell lines.[12] UDS was also found after exposure to X-rays, but only after relatively high doses.[42] Quantitation of UDS by means of ARG grain counting over cell nuclei showed that the phenomenon was dosage dependent with increasing UV fluxes, but the maximum rate of UDS achieved was a small fraction (1 to 5%) of the rate of normal replicative DNA synthesis.[12,43] UDS is also stimulated by many DNA alkylating agents including mutagens and carcinogens.[44,45] It has been proposed that UDS in mammalian cells be used as an indicator of potential mutagenicity or carcinogenicity of new chemicals and environmental pollutants.[46,47] Studies have shown that the correlation between stimulation of UDS and mutagenicity or carcinogenicity for many compounds is quite good and the assay is as readily applied as the Ames test for mutagenesis in *Salmonella*.[46,48] Since many potentially carcinogenic chemicals require metabolic activation, it is sometimes necessary to supplement the test cell cultures with exogenous enzymes (e.g., liver homogenate or microsomes) in order to activate the compounds to chemical forms that will interact with DNA.[46]

b. Excision-type DNA Repair

With bacterial studies as a guide, experiments were carried out with mammalian cells to determine the nature of UDS. Using ³H-bromodeoxyuridine (³H-BrUdR) as a combined buoyant density and radioactive label, it was shown that, in UV-exposed cells, ³H-BrUdR was incorporated into preexisting, unreplicated DNA strands.[12] Isopycnic sedimentation of ³H-BrUdR-labeled DNA in alkaline CsCl[43,49] led to the conclusion that the repair synthesis involved runs of nucleotides that were very short in relation to the size of the isolated DNA molecules. This was in contrast to the case in bacterial cells, where substantial breakdown and resynthesis of DNA occurs during repair.[29,50]

The size of the repair "patch" depends on the nature of the induced damage. In a continuing series of studies, Regan and Setlow, and co-workers have shown that DNA damage can, in most cases, be classified as "UV-like" or long-patch repair or "X-ray-like" or short-patch repair.[51] In the former case, the repair patch appears to consist of about 100 nucleotides, and short-patch repair to require about 3 nucleotides. Most chemical agents stimulate one or the other type of repair. For example, monofunctional alkylating agents (methylmethane sulfonate, MMS, ethylmethane sulfonate, EMS) mimic ionizing radiation and stimulate short-patch repair.[51,52] However, it should be noted that some chemicals stimulate both kinds of repair (e.g., 4-nitroquinoline-1-oxide, 4NQO),[51] and ionizing radiation may, under anoxic conditions, produce base modification or other adducts in DNA that may stimulate long-patch repair.[53] The relative role of short - and long-patch repair in mutagenesis and carcinogenesis is not known, but in the DNA repair-deficient disease xeroderma pigmentosum (see below) it is the ability to initiate the excision repair function that is defective.[54,55]

Following excision-type repair, the DNA of both bacteria[57] and mammalian cells[56] is capable of normal replication. This was inferred from the observation that UDS was seen in HeLa cell cultures after as little as 1.5 Jm^{-2} where there was substantial cell survival,[12] and subsequently more direct evidence was obtained in human fibroblasts (WI-38) and in *E. coli* using density labeling methods to follow the progression of repaired DNA strands through semiconservative replication to new double-strand DNA molecules.[56,57]

c. Photoreactivation

Photoreactivation (PR) is a well-established DNA repair mechanism in prokaryotic organisms and some PR activity has now been demonstrated in most metazoa.[34] The human PR enzyme has been demonstrated in lymphocytes and in fibroblasts in culture[22,58] and purified to a substantial degree.[59] The importance of PR in human cancer has not been established, although a lower than normal level of PR activity in xeroderma pigmentosum fibroblasts has been reported.[58] Photoreactivation of UV-induced tumor formation has been reported in a species of fish by Hart and Setlow.[60] This remarkable finding strongly suggests that UV-induced pyrimidine dimers can lead to malignant transformation, and therefore it has important implications for humans chronically exposed to sunlight.

d. Postreplication Repair (PRR)

It appears that some kinds of DNA damage such as pyrimidine dimers, even though disruptive of the secondary structure of the double helix, do not serve as absolute blocks to DNA replication, and may be, in some manner, bypassed during semiconservative replication. Some evidence suggests that a "gap" may be left in the daughter strand opposite the dimer (or other damage), which is subsequently filled by "postreplication repair." Other ingenious schemes for bypassing damaged regions have been proposed which include synthesis past the damaged region, followed by excision repair or recombination events between the daughter strands. An interesting model has been proposed by Higgins et al.[62] in which DNA replication is blocked on the parental strand containing a pyrimidine dimer, but not blocked on the opposite strand. This results in unequal synthesis of daughter strands. The model, called "branch migration," suggests that the parental strands dissociate from the newly synthesized daughter strands, and rewind themselves, leading to the opportunity for complementary association of the daughter strands. The missing region of that daughter strand which was coded by the parental strand containing the pyrimidine dimer can then be correctly synthesized presumably by a repair polymerase using the other daughter strand as the template. The daughter strands may then dissociate from each other and reassociate with their original parental strand, the net effect being a shift or migration of the growing point region past the pyrimidine dimer.

PRR forms a significant part of the DNA repair system in rodents, and may also be of considerable importance in humans. The presence of PRR in rodent cells was inferred from studies of the effects of caffeine and other methylated xanthines on cell survival after UV-irradiation.[64,65] In bacteria, caffeine inhibits excision-type repair, and shows a synergistic killing effect with UV.[66] A similar effect on survival is seen in rodent cells in culture, but excision repair is not affected as judged by studies of UDS and incorporation of thymidine after irradiation.[67] Further, this effect of caffeine can be seen when it is added to irradiated rodent cells at a time when most excision-type repair has been completed.[68] Normal human cells in culture show little effect of caffeine either with or wihout UV-irradiation, but a strain of fibroblasts from a xeroderma pigmentosum patient (XP-variant) which shows nearly normal excision repair is susceptible to the synergistic killing efect of caffeine after UV-irradiation.[69] Caffeine also potentiates UV-induced cell mutagenesis in the latter cell strain.[69]

The role of recombination in postreplication repair of mammalian cell DNA damage is not yet clear. In bacterial systems, it is an important component of DNA repair,[32] but in mammalian cells, evidence for this activity has been difficult to obtain. The problem may lie in the difficulty in detecting very small exchanges, which would be below the sensitivity of the methods available. Recent reports have provided some evidence for the transfer of pyrimidine dimers from parental to daughter DNA strands in UV-irradiated cells. When UV-irradiated cells are labeled with ^{3}H-TdR following irradiation, the labeled daughter strands contain sites that are sensitive to T4 endonuclease V, which specifically nicks DNA strands adjacent to pyrimidine dimers.[70,71] The nicked strands are detected by their reduced sedimentation rate in alkaline sucrose gradients.[71]

B. Mammalian DNA Repair Enzymes and their Substrates
1. Substrates for DNA Repair Formed by Carcinogens
a. Physical Agents

The predominant lesion formed by UV light in DNA is the pyrimidine dimer,[72] but additional damage occurs through formation of DNA-protein cross-links,[73] and photohydrates of pyrimidines.[74] The latter are subject to repair by enzymes that are distinct from excision-type enzymes that act on pyrimidine dimers or chemical adducts involving large molecules.[74,75]

The greater portion of DNA damage produced by ionizing radiation has been attributed to the production (in oxygenated media) of hydroxy radicals (OH.) which then can interact with DNA to cause strand breaks[75] or with the bases, especially thymine and cytosine, giving rise to products in which the 5,6 double bond is reduced.[75] It has been recently suggested that active oxygen radicals may also be generated during the metabolism of polycyclic hydrocarbons such as benzo(a)pyrene.[75] Thus the repair of this class of damage may be of relatively great importance, since production of active intermediates leading to the damage can be initiated by several different environmental agents.

Direct base damage, resulting in the loss of the base would produce apurinic or apyrimidinic sites repairable by the enzymes specific for this lesion (see below). Under anoxic conditions, ionizing radiation produces less strand breakage, but more excision-type repair is apparent, indicating the formation of radiation products which cause distortion of the double helix without strand breakage.[75]

b. Chemical Agents

A very wide variety of chemicals has been shown to bind to DNA and to stimulate DNA repair, and the correlation between stimulation of UDS and carcinogenicity and mutagenicity has been noted above.[46,47] The chemicals include monofunctional alkylating agents such as methylmethane sulfonate (MMS) which does not require metabolic activation, polynuclear hydrocarbons which do, and multi-functional agents such as mitomycin C which can cross-link DNA strands.[76] Benzo(a)pyrene (BP) is particularly interesting because it requires two or three distinct enzymatic steps for activation to forms that can exist in an electrophilic state capable of binding to DNA.[77-79] Further, there are at least three, and possibly as many as six chemical forms capable of generating these electroihilic reactants.[80] They include the 4,5-oxide,[81] the *cis* and *syn* isomers of the 7,8-dihydroxydihydro-9,10-oxide,[82] and 6-hydroxy-BP.[83] Once bound to DNA bases these compounds introduce a distortion into the double helix which serves as a stimulus for repair. In some cases the interaction may result in strand breakage, which also serves to stimulate repair.[84] Studies with N-acetylaminofluorene (AAF),[85] indicate that it also stimulates a repair process similar to that following UV-irradiation. There is evidence that these large molecules may remain associated with DNA for relatively long periods, and even remain bound when the DNA replicates.[86,87] The molecular details of this binding that allow such behavior are not clear.

Agents such as MMS and related compounds are capable of reacting with essentially all nucleophilic sites in DNA, but there is a preference for some sites over others.[88] The major alkylated base found after both in vitro and in vivo treatment with methyl- or ethylating agents is 7-alkyl guanine, with much smaller amounts of 0-6-alkyl guanine, and other alkylated bases. 7-alkyl-guanine itself does not significantly distort the DNA helix, and it does not stimulate DNA repair. However, this alkylation does lead to destabilization of the base-sugar bond, and the base is therefore more subject to spontaneous loss. Also, nonalkylated bases are lost spontaneously from mammalian DNA. Lindahl[89] has estimated that 10^4 purines are lost by hydrolysis during a twenty hour replication cycle. The apurinic site left behind is then a substrate for specific repair enzymes. Studies of the loss of alkylated bases with time in vivo, and in the target organs for carcinogenesis by the agent have produced some interesting correlations. Ethylnitrosourea causes brain tumors if injected into juvenile rats. If the time course of alkylation of guanine and the relative rates of loss of the alkylated bases is followed, 0-6-ethyl guanine is lost from brain DNA at a much slower rate than is 7-ethyl guanine.[90] This has been interpreted as due to the lack of a specific repair enzyme in brain tissue.[91] Also there are cases where the ratio of 0-6-methyl-guanine to 7-methyl guanine correlates with the carcinogenic potency of the methylating agent.[92]

2. Demonstration of Specific Enzymatic Activity Concerned with DNA Repair in Mammalian Cells

During the past few years, mammalian DNAs that may participate in DNA repair have been demonstrated in a number of species and tissues.[93] In only a few cases, however, have any been purified to a reasonable extent. Among these, the apurinic/apyrimidinic site-specific endonucleases purified by Ljungquist and Lindahl[94] and Verly et al.[95] are good examples. The enzymes have a molecular weight of about 32,000 daltons, and cleave double-stranded DNA at apurinic sites to give deoxyribose-5′-phosphate and 3′-hydroxyl ends.[96] They are not active toward pyrimidine dimers or other chemical agents binding to DNA which do not induce loss of bases.[94] This enzyme activity has been shown in extracts of cultured human cells, including cells from XP patients of four complementation groups (see below). In the latter studies, extracts from the XP cells had similar activities among the complementation groups, but all were lower than extracts from HeLa cells or WI-38 human fibroblasts.[97] An enzyme with this activity has also been purified from calf thymus.[98] The UV light or ionizing radiation base damage to DNA which results in the appearance of apurinic sites that are the substrate for this enzyme is not known, but it seems to be a minor product, compared to pyrimidine dimer formation. Using phage PM2 DNA, it was found that one apurinic site was produced for every 100 to 150 pyrimidine dimers.[99]

Recent evidence suggests that there may be a number of endonucleases with overlapping activities in human cells. A report by Linsley et al.[100] indicated at least six chromatographically separate apurinic site endonucleases could be demonstrated in extracts of human placenta. Also Cook and Freidberg[101] have shown three chromatographically separable activities in extracts of human KB cells which are able to excise pyrimidine dimers from UV-irradiated *E. coli* DNA. The role of these various activities in vivo is unknown, however preliminary evidence suggests that group D XP cells may be deficient or defective in some of these endonuclease activities.[102]

Although its true role is uncertain, the correxonuclease isolated from human placenta by Doniger and Grossman[103] may represent the repair step following endonuclease action. Similarly, the role in repair of the several mammalian DNA polymerases remains to be determined.

A number of recent studies have suggested that a very high degree of specificity may exist in the repair of individual damaged DNA bases. In *E. coli,* Lindahl and co-workers[104] have demonstrated specific glycosylases which cleave damaged or improper (i.e., uracil rather than thymine) bases from double-stranded DNA, leaving an apurinic/apyrimidinic site which can then be attacked by the appropriate endonucleases. Preliminary studies by Linn et al.[105] suggest that mammalian cells may contain an "insertase" which can replace the appropriate base at an apurinic site after spontaneous loss or glycosylase action.

C. Genetic Control of DNA Repair

1. Human Diseases with DNA Repair or DNA Replication Defects

The discovery of defective DNA repair in cells from xeroderma pigmentosum patients[106] stimulated the examination of a variety of other diseases in which sensitivity to sunlight or X-radiation had been noticed for evidence of DNA repair deficiencies. There are now several conditions in which some preliminary evidence for abnormalities in DNA repair or DNA replication has been discovered. Some of these are listed in Table 1, and are discussed in more detail in the text.

a. Xeroderma Pigmentosum

This recessive, hereditary disease was the first to be shown to have an associated DNA repair defect. This discovery was made by Cleaver[106] who at the time was searching for a mammalian analog of the repair deficient bacterial mutants which were proving to be so useful in genetic studies. The clinical features of this disease have been well described elsewhere and will only be summarized here. On exposure to sunlight, XP patients develop extensive irregular freckles and skin lesions. With continued exposure, skin cancers of various types occur which may metastasize and cause death. The more severe cases also show neurological symptoms, and defects in the immune surveillance systems as indicated by increased susceptibility to infection. There is also some suggestion of increased sensitivity to X-rays.[108] DNA repair activity in cells from XP patients is usually subnormal as measured by the stimulation by UV light of incorporation of ^{3}H-thymidine in cell cultures.[109]

XP patients can be assigned to complementation groups on the basis of the restoration of UDS in heterokaryons formed between cell strains by fusion of cells with inactivated Sendai virus.[110] Seven complementation groups, designated A-G have now been defined. Each shows a characteristic level of subnormal UDS after UV exposure. Groups B, F, and G are presently represented by single individuals. Recent studies by

TABLE 1

Some Human Diseases in Which Evidence for DNA Repair or Replication Defects Has Been Found

Disease	Inheritance	Associated cancers	Other	Evidence for defect in DNA repair	Ref.
Xeroderma pigmentosum (XP)	Autosomal recessive; 7 complementation groups, A-F	Miscellaneous skin, squamous & basal carcinoma, sarcoma, melanoma, with metastsis after sunlight.	Neurological disorders, in groups A, B, D	Lack of initiation of excision repair after UV light damage to DNA	106 107 109 111
Xeroderma pigmentosum, variant	Autosomal recessive	As other XP	No neurological signs	Defective postreplication repair	117
Ataxia telangiectasia (AT)	Autosomal recessive; at least 2 complementation groups	Lymphoid neoplasms	Neurological and immunological deficiencies	Excess chromosomal abnormalities; anoxic gamma-ray products in DNA not repaired	129 130 131 132 133
Fanconi's anemia (FA)	Autosomal recessive	Leukemia, and other specific sites; excess cancer risk also in heterozygotes	Neurological disorders	Failure to repair DNA crosslinks excess chromosomal aberrations	135 136 137 138 139
Bloom's syndrome	Autosomal recessive	Leukemia	Sun sensitive	Excess sister chromatid exchanges in peripheral leukocytes	121 145
Progeria (Hutchinson-Gilford syndrome)	Autosomal recessive	?	Premature senility	?	148 149 150
Down's syndrome	Autosomal recessive	leukemia		Excess chromosomal aberrations on exposure to ionizing radiation	154 155 156

TABLE 1 (continued)
Some Human Diseases in Which Evidence for DNA Repair or Replication Defects Has Been Found

Disease	Inheritance	Associated cancers	Other	Evidence for defect in DNA repair	Ref.
Dyskeratosis congenita	X-linked recessive	Leukemia	Pancytopenia, hyperpigmentation	Excess sister chromatid exchanges with psoralen plus light	157 158
Cockayne's syndrome	Autosomal recessive	?	Dwarfism, premature aging	Sun sensitivity; fibroblasts in vitro sensitive to killing by UV light	113 160 161
Photosensitive diseases: Polymorphic light eruption	?	?	?	Lower than normal UDS in peripheral leukocytes after UV light	162 163
Actinic keratosis	?	Skin	?	Low UDS in peripheral leukocytes after UV light exposure	164
D-deletion retinoblasoma	Dominant with high penetrance	Retinoblastoma	Microcephaly, other somatic defects	Fibroblasts in vitro abnormally sensitive to X-rays	174 175 176
Cutaneous malignant melanoma	Dominant; ethnic clustering	Melanoma with metastasis	?	Tumor cells resistant to UV light; skin fibroblasts show normal UDS	169 172 173

Andrews and co-workers[111,112] have indicated that the severity and age of onset of neurological symptoms in XP patients are correlated with the UV light sensitivity (in terms of in vitro colony forming ability, CFA) of skin fibroblasts. An apparent exception to this correlation exists in the group B individual whose fibroblasts showed an intermediate level of CFA after UV light but had severe neurological problems. However, this indiviual also had neurological symptoms characteristics of another rare disorder, Cockayne's syndrome, which also has associated UV sensitivity.[113] It was concluded by Andrews et al. that this individual had both XP and Cockayne's syndrome, and that the neurological symptoms were not due to XP.[112] Groups C and E which showed the highest CFA after UV had no neurological problems, while group D which had slightly lower CFA, also had neurological problems, but they appeared at a later chronological age (7 to 14 years) than in group A. A possible interpretation is that neurones in the CNS require that their DNA be maintained, even though they have no proliferative potential.

Studies of the geographical distribution of XP indicate that it is world-wide, but the various complementation groups are not spread uniformly. In Japan, by far the predominant group is A,[114] and the single group F patient was also found there. In Europe and America, group C is most common, but A and D are also found. These findings suggest very rare gene mutations that become established in the population, and in which there is no significant disadvantage in the heterozygotes. The incidence of the disease is also higher in Japan ($1/4 \times 10^4$) compared to Europe and America ($1/2.5 \times 10^5$).[115]

The biochemical defect in XP groups A-G is associated with the initiating steps in excision repair. At first it was thought that an endonuclease that makes the first incision might be defective[54,55] but recent studies with cell homogenates have shown that endonuclease activity is present in XP cells,[97] although for some reason the enzymes do not act on the damaged DNA in vivo. The DNA damage is accessible to endonuclease action because the endonuclease isolated from T4 bacteriophage will make the first cut in UV-damaged DNA in isolated XP nuclei and permit UDS to occur.[116]

An additional group of XP patients shows many of the clinical symptoms of XP, but has apparently normal excision-type DNA repair. This group has been called XP variant.[117] Studies by Lehmann et al.[26] and Maher et al.[69,118] have indicated a defect in postreplication repair (PRR) in cells from patients of this group. At the molecular level in normal cells, DNA replicated immediately following UV-irradiation appears first as relatively low molecular size (30 to 100×10^6 daltons) and within a few hours as higher molecular weight molecules (150×10^6 daltons).[26] In cells of XP variant XP4BE, the size of the initially synthesized DNA is smaller than that found in normal controls (about 40×10^6 daltons) and also it is converted to higher molecular weight at a slower rate. In the presence of caffeine, which has no effect in normal cells, the conversion to high molecular weight in UV-irradiated XP4BE cells is greatly inhibited,[26] as is also the case in rodent cells. In nonvariant XP cells, caffeine has some effect on the conversion of new DNA from low to high molecular weight, suggesting that excision repair and PRR are not entirely independent processes.

Maher and co-workers[118] have studied cell survival and mutagenesis in XP strains and have found that caffeine potentiated both cell killing and mutagenesis in an XP variant[118] but not in other XP groups. An important finding was that there was a constant relationship between cell killing and mutant production which was the same whether caffeine was present or not. This suggests a common factor or process exists which may result in either cell death or mutation, and which occurs in association with PRR. Studies with nonvariant XP strains have shown that even though XP cells are more sensitive to killing by UV and production of mutants is greater per unit of UV dose, the ratio of mutants to survivors is constant for both normal and XP cells. This indicates that excision repair is relatively error free, since a higher level of excision repair occurs in normal cells than in XP cells at a given UV dose, but the ratio of mutants to survivors is the same.[118]

Examinations of the karyotype of XP patients have shown no marker chromosomes, or any excess of chromosome abnormalities,[119] or increased incidence of aberrations,[112] such as in Bloom's syndrome.[121] However, XP skin fibroblasts in culture show increased susceptibility to induction of sister chromatid exchanges (SCEs) by monofunctional alkylating agents.[122] This is an interesting finding because excision-type repair and UDS are stimulated in normal and XP cells by direct-acting alkylating agents to about the same extent. Since SCEs are thought to be due to unrepaired damage, the implication is that the kind of damage leading to SCEs is not the same as that which stimulates excision repair in XP cells. Comparative chemical studies of alkylated DNA from XP and normal cells after completion of excision repair might provide evidence for the nature of the lesion that causes SCEs.

It is, of course, of great interest to be able to detect XP heterozygotes in order to provide genetic counseling for carriers, but methods presently available are not readily applied on a routine basis. It has been shown that cells from heterozygotes are susceptible to mutation to DNA repair deficiency at a higher rate than normal homozygous repair-competent cells.[123] Also, cell fusion techniques can be used to show that the repair enzymes produced by a heterozygous nucleus have less ability (or are lesser in amount) to deal with damage in homozygous XP nuclei in the heterokaryon, than does a homozygous normal nucleus.[124] More definitive tests for heterozygosis will be facilitated when the defective gene products responsible for XP are known.

The possible role of virus in the etiology of cancer in XP patients is not settled. Evidence regarding increased susceptibility to transformation of XP fibroblasts by SV40 is inconclusive.[125,126] A study of susceptibility of XP and normal fibroblasts to transformation by RNA feline sarcoma virus and Kirsten murine sarcoma virus (KiMSV) showed wide variation in susceptibility among both XP and normal cells.[127] There was no consistent association of susceptibility among XP complementation groups or between XP patients and controls. However, cells from older normal persons seemed to be somewhat more susceptible to infection with KiMSV. A study is presently underway among XP patients in North Africa to determine the distribution of certain viral antigens among XP patients, and their families.[128]

b. Ataxia Telangiectasia

This rare autosomal recessive condition has been termed the γ-ray analog of XP.[129] Like XP, AT patients have neurological symptoms that appear at an early age, and become progressively more severe with age.[130] AT patients do not show the extreme sensitivity to sunlight as do XP patients, but instead many are sensitive to ionizing radiation damage. This discovery was made following therapeutic radiation treatment for tumors.[131] While XP tumors are predominantly of cutaneous origin, those of AT patients are often of the lymphoreticular system.[130] A detailed comparison of the clinical and DNA repair features of XP and AT has been presented by Kraemer.[132]

The frequency of AT, while rare, is still much higher than XP, with about 1/40,000 being affected.[130] This indicates that the heterozygous carrier frequency may be as high as 1% of the population.[133]: Among blood relatives of AT patients, including heterozygotes, the cancer incidence is significantly greater than among spouses and matched controls.[133] This increased risk ranged from sevenfold for lymphoproliferative neoplasms to tenfold for ovarian cancer. Calculations indicated that cancer deaths among AT heterozygotes may make up 5% of all cancer deaths before age 45.[133] These findings indicate the desirability of screening tests, at least among AT families, to detect heterozygosis and to provide appropriate counseling.

The DNA repair defect in AT is apparently concerned with repair of γ-ray-induced base damage, and is distinct from defects in UV-induced pyrimidine dimer excision as in XP or repair of DNA strand breakage produced by chemicals or ionizing radiation.[134] The latter kinds of damage seem to be repaired normally in AT. The specific damage that goes unrepaired has not been defined, but it seems not to be the thymine-5,6-glycol formed under aerobic irradiation conditions,[134] and for which a repair defect has been found in some strains of Fanconi's anemia (see below).[135] Under anoxic conditions, γ-rays stimulate less UDS or repair replication in AT cells than in normal controls[134] suggesting that a unique radiation product is involved.

Experiments concerned with survival of colony forming ability (CFA) after ionizing radiation exposure have shown lower survival of cells from AT patients and also from some known heterozygotes. It is significant that when reduced survival is observed, it is paralleled by reduced repair replication after a given dose of ionizing radiation, compared to normal controls.[136] This finding further reinforces the association between DNA repair and cell survival.

c. Fanconi's Anemia

Also called Fanconi's syndrome or pancytopenia, FA is along with XP and AT an autosomal recessive condition showing evidence of a DNA repair defect. As in XP and AT, the disease is clinically defined by characteristic neurological signs, immunodeficiency, congenital anomalies, and increased cancer risk.[137] Heterozygotes also show increased cancer risk, especially of specific sites. For example, it has been estimated by Swift that of all cancer deaths, perhaps 1% of the patients carried the FA gene, but among deaths from acute leukemia, 4% carried the FA gene.[138]

At the cellular level, increased chromosomal aberrations are seen, both spontaneously and after treatment of cell cultures with DNA cross-linking agents such as mitomycin C (MMC).[139] In cells from heterozygotes, there is also some indication of increased chromosome instability when treated with diepoxybutane compared to normal controls.[140] This finding may lead to a method for heterozygote detection.

The DNA repair defect in FA differs from that in XP and AT. The CFA of FA fibroblasts exposed to UV light, ionizing radiation or chemicals which mimic ionizing radiation (e.g., MMS, EMS) does not differ from that of normal controls.[141] However, FA fibroblasts are more readily killed by chemical agents which introduce cross-links in DNA.[142,143] In a continuing series of studies on the DNA repair activity of cell-free preparations toward γ-ray-induced 5,6-dihydroxydihydrothymine in DNA, Cerutti and co-workers have found that whole cell sonicates from FA fibroblasts are less active than those of either normal cells or AT cells in removing this lesion from DNA in vitro.[144] Since a cross-linkage of the molecule is not involved in this lesion, it may be that two or more DNA repair defects are present in FA.

The three diseases discussed above (AT, XP, and FA) are the only ones in which reasonably clear evidence has been presented for a DNA repair defect involving a specific kind or group of lesions. There are, however, several more hereditary and spontaneous conditions in which chromosome abnormalities have been demonstrated and where there is presumptive evidence for DNA repair or DNA replication anomalies. The more prominent of these will be reviewed briefly.

d. Bloom's Syndrome

Primarily restricted to European Jews of the Ashkenazim and their descendants,[145] Bloom's syndrome is an autosomal recessive disease with characteristic facial and somatic features. Clinical features suggesting a DNA repair defect are sun sensitivity and a higher than normal risk of acute leukemia.[145] The observation of an extraordinarily high spontaneous level of SCEs in a fraction of peripheral lymphocytes and in fibroblast cultures in vitro also suggested difficulties in DNA repair.[121] However, studies of UDS and repair replication after treatment of cells with a number of different DNA-damaging agents showed their response to be the same as that of normal controls. An interesting recent study suggests that the increase in SCEs in Bloom's cells may be due to the endogenous production of a substance that induces SCEs, and that no DNA repair defect exists as such.[147]

e. Progeria (Hutchinson-Gilford Syndrome)

This disease is characterized by precocious aging and early death due to conditions usually associated with normal old age.[148] This is an extremely rare disease, and the mode of inheritance is autosomal recessive.[148] Its importance in DNA repair studies stems from the controversy surrounding the role of DNA repair in the normal process of aging. Initial studies of DNA strand break rejoining appeared to show a deficiency in rejoining in skin fibroblasts from a progeria patient[149] but this finding could not be confirmed by others. The problem has apparently been resolved by recent studies of Williams[151] who has show a very marked dependence on passage number of the ability of human skin fibroblasts to rejoin X-ray-induced DNA strand breaks provided that the DNA is examined within the first few minutes after irradiation. If the cells are allowed 30 min or so for repair, then no difference in the ability to rejoin breaks is indicated. Studies of progeroid cells have been repeated in which these and other factors[152] are accounted for, and it seems likely that progeroid cells can repair strand breaks normally.

A condition similar to progeria, *Werner's Syndrome,* also shows characteristics of premature aging, but no DNA repair defects have been reported.[153]

f. Down's Syndrome

This is another recessive condition in which is found an excess of leukemia[154] and an increased frequency of chromosomal aberrations compared to controls when cultured cells are exposed to ionizing radiation or certain chemicals which mimic such radiation.[155] A recent study has indicated a reduced level of UDS in peripheral lymphocytes exposed to UV light.[156] Over a range of UV doses of 3.2 to 19.2 Jm^{-2}, the incorporation of ^3H-thymidine in the presence of hydroxyurea was about 70 to 75% that of normal controls. Similar results with other cell types have not been reported.

g. Dyskeratosis Congenita

This is an X-linked recessive condition, resembling FA in certain respects such as pancytopenia, hyperpigmentation, and excess risk of malignancy, but a similar DNA repair defect has not been shown.[157] A recent report by Carter[158] indicated that an excess of SCEs of approximately 50% over controls was found after in vitro exposure of peripheral leukocytes to trimethylpsoralen plus long-wave UV light of 365 nm. The conditions of exposure were such that significant interstrand cross-linking of DNA would be expected, and therefore it was suggested that a defect in repair of these cross-links might be present.

h. Cockayne's Syndrome

This is an autosomal recessive condition characterized by dwarfism, premature aging, and optic and aural degeneration.[159] A DNA repair defect is suggested by abnormal sun sensitivity. Skin fibroblasts from a number of patients have been shown to be abnormally sensitive to killing by UV light (254 nm) but not by X-rays.[160] Quantitation of UDS and repair replication after UV exposure as well as studies of pyrimidine dimer excision showed these functions to be within normal limits.[161] The nature of the repair defect is not presently known, but appears to differ from that found in XP.

i. Photosensitive Conditions

Because the most common cancer is produced in the skin by excessive exposure to sunlight, it is of some concern to be able to identify those persons who may be more susceptible. Studies have been done in a number of laboratories using peripheral leukocytes and skin fibroblasts obtained from patients with sunlight-induced premalignant lesions. The results of these studies have led to some controversy. Using peripheral leukocytes from patients with *polymorphic light eruption* it was found that UV-stimulated incorporation of ^{3}H-thymidine was lower than in cells from normal controls.[162] A later report of results from another laboratory in which skin fibroblasts from different group of patients were studied, indicated no difference in UDS from controls after exposure to UV light as judged by autoradiography.[163] In patients with *actinic keratosis*, peripheral leukocytes have been reported to have lower than normal UDS after UV light exposure.[164] This has apparently not been confirmed in skin fibroblast cultures, and there is some doubt whether lower UDS is present in all patients.[165] Studies of fibroblasts from another photosensitive disease, *actinic reticuloid*[166] showed normal UDS after UV exposure.[163]

Until confirmatory results with other cell types are obtained, findings of reduced UDS after DNA damage in peripheral leukocytes from diseased patients should probably be regarded only as suggestive of a DNA repair defect. Because of the well-known variation in response of leukocytes to in vitro culture conditions, to PHA and different batches of PHA, different sera, and various media formulations, this kind of assay is subject to many unknowns, but with further study may have some usefulness for screening for DNA repair capacity.[167] Those readers familiar with the continuing efforts to study aryl hydrocarbon hydroxylase (AHH) in human leukocyte cultures will recognize the many pitfalls.[168]

j. Cutaneous Malignant Melanoma

Although this is a rather rare cancer, it is of interest because of its often poor prognosis and certain factors suggesting a possible DNA repair defect. This disease shows both ethnic clustering and familial inheritance, probably as a dominant trait with reduced penetrance.[169] It most often occurs in light-skinned caucasians on sun-exposed areas of the body, and with some excess in males.[170] It is rarely found in blacks.

Studies of DNA repair in cell cultures from CMM patients have been done principally by investigators in Queensland, Australia where the incidence of CCM is particularly high due to a combination of high sunlight intensity and the presence of a susceptible ethnic population.[171] At normal body temperature, no difference was noted in UDS or repair replication between normal fibroblasts and melanoma tumor cells in vitro. At higher, but nonlethal temperatures of 40 to 42°C, there was inhibition of DNA repair, but not specifically in either cell type.[172] Preliminary studies of the ability of fibroblasts from melanoma patients to reactivate intracellular UV-irradiated virus have suggested that they are normal in this function.[205] Earlier studies of melanoma tumor cells showed that they were more resistant to inactivation by UV light and also that DNA replication was less inhibited by UV than in normal cells.[173] Whether these qualities contributed to the development of the tumors is not known.

In our laboratory, we have examined about forty skin fibroblast cell strains from melanoma families including patients, blood relatives, and spouses, as well as strains from unrelated presumed normal individuals. Autoradiographic experiments have revealed no significant differences in UDS among this group after exposure of cells to UV light.[206]

k. Retinoblastoma

This condition occurs both as a familial disease and spontaneously. The hereditary form is an autosomal dominant with high penetrance.[174] A characteristic deletion (D-deletion) is sometimes present on the long arm of chromosome 13 (13q-).[175] A study of the X-ray sensitivity of skin fibroblasts in culture from a patient with this deletion showed that the CFA was less than normal with a D_o of 94 ± 5 rad* for colony formation after irradiation compared to 149 rads for normal controls.[176] The D_o for fibroblasts from patients with the nondeletion familial disease was 121 to 132 rads. The suggestion was made that the deleted portion of chromosome 13 may carry information related to the repair of X-ray damage.[176]

In addition to the genetically controlled conditions noted here as having some indication of DNA repair defects, there are many other hereditary conditions which predispose to neoplasia. Mulvihill has recently listed 200 of these, of which only a small fraction have been examined for DNA repair activities.[177] Many of these conditions affect the skin, and hence affected persons may be more susceptible than normal to tumor initiation by environmental agents such as sunlight or chemicals. A number of these have been reviewed by Lutzner.[178]

2. Inter- and Intraspecies Comparative Studies of DNA Repair

It was recognized very early that substantial differences existed between human and rodent cells in regard to UDS and repair replication. After a given dose of UV light rodent cell lines showed much less UDS than human derived cells,[40] but it is worth noting that no normal mammalian species so far studied lacks UDS entirely. More recent studies have established that excision of pyrimidine dimers from the macromolecular DNA of rodent cells in culture is very low or absent[8,179] while human fibroblasts may excise 50% or more of the dimers within 24 hr.[180]

Human and rodent cells differ in the way that DNA damage is handled. In human cells, excision repair is much more active, and may be the dominant mode of repair. In rodents, postreplication repair (PRR) makes up an important part of the repair process as indicated by experiments showing inhibition of PRR in rodent cells but not in human cells by caffeine.[27,64]

Photoreactivation (PR) may be of some importance in humans, but this is not yet clearly established.[22] In rodents PR is probably of very little importance because of their predominantly nocturnal habits. In other lower animals PR may have an important survival value. Among marsupials, PR of cell killing and reversal of thymine dimers has been shown in *Potorous*.[181] In chick embryo cells PR enzymatic activity has been demonstrated,[182] and PR of UV light-induced tumors in fish has been noted above.

In an interesting study by Hart and Setlow,[183] in which they compared UDS among skin fibroblast cultures from several mammalian species, there appeared a correlation between the amount of UDS after exposure to UV light and the average expected lifespan of the species. While this is certainly an intriguing finding, there are some problems in interpretation. It has already been noted that low UDS in rodent cells may

* D_o = the dose which will reduce survival by e^{-1} on the exponential portion of the survival curve.

indicate that they repair their DNA via other pathways than excision repair or repair replication. Also, it has been reported that mouse cells lose much of their ability to perform UDS after only a few passages or divisions in culture.[184] It is not clear whether this may have happened in the reported experiments.[183]

Regarding intraspecies differences in DNA repair (excluding bacteria), man appears to be the only animal where differences in DNA repair have been clearly shown, as evidenced by the examples presented above. It would be of great benefit to have an animal model of XP, for example, but none is known.

A recent study by Paffenholz[185] indicated that differences in UV-light-induced UDS exist among mouse embryo fibroblasts prepared from 10 day fetuses of three different strains, and that a positive correlation was found between the level of UDS and the average normal life-span of the strains. If these results are confirmed for other mouse strains, then breeding experiments may be possible to elucidate the genetic control of DNA repair in mice.

3. Developmental Aspects of DNA Repair
a. Differentiated Tissues

Studies of DNA repair in differentiated tissues have shown that some DNA repair potential is generally present. Repair activity has been shown in vivo in nervous tissues where proliferative activity is minimal,[186] and in quiescent rat liver after treatment with dimethylnitrosamine.[187] Rejoining of DNA strand breakage has been shown after labeling regenerating rat liver with ^{3}H-thymidine.[188] In quiescent rat liver, some of the repair enzymes are undoubtedly present, but a complete array may not be. This is also true of kidney, and some other organs and tissues. This conclusion is based on studies involving short-term organ cultures in which tissue fragments were challenged with MMS, and the stimulation of incorporation of ^{3}H-thymidine into DNA in the presence of hydroxyurea was measured.[189] The tissues where proliferative activity is normally present showed varying levels of ^{3}H-thymidine incorporation, and normally quiescent tissues showed little or none. The highest incorporation level was found in testes, with intermediate levels in lung, spleen, and skin, but was undetectable in liver and kidney under the conditions of these experiments. It may be that the latter tissues can repair only certain kinds of DNA damage.[187,188]

In a recent series of experiments, Swenberg and Petzold[190] devised a method for measuring repair of DNA strand breaks in vivo. They prelabeled newborn mice over a period of 3 weeks with ^{3}H-thymidine and then treated the animals with various carcinogens and procarcinogens. The appearance and disappearance of DNA damage in target and nontarget organs was followed by a modification of the alkaline elution technique applied to tissue homogenates.[191] They found a significant excess of DNA damage in the target organs for the various carcinogens tested. A similar correlation has been shown by Stich et al.[192]

b. Influence of Age and Aging on DNA Repair

The hypothesis that accumulation of DNA damage and the concomitant loss of DNA repair capacity are contributory factors in aging is very attractive, but supporting evidence is limited. Studies of DNA repair in aging cell cultures have not permitted any firm conclusions, primarily because in the transition from in vivo growth to in vitro culture, cells undergo adaptational and other changes which have undefined effects on DNA repair capability. The studies referred to above[184,185] which showed changes in repair with age of embryos used for culture preparation and also with the passage number in vitro are examples.

Studies of DNA repair in animals as they age are as yet incomplete. The observation that ionizing radiation exposure seems to accelerate the normal process has been used as an argument that the radiation damage is an unrepaired addition to normally accumulated damage.[193] A similar accumulation of DNA damage could be mediated through environmental chemicals.[194,195] The present status of this problem is, that while DNA damage may accumulate and participate in the aging process, there is no evidence that DNA repair capability declines with age.

4. Inhibition of DNA Repair and its Relationship to Tumorigenesis

At this writing, there is only one inhibitor of DNA repair which shows significant specificity and that is caffeine (see above).[26] This is not to say that other materials which have been shown to inhibit DNA repair (either UDS or repair replication) in a nonspecific manner have no influence on carcinogenesis as result. The attractiveness of the proposal that some tumor promoters and cocarcinogens may act by inhibiting repair of DNA damage caused by the primary carcinogen continues to stimulate experimental tests of this hypothesis. A large number of such materials has been examined for effects on DNA repair. Included have been hormones,[196] detergents,[197] croton oil and its active principle tetradecanoyl phorbol-13-acetate (TPA),[198] hydroxyurea,[199] arabinocytosine,[200] tobacco tar fractions,[201] and various metabolic poisons including cyanide and methylsulfoxide.[202] In no case was there an indication of specificity of inhibition of DNA repair synthesis[203,204] although many of the materials did strongly inhibit both replicative and repair synthesis. Therefore, the question of whether inhibition of DNA repair may enhance tumorigenesis following DNA damage by a carcinogen remains open.

ACKNOWLEDGMENTS*

I thank B. Wagner and J. DeMint for aid in preparation of this review.

REFERENCES

1. Pott, P., reprinted in U.S. National Cancer Institute Monograph No. 10, 7, 1963.
2. Cook, J. W., Hewett, C. L., and Hieger, I., The isolation of a cancer-producing hydrocarbon from coal tar, *Chem. Soc. London*, 1, 395, 1933.
3. Furth, J. and Lorenz, E., Carcinogenesis by ionizing radiations, in *Radiation Biology*, Vol. 1 (Part 2), Hollaender, A., Ed., McGraw-Hill, New York, 1954, 1145.
4. Heath, C. W., Jr., Caldwell, G. G., and Feorino, P. C., Viruses and other microbes, in *Persons at High Risk of Cancer*, Fraumeni, J. F., Jr., Ed., Academic Press, New York, 1975, 241.
5. Higginson, J., Present trends in cancer epidemiology, *Can. Cancer Conf.*, 8, 40, 1969.
6. Prehn, R. T., A clonal selection theory of chemical carcinogenesis, *J. Nat. Cancer Inst.*, 32, 1, 1964.
7. Heidelberger, C., Chemical oncogenesis in culture, *Adv. Cancer Res.*, 18, 317, 1973.
8. Cleaver, J. E., Repair processes for photochemical damage in mammalian cells, in *Advances in Radiation Biology*, Vol. 4, Lett, J. T., Adler, H., and Zelle, M. R., Eds., Academic Press, New York, 1974, 1.
9. Strauss, B. S., Repair of DNA in mammalian cells, *Life Sci.*, 15, 1685, 1975.

*   Support from the Council for Tobacco Research, U.S.A., the National Cancer Institute (Grant No. CA-15079), and the U.S. Air Force Office of Scientific Research (Grant No. 77-3343 and Contract AF-33615-76-C-5005) is gratefully acknowledged.

10. Grossman, L., Enzymes involved in the repair of DNA, in *Advances in Radiation Biology*, Vol. 4, Lett, J. T., Adler, H., and Zelle, M. R., Eds., Academic Press, New York, 1974, 77.

11. Pettijohn, D. and Hanawalt, P. C., Evidence for repair replication of ultraviolet damaged DNA in bacteria, *J. Mol. Biol.*, 9, 395, 1964.

12. Rasmussen, R. E., and Painter, R. B., Radiation-stimulated DNA synthesis in cultured mammalian cells, *J. Cell Biol.*, 29, 11, 1966.

13. McGrath, R. A. and Williams, R. W., Reconstruction in vivo of inactivated Escherichia coli deoxyribonucleic acid; the rejoining of broken pieces, *Nature*, 212, 534, 1966.

14. Lett, J. T., Caldwell, I., Dean, C. J., and Alexander, P., Rejoining of X-ray induced breaks in the DNA of leukemia cells, *Nature*, 214, 790, 1967.

15. Boyce, R. P. and Howard-Flanders, P., Release of ultraviolet light-induced thymine dimers from DNA in E. coli K-12, *Proc. Nat. Acad. Sci., U.S.A.*, 51, 293, 1964.

16. Setlow, R. B. and Carrier, W.L., The disappearance of thymine dimers from DNA: an error-correcting mechanism, *Proc. Nat. Acad. Sci. U.S.A.*, 51, 226, 1964.

17. Regan, J. D., Trosko, J. E., and Carrier, W. L., Evidence for excision of ultraviolet-induced pyrimidine dimers from the DNA of human cells in vitro, *Biophys. J.*, 8, 319, 1968.

18. Hanawalt, P. C. and Haynes, R. H., Repair replication of DNA in bacteria: irrelevance of chemical nature of base defect, *Biochem. Biophys. Res. Commun.*, 19, 462, 1965.

19. Roberts, J. J., Crathorn, A. R., and Brent, T. P., Repair of alkylated DNA in mammalian cells, *Nature*, 218, 970, 1968.

20. Lindahl, T., Mammalian deoxyribonucleases acting on damaged DNA, in *Molecular and Cellular Repair Processes*, Beers, R. F., Jr., Herriott, R. M., and Tilghman, R. C., Eds., Johns Hopkins University Press, Baltimore, 1972, 3.

21. Kelner, A., Effect of visible light on the recovery of *Streptomyces griseus* conidia from ultraviolet irradiation injury, *Proc. Nat. Acad. Sci. U.S.A.*, 35, 73, 1949.

22. Sutherland, B. M., Photoreactivating enzyme from human leukocytes, *Nature*, 248, 109, 1974.

23. Lindahl, T., DNA N-glycosidases, a new class of DNA-repair enzymes, *Hereditas*, 1 (Abstr.), 128, 1976.

24. Witkin, E. M., Ultraviolet mutagenesis and inducible DNA repair in Escherichia coli, *Bacteriol. Rev.*, 40, 869, 1976.

25. Maher, V. M. and Mc McCormick, J. J., Effect of DNA repair on the cytotoxicity and mutagenicity of ultraviolet irradiation and of chemical carcinogens in normal and xeroderma pigmentosum cells, in *Biology of Radiation Carcinogenesis*, Yuhas, J. M., Tennant, R. W., and Regan, J. D., Eds., Raven Press, New York, 1976, 129.

26. Lehmann, A. R., Postreplication repair of DNA in ultraviolet-irradiated mammalian cells, in *Molecular Mechanisms for Repair f DNA*, Hanawalt, P. C. and Setlow, R. B., Eds., Plenum Press, New York, 1976, chap. 87.

27. Lehmann, A. R., Kirk-Bell, S., Arlett, C. F., Paterson, M. C., Lohman, P. H. M., de Weerd-Kastelein, L. A., and Bootsma, D., Xeroderma pigmentosum cells with normal levels of excision repair have a defect in DNA synthesis after ultraviolet-irradiation, *Proc. Nat. Acad. Sci. U.S.A.*, 72, 219, 1975.

28. Hollaender, A. and Curtis, J. T., Effect of sublethal doses of monochromatic ultraviolet radiation on bacteria in liquid suspensions, *Proc. Soc. Exp. Biol. Med.*, 33, 61, 1935.

29. Boyce, R. P. and Howard-Flanders, P., Genetic control of DNA breakdown and repair in E. coli K-12 treated with mitomycin C or ultra-violet light, *Z. Vererbungsl*, 95, 345, 1964.

30. Hill, R. F. and Feiner, R. R., Further studies of ultraviolet-sensitive mutants of *Escherichia coli* strain B, *J. Gen. Microbiol.*, 35, 105, 1964.

31. Lawley, P. D. and Brookes, P., Cytotoxicity of alkylating agents towards sensitive and resistant strains of *Escherichia coli* in relation to extent and mode of alkylation of cellular macromolecules and repair of alkylation lesions in deoxyribonucleic acids, *Biochem. J.*, 109, 433, 1968.

32. Clark, A. J., Chamberlin, M., Boyce, R. P., and Howard-Flanders, P., Abnormal metabolic response to ultraviolet light of a recombination-deficient mutant of *Escherichia coli* K 12, *J. Mol. Biol.*, 19, 442, 1966.

33. Radman, M., Phenomenology of an inducible DNA repair which is accompanied by mutagenesis, in *Molecular Mechanisms for Repair of DNA*, Hanawalt, P. C. and Setlow, R. B., Eds., Plenum Press, New York, 1975, 355.

34. Rupert, C. S., Enzymatic photoreactivation: overview, in *Molecular Mechanisms for the Repair of DNA*, Part B, Hanawalt, P. C. and Setlow, R. B., Eds., Plenum Press, New York, 1975, chap. 11.

35. Harm, W., Analysis of photoenzymatic repair of UV lesions in DNA by single light flashes, VIII. Inhibition of photoenzymatic repair of UV lesions in E. coli DNA by caffeine, *Mutat. Res.*, 10, 319, 1970.

36. **Garen, A. and Zinder, N. D.**, Radiological evidence for partial genetic homology between bacteriophage and host bacteria, *Virology*, 1, 347, 1955.

37. **Kaplan, J. C., Kushner, S. R., and Grossman, L.**, Enzymatic repair of DNA. I. Purification of two enzymes involved in the excision of thymine dimers from ultraviolet-irradiated DNA, *Proc. Nat. Acad. Sci., U.S.A.*, 63, 144, 1969.

38. **Olivera, B. M. and Lehman, I. R.**, Linkage of polynucleotides through phosphodiester bonds by an enzyme from *E. coli, Proc. Nat. Acad. Sci. U.S.A.*, 57, 1426, 1967.

39. **Heflich, R. H., Dorney, D. J., Maher, V. M., and McCormick, J. J.**, Reactive derivations of benzo(a)pyrene and 7,12 dimethyl benz(a)anthracene cause S1 nuclease sensitive sites in DNA and UV-like repair, *Biochem. Biophys. Res. Commun.*, 77, 634, 1977.

40. **Rasmussen, R. E. and Painter, R. B.**, Evidence for repair of ultra-violet damaged deoxyribonucleic acid in cultured mammalian cells, *Nature*, 203, 1360, 1964.

41. **Evans, R. G. and Norman, A.**, Radiation stimulated incorporation of thymidine into the DNA of human lymphocytes, *Nature*, 217, 455, 1968.

42. **Painter, R. B. Cleaver, J. E.**, Repair replication in HeLa cells after large doses of x-irradiation, *Nature*, 216, 369, 1967.

43. **Painter, R. B. and Cleaver, J. E.**, Repair replication, unscheduled DNA synthesis and the repair of mammalian DNA, *Radiat. Res.*, 37(3), 451, 1969.

44. **Stich, H. F., San, R. H. C., Miller, J. A., and Miller, E. C.**, Various levels of DNA repair synthesis in xeroderma pigmentosum cells exposed to the carcinogens N-hydroxy and N-acetoxy-2-acetylaminofluorene, *Nature (London)*, 238, 9, 1972.

45. **Stich, H. F. and San, R. H. C.**, DNA repair synthesis and survival of repair deficient human cells exposed to the K-region epoxide of benz(a)anthracene, *Proc. Soc. Exp. Biol. Med.*, 142, 155, 1973.

46. **Stich, H. F., Kieser, D., Laishes, B. A., San, R. H. C., and Warren, P.**, DNA repair of human cells as a relevant, rapid, and economic assay for environmental carcinogens, in *Recent Topics in Chemical Carcinogenesis*, Odashima, S., Takayama, S. and Sato, H., Eds., University Park Press, Baltimore, 1975, 3.

47. **Williams, G. M.**, Use of liver epithelial cultures for study of chemical carcinogenesis, *Am. J. Pathol.*, 85(3), 739, 1976.

48. **Ames, B. N., Lee, F. D., and Durston, W. E.**, An improved bacterial test for the detection and classification of mutagens and carcinogens, *Proc. Nat. Acad. Sci. U.S.A.*, 70, 782, 1973.

49. **Lee, Y. C., Byfield, J. E., Bennett, L. R., Chan, P. Y. M.**, X-ray repair replication in L1210 leukemia cells, *Cancer Res.*, 34, 2624, 1974.

50. **Little, J. B.**, Radiation-induced DNA degradation in human cells: lack of evdence following moderate doses of X-rays, *Int. J. Radiat. Biol.*, 13, 591, 1968.

51. **Regan, J. D. and Setlow, R. B.**, Two forms of repair in the DNA of human cells damaged by chemical carcinogens and mutagens, *Cancer Res.*, 34, 3318, 1974.

52. **Painter, R.**, Repair in mammalian cells: overview, in *Molecular Mechanisms for Repair of DNA*, Hanawalt, P. C. and Setlow, R. B., Eds., Plenum Press, New York, 1975, 595.

53. **Cerutti, P.**, Excision repair of DNA base damage, *Life Sci.*, 15, 1567, 1975.

54. **Cleaver, J. E.**, Xeroderma pigmentosum: a human disease in which an initial stage of DNA repair is defective, *Proc. Nat. Acad. Sci. U.S.A.*, 63(2), 428, 1969.

55. **Setlow, R. B., Regan, J. D., German, J., Carrier, W. L.**, Evidence that xeroderma pigmentosum cells do not perform the first step in the repair of ultraviolet damage to their DNA, *Proc. Nat. Acad. Sci. U.S.A.*, 64, 1035, 1969.

56. **Rasmussen, R. E., Reisner, B. L., and Painter, R. B.**, Normal replication of repaired human DNA, *Int. J. Radiat. Biol.*, 17(3), 285, 1970.

57. **Hanawalt, P. C.**, Normal replication of DNA after repair replication in bacteria, *Nature*, 214, 269, 1967.

58. **Sutherland, B. M., Rice, M., and Wagner, E. K.**, Xeroderma pigmentosum cells contain low levels of photoreactivating enzyme, *Proc. Nat. Acad. Sci. U.S.A.*, 72, 103, 1975.

59. **Sutherland, B. M.**, The human leukocyte photoreactivating enzyme, in *Molecular Mechanisms for Repair of DNA, Part A.*, Hanawalt, P. C. and Setlow, R. B., Eds., Plenum Press, New York, 1975, 107.

60. **Hart, R. W. and Setlow, R. B.**, Direct evidence that pyrimidine dimers in DNA result in neoplastic transformation, in *Molecular Mechanisms for Repair of DNA*, Hanawalt, P. C. and Setlow, R. B., Eds., Plenum Press, New York, 1975, 719.

61. **Howard-Flanders, P.**, Repair by genetic recombination in bacteria: overview, in *Molecular Mechanisms for Repair of DNA*, Hanawalt, P. C. and Setlow, R. B., Eds., Plenum Press, New York, 1975, 265.

62. **Higgins, N. P., Kato, K., and Straus, B.**, A model for replication repair in mammalian cells, *J. Mol. Biol.*, 101, 417, 1976.

63. **Lehmann, A. R., Kirk-Bell, S., and Jaspers, N. G. J.,** Postreplication repair in normal and abnormal human fibroblasts, in *DNA Repair Processes,* Nichols, W. W. and Murphy, D. G., Eds., Symposia Specialists, Miami, Fla., 1977, 203.

64. **Rauth, A. M.,** Evidence for dark-reactivation of ultraviolet light damage in mouse L cells, *Radiat. Res.,* 31, 121, 1967.

65. **Doneson, I. N. and Shankel, D. M.,** Mutational synergism between radiations and methylated purines in *Escherichia coli, J. Bacteriol.,* 87, 61, 1964.

66. **Shimada, K. and Takagi, Y.,** The effect of caffeine on the repair of ultraviolet-damaged DNA in bacteria, *Biochem. Biophys. Acta,* 145, 763, 1967.

67. **Trosko, J. E. and Chu, E. H. Y.,** Inhibition of repair of UV-damaged DNA by caffeine and mutation induction in Chinese hamster cells, *Chem. Biol. Interact.,* 6, 317, 1973.

68. **Roberts, J. J., Sturrock, J. E., and Ward, K. N.,** The enhancement by caffeine of alkylation-induced cell death, mutations and chromosomal aberrations in Chinese hamster cells, as a result of inhibition of postreplication DNA repair, *Mutat. Res.,* 26, 129, 1974.

69. **Maher, V. M., Ouellette, L. M., Curren, R. D., and McCormick, J. J.,** Caffeine enhancement of the cytotoxic and mutagenic effect of ultraviolet irradiation in a xeroderma pigmentosum variant strain of human cells, *Biochem. Biophys. Res. Commun.,* 71, 228, 1976.

70. **Fujiwara, Y. and Tatsumi, M.,** Low-level DNA exchanges in normal human and xeroderma pigmentosum cells after UV irradiation, *Mutat. Res.,* 43, 279, 1977.

71. **Meneghini, R. and Hanawalt, P. C.,** T4-Endonuclease V sites in DNA from ultraviolet irradiated human cells, *Biochem. Biophys. Acta,* 425, 428, 1976.

72. **Setlow, R. B. and Setlow, J. K.,** Evidence that ultraviolet-induced thymine dimers in DNA cause biological damage, *Proc. Nat. Acad. Sci. U.S.A.,* 48, 1250, 1962.

73. **Todd, P. and Han, A.,** UV-Induced DNA to protein cross-linking in mammalian cells, in *Aging, Carcinogenesis and Radiation Biology,* Smith, K. C., Ed., Plenum Press, New York, 1976, 83.

74. **Yamane, T., Wyluda, B., and Shulman, R.,** Dihydrothymine from UV-irradiated DNA, *Proc. Nat. Acad. Sci. U.S.A.,* 58, 439, 1967.

75. **Cerutti, P. A. and Remsen, J. F.,** Formation and repair of DNA damage induced by oxygen radical species in human cells, in *DNA Repair Processes,* Nichols, W. W. and Murphy, D. G., Eds., Symposia Specialists, Miami, Fla., 1977, 147.

76. **Iyer, V. N. and Szybalski, W.,** A molecular mechanism of mitomycin action: linking of complementary DNA strands, *Proc. Nat. Acad. Sci. U.S.A.,* 50, 355, 1963.

77. **Borgen, A., Darvey, H., Castagnoli, N., Crocker, T. T., Rasmussen, R. E., and Wang, I. Y.,** Metabolic conversion of benzo(a)pyrene by Syrian hamster liver microsomes and binding of metabolites to DNA, *J. Med. Chem.,* 16, 502, 1973.

78. **Sims, P., Grover, P. L., Swaisland, A., Pal, K., and Hewer, A.,** Metabolic activation of benzo(a)pyrene proceeds by a diol-epoxide, *Nature,* 252, 326, 1974.

79. **Grover, P. L., Hewer, A., and Sims, P.,** Formation of K-region epoxides as microsomal metabolites of pyrene and benzo(a)pyrene, *Biochem. Pharmacol.,* 21, 2713, 1972.

80. **Miller, J. A. and Miller, E. C.,** Some current thresholds of research in chemical carcinogenesis, in *Chemical Carcinogenesis,* Part A, Ts'o, P. O. P., and DiPaolo, J. A., Eds., Marcel Dekker, New York, 1974, 61.

81. **Miyata, N., Shudo, K., Kitahara, Y., Huang, G. F., and Okamata, T.,** Mutagenicity of K-region epoxides of polycyclic aromatic compounds-structure-activity relationship, *Mutat. Res.,* 37, 187, 1976.

82. **Wood, A. W., Wislocki, P. A., Chang, R. L., Levin, W., Lu, A. Y. H., Yagi, H., Hernandez, O., Jerina, D., and Conney, A. H.,** Mutagenicity and cytotoxicity of benzo(a)pyrene benzo-ring epoxides, *Cancer Res.,* 36, 3358, 1976.

83. **Ts'o, P. O. P. and Lu, P.,** Interaction of nucleic acids. II. Chemical linkage of the carcinogen 3, 4 — benzpyrene to DNA induced by photoradiation, *Proc. Nat. Acad. Sci. U.S.A.,* 51, 272, 1964.

84. **Gamper, H. B., Lung, A. S. C., Straub, K., Bartholomew, J. C., and Calvin, M.,** DNA strand scission by benzo(a)pyrene diol epoxides, *Science,* 197(4304), 671, 1977.

85. **Lieberman, M. W., Baney, R. N., Lee, R. E., Sell, S., and Farber, E.,** Studies on DNA repair in human lymphocytes treated with proximate carcinogens and alkylating agents, *Cancer Res.,* 31, 1297, 1971.

86. **Rasmussen, R. E.,** Binding of Benzo(a)pyrene to DNA: Relevance of DNA Synthesis in Cultured Mouse Embryo Cells, Proc. 10th Int. Cancer Congr., Houston, Texas, 1970.

87. **Bates, R. R., del Ande Eaton, S., Morgan, D. L., and Yuspa, S. H.,** Replication of DNA after binding of the carcinogen 7, 12-dimethylbenz(a)anthracine, *J. Nat. Cancer Inst.,* 45(6), 1223, 1970.

88. **Singer, B.,** Sites in nucleic acids reacting with alkylating agents of differing carcinogenicity or mutagenicity, *J. Toxicol. Environ. Health,* 2, 1279, 1977.

89. **Lindahl, T.**, DNA repair enzymes acting on spontaneous lesions in DNA, in *DNA Repair Processes*, Nichols, W. W. and Murphy, D. G., Eds., Symposia Specialists, Miami, Fla., 1977, 225.

90. **Goth, R. and Rajewsky, M. F.**, Ethylation of nucleic acids by ethylnitrosourea-1-^{14}C in the fetal and adult rat, *Cancer Res.*, 32, 1501, 1972.

91. **Kleihues, P. and Cooper, H. K.**, Repair excision of alkylated bases from DNA in vivo, *Oncology*, 33, 86, 1976.

92. **Goth, R. and Rajewsky, M. F.**, Persistence of O^6-ethylguanine in rat brain DNA: correlation with nervous system specific carcinogenesis by ethylnitrosourea, *Proc. Nat. Acad. Sci. U.S.A.*, 71, 639, 1974.

93. **Van Lancker, J. L.**, DNA injuries, their repair and carcinogenesis, *Curr. Top. Pathol.*, 64, 65, 1977.

94. **Ljungquist, S. and Lindahl, T.**, A mammalian endonuclease specific for apurinic sites in double-stranded deoxyribonucleic acid. I. Purification and general properties, *J. Biol. Chem.*, 249, 1530, 1974.

95. **Verly, W. F. and Paquette, Y.**, An endonuclease for depurinated DNA in *Escherichia coli* B., *Can. J. Biochem.*, 50, 217, 1972.

96. **Gossard, F. and Verly, W. G.**, Action mechanism of *Escherichia coli* endonuclease for apurinic sites, *Fed. Proc.*, 35, 1589, 1976.

97. **Cook, K. H. and Freidberg, E. C.**, *Biochemistry*, 1978, in press.

98. **Bacchetti, S. and Benne, R.**, Purification and characterization of an endonuclease from calf thymus acting on irradiated DNA, *Biochem. Biophys. Acta*, 390, 285, 1975.

99. **Teebor, G. W., Goldstein, M. S., Duker, N. J., and Brent, T. P.**, On the nature of the human endonuclease activity directed against ultraviolet-irradiated DNA, *J. Supramol. Struct.*, Suppl. 2, 11, 1978.

100. **Linsley, W. S., Penhoet, E. E., and Linn, S.**, Human endonuclease specific for apurinic/apyrimidinic sites in DNA. Partial purification of multiple forms from placenta, *J. Biol. Chem.*, 252, 4, 1235, 1977.

101. **Cook, K. H. and Freidberg, E. C.**, Partial purification, isolation and characterization of three nuclease activities from human KB cells which can excise thymine-containing pyrimidine dimers, *J. Supramol. Struct.*, Suppl. 2, 10, 1978.

102. **Linn, S., Linsley, W. S., Kuhnlein, U., Penhoet, E. E., and Deutsch, W. A.**, Enzymes for the repair of apurinic/apyrimidinic sites in human cells, *J. Supramol. Struct.*, Suppl. 2, 11, 1978.

103. **Doniger, J. and Grossman, L.**, Human correxonuclease: purification and properties of a DNA repair exonuclease from placenta, *J. Biol. Chem.*, 251, 4579, 1976.

104. **Lindahl, T., Karran, P., and Riazuddin, S.**, DNA glycosylases of *Escherichia coli*, *J. Supramol. Struct.*, Suppl. 2, 12, 1978.

105. **Linn, S., et al.**, unpublished data, reported at Conf. on Mechanisms for Repair of DNA, Keystone, Colo., March, 1978.

106. **Cleaver, J. E.**, Defective repair replication of DNA in xeroderma pigmentosum, *Nature*, 218, 652, 1968.

107. **Robbins, J. H., Kraemer, K. H., Lutzner, M. A., Festoff, B. W., and Coon, H. G.**, Xeroderma pigmentosum. An inherited disease with sun sensitivity, multiple cutaneous neoplasms and abnormal DNA repair, *Ann. Intern. Med.*, 80, 221, 1974.

108. **Setlow, R. B., Faulcon, F. M., and Regan, J. D.**, Defective repair of gamma-ray induced DNA damage in xeroderma pigmentosum cells, *Int. J. Radiat. Biol.*, 29, 125, 1976.

109. **Cleaver, J. E. and Bootsma, D.**, Xeroderma pigmentosum: biochemical and genetic characteristics, *Ann. Rev. Genet.*, 9, 19, 1975.

110. **de Weerd-Kastelein, E. A., Keijzer, W., and Bootsma, D.**, Genetic heterogeneity of xeroderma pigmentosum demonstrated by somatic cell hybridization, *Nature*, 238, 80, 1972.

111. **Andrews, A. D., Barrett, S. F., and Robbins, J. H.**, Relation of DNA repair processes to pathological aging of the nervous system in xeroderma pigmentosum, *Lancet*, 1, 1318, 1976.

112. **Andrews, A. D., Barrett, S. F., and Robbins, J. H.**, The relationship between neurologic disease, acute sun sensitivity and post-ultraviolet colony-forming ability in xeroderma pigmentosum, *J. Supramol. Struct.*, Suppl. 2, 29, 1978.

113. **Cockayne, E. A.**, Dwarfism with retinal atrophy and deafness, *Arch. Dis. Child.*, 21, 52, 1946.

114. **Takebe, H., Miki, Y., Kozuka, T., Furuyama, J., Tanaka, K., Sasaki, M. S., Fujiwara, Y., and Akiba, H.**, DNA-Repair characteristics and skin cancers of xeroderma pigmentosum patients in Japan, *Cancer Res.*, 37(2), 490, 1977.

115. **Takebe, H.**, Relationship between DNA repair defects and skin cancers in xeroderma pigmentosum, *J. Supramol. Struct.*, Suppl. 2, 30, 1978.

116. **Tanaka, K., Sekiguchi, M., and Okada, Y.**, Restoration of ultraviolet-induced unscheduled DNA synthesis of xeroderma pigmentosum cells by the concomitant treatment with bacteriophage T4 endonuclease V and HVJ (Sendai virus), *Proc. Nat. Acad. Sci. U.S.A.*, 72, 4071, 1975.

117. **Cleaver, J. E.**, Xeroderma pigmentosum: variants with normal DNA repair and normal sensitivity to ultraviolet light, *J. Invest. Dermatol.*, 58, 124, 1972.

118. **Maher, V. M., McCormick, J. J., Grover, P. L., and Sims, P.**, Effect of DNA repair on the cytotoxicity and mutagenicity of polycyclic hydrocarbon derivatives in normal and XP human fibroblasts, *Mutat. Res.*, 43, 117, 1977.

119. **McKusick, V. A.**, *Mendelian Inheritance in Man. Catalogs of Autosomal Dominant, Autosomal Recessive, and X-linked Phenotypes*, 3rd Ed., Johns Hopkins University Press, Baltimore, 1971.

120. **Sasaki, M. A.**, DNA repair capacity and susceptibility to chromosome breakage in xeroderma pigmentosum cells, *Mutat. Res.*, 20, 291, 1973.

121. **Chaganti, R. S. K., Schonberg, S., and German, J.**, A manyfold increase in sister chromatid exchanges in Bloom's syndrome lymphocytes, *Proc. Nat. Acad. Sci. U.S.A.*, 71, 4508, 1974.

122. **Wolff, S., Rodin, B., and Cleaver, J. E.**, Sister chromatid exchanges induced by mutagenic carcinogens in normal and xeroderma pigmentosum cells, *Nature*, 265, 347, 1977.

123. **Cleaver, J. E., Bootsma, D., and Freidberg, E. C.**, Human diseases with genetically-altered DNA repair processes, *Genetics*, Suppl. 79, 215, 1975.

124. **Giannelli, F. and Pawsey, S. A.**, DNA repair synthesis in human heterokaryons. II. A test for heterozygosity in xeroderma pigmentosum and some insight into the structure of the defective enzyme, *J. Cell Sci.*, 15, 163, 1974.

125. **Veldhuisen, G. and Pouwels, P. H.**, Transformation of xeroderma pigmentosum cells by SV40, *Lancet*, 2, 529, 1970.

126. **Key, D. J. and Todaro, G. J.**, Xeroderma pigmentosum cell susceptibility to SV40 virus transformation. Lack of effect of low dosage ultraviolet radiation in enhancing viral-induced transformation, *J. Invest. Dermatol.*, 62, 7, 1974.

127. **Chang, K. S. S.**, Susceptibility of xeroderma pigmentosum cells to transform by murine and feline sarcoma viruses, *Cancer Res.*, 36, 3294, 1976.

128. **Giraldo, G.**, personal communication.

129. **Paterson, M., Smith, B., Lohman, P., Anderson, A., and Fishman, L.**, Defective excision repair of gamma-ray damaged DNA in human (ataxia telangiectasia) fibroblasts, *Nature*, 260, 444, 1976.

130. **Sedgwick, R. P. and Boder, E.**, Ataxia telangiectasia, in *Handbook of Clinical Neurology*, Vol. 14, Vinken, P. J. and Bruyn, G. W., Eds., North-Holland, Amsterdam, 1972, 267.

131. **Gotoff, S. P., Amirmokri, E., and Liebner, E.**, Ataxia telangiectasia-neoplasia, untoward response to x-irradiation and tuberous sclerosis, *Am. J. Dis. Child.*, 114, 617, 1967.

132. **Kraemer, K. H.**, Progressive degenerative diseases associated with defective DNA repair: xeroderma pigmentosum and ataxia telangiectasia, in *DNA Repair Processes*, Nichols, W. W. and Murphy, D. G., Eds., Symposia Specialists, Miami, Florida, 1977, 37.

133. **Swift, M., Sholman, L., Perry, M., and Chase, C.**, Malignant neoplasms in the families of patients with ataxia telangiectasia, *Cancer Res.*, 36, 209, 1976.

134. **Paterson, M. C., Smith, B. P., Lohman, P. H. M., Anderson, A. K., and Fishman, L.**, Defective excision repair of gamma ray damaged DNA in human (ataxia telangiectasia) fibroblasts, *Nature (London)*, 260, 444, 1976.

135. **Poon, P. K., O'Brien, R. L., and Parker, J. W.**, Defective DNA repair in Fanconi's anaemia, *Nature (London)*, 250, 223, 1974.

136. **Taylor, A. M. R., Harnden, D. G., Arlett, C. F., Harcourt, S. A., Lehmann, A. R., Stevens, S., and Bridges, B. A**, Ataxia telangiectasia: a human mutation with abnormal radiation sensitivity, *Nature (London)*, 258, 427, 1975.

137. **Nilsson, L. R.**, Chronic pancytopenia with multiple congenital abnormalities (Fanconi's anaemia), *Acta Paediatr.*, 49, 518, 1960.

138. **Swift, M.**, Fanconi's anemia in the genetics of neoplasia, *Nature*, 230, 370, 1971.

139. **Sasaki, M. S.**, Cytogenetic evidence for the repair of DNA cross-links: its normal functioning in xeroderma pigmentosum and its impairment in Fanconi's anemia, *Mutat. Res.*, 46, 152, 1977.

140. **Auerbach, A. D. and Wolman, S. R.**, Susceptibility of Fanconi's anemia fibroblasts to chromosome damage by carcinogens, *Nature*, 261, 494, 1976.

141. **Finkelberg, R., Thompson, M., and Siminovitch, L.**, Survival after treatment with EMS, gamma rays and mitomycin C of skin fibroblasts from patients with Fanconi's anemia, *Am. J. Hum. Genet.*, 26, A30, 1974.

142. **Lehman, A., Kirk-Bell, S., Arlett, C., Harcourt, S. A., de Weerd-Kastelein, E. A., Keijzer, W., and Hall-Smith, P.**, Repair of ultraviolet light damage in a variety of human fibroblast cell strains, *Cancer Res.*, 37, 904, 1977.

143. **Fujiwara, Y. and Tatsumi, M.**, Repair of mitomycin C damage to DNA in mammalian cells and its impairment in Fanconi's anemia cells, *Biochem. Biophys. Res. Commun.*, 66, 592, 1975.

144. **Cerutti, P., Shinohara, K., and Remsen, J.**, Repair of DNA damage induced by ionizing radiation and benzo(a)pyrene in mammalian cells, *J. Toxicol. Environ. Health*, 2, 1375, 1977.

145. **German, J.,** Bloom's syndrome. II. The prototype of human genetic disorders predisposing to chromosome instability and cancer, in *Chromosomes and Cancer,* German, J., Ed., John Wiley & Sons, New York, 1974, 601.
146. **Cleaver, J. E.,** DNA damage and repair in light-sensitive human skin disease, *J. Invest. Dermatol.,* 54, 181, 1970.
147. **Tice, R., Rary, J. M., and Bender, M. A.,** An investigation of DNA repair potential in Bloom's syndrome, *J. Supramol. Struct.,* Suppl. 2, 82, 1978.
148. **Nyhan, W. L. and Sakati, N. O.,** Progeria — the Hutchinson-Gilford syndrome, in *Genetic & Malformation Syndromes in Clinical Medicine,* Year Book Medical Publishers, Chicago, 1976, 197.
149. **Epstein, J., Williams, J. R., and Little, J. B.,** Deficient DNA repair in human progeroid cells, *Proc. Natl. Acad. Sci., U.S.A.,* 70, 977, 1973.
150. **Regan, J. D. and Setlow, R. B.,** DNA repair in human progeroid cells, *Biochem. Biophys. Res. Commun.,* 59, 858, 1974.
151. **Williams, J. R.,** DNA strand breaks: patterns of induction and rejoining in mammalian cells, in *DNA Repair Processes,* Nichols, W. W. and Murphy, D. G., Eds., Symposia Specialists, Miami, Fla., 1977, 73.
152. **Lett, J. T.,** Cellular senescence and the capacity for rejoining DNA strand breaks, in *DNA Repair Processes,* Nichols, W. W. and Murphy, D. G., Eds., Symposia Specialists, Miami, Fla., 1977, 89.
153. **Fujiwara, Y., Higashik, T., Tatsumi, M.,** Retarded rate of DNA-replication and normal level of DNA-repair in Werner's Syndrome fibroblasts in culture, *J. Cell Physiol.,* 92(3), 365, 1977.
154. **Benda, C. E.,** *Down's Syndrome. Mongolism and its Management,* Grune & Stratton, New York, 1969.
155. **Sasaki, H. S. and Tonomura, A.,** Chromosomal radiosensitivity in Down's Syndrome, *Japn. J. Hum. Genet.,* 14, 81, 1969.
156. **Lambert, B., Hansson, K., Bui, T. H., Funes-Cravioto, Lindsten, J., Holmberg, M., and Strausmanis, R.,** DNA repair and frequency of X-ray and UV-light induced chromosome aberrations in leukocytes from patients with Down's syndrome, *Ann. Hum. Genet.,* 39, 293, 1976.
157. **Zeligman, I.,** Dyskeratosis congenita, in *Clinical Dermatology,* Vol. 1, Harper and Row, New York, 1972, Unit 1-34.
158. **Carter, D. M., Gaynor, A., and McGuire, J.,** Sister chromatid exchanges in dyskeratosis congenita after exposure to trimethyl psoralen and UV light, *J. Supramol. Struct.,* Suppl. 2, 84, 1978.
159. **Levinson, A. and Bigler, J. A.,** *Mental Retardation in Infants and Children,* The Yearbook Publishers, Chicago, 1960, 193.
160. **Schmickel, R. D., Chu, E. H. Y., Trosko, J. E., and Chang, C. C.,** Cockayne Syndrome: a cellular sensitivity to ultraviolet light, *Pediatrics,* 60, 135, 1977.
161. **Andrews, A. D., Yoder, F. W., Barrett, S. F., Petinga, R. A., and Robbins, J. H.,** Cockayne's syndrome fibroblasts have decreased colony-forming ability but normal rates of unscheduled DNA synthesis after ultraviolet irradiation, *Clin. Res.,* 24, 624A, 1976.
162. **Horkay, I., Tamasi, P., and Csongor, J.,** UV light-induced DNA damage and repair in lymphocytes in photodermatoses, *Acta Dermat. Venereol.,* 53, 105, 1973.
163. **Ichibashi, M. and Ramsay, C. A.,** Excision repair of DNA in some photodermatoses, *Br. J. Dermatol.,* 95, 13, 1976.
164. **Lambert, B., Ringborg, U., and Swanbeck, G.,** Ultraviolet-induced DNA repair synthesis in lymphocytes from patient with actinic keratosis, *J. Invest. Dermatol. ,* 67, 594, 1976.
165. **Cleaver, J. C.,** Human disease with *in vitro* manifestations of altered repair and replication of DNA, in *Progress in Cancer Research and Therapy,* Mulvihill, J. J., Miller, R. W., and Fraumeni, J. F., Eds., Raven Press, New York, 1977, 355.
166. **Ive, F. A., Magnus, I. A., Warin, R. P., and Wilson-Jones, E.,** Actinic reticuloid. A chronic dermatosis associated with severe photosensitivity and the histological resemblance to lymphoma, *Br. J. Dermatol.,* 81, 469, 1969.
167. **Lavin, M. F. and Kidson, C.,** Repair of ionizing radiation induced DNA damage in human lymphocytes, *Nucleic Acids Res.,* 4, 4015, 1977.
168. **Paigen, B., Minowada, J., Gurtoo, H. L., Paigen, K., Parker, N. B., Ward, E., Hayner, N. T., Bross, I. D. J., Bock, F., and Vincent, R.,** Distribution of aryl hydrocarbon hydroxylase inducibility in cultured human lymphocytes, *Cancer Res.,* 37, 1829, 1977.
169. **Lynch, H. T.,** Skin, heredity and cancer, in *Cancer Genetics,* Lynch, H. T., Ed., Charles C Thomas, Springfield, Ill., 1976, chap. 21.
170. **McNeer, G. and Das Gupta, T.,** Life history of melanoma, *Am. J. Roentgenol.,* 93, 686, 1965.
171. **Beardmore, G. L.,** The epidemiology of malignant melanoma, in *Melanoma and Skin Cancer,* McCarthy, W. H., Ed., Government Printer, Sydney, Aust., 1972, 39.
172. **Goss, P. and Parsons, P. G.,** Temperature-sensitive DNA repair of ultraviolet damage in human cell lines, *Int. J. Cancer,* 17, 296, 1976.

173. Lavin, M. F., Willett, G. M., Chalmers, A. H., and Kidson, C., DNA replication and repair in a human melanoma cell-line resistant to ultraviolet-radiation, *Int. J. Radiat. Biol.*, 31, 101, 1977.

174. Falls, H. F., The genetics of retinoblastoma, in *Cancer Genetics*, Lynch, H. T., Ed., Charles C Thomas, Springfield, Ill., 1976, chap. 16.

175. Jensen, R. D. and Miller, R. W., Retinoblastoma: epidemiologic characteristics, *N. Engl. J. Med.*, 285, 307, 1971.

176. Weichselbaum, R. R., Nove, J., and Little, J. B., Skin fibroblasts from a D-deletion type retinoblastoma patient are abnormally X-ray sensitive, *Nature*, 266, 726, 1977.

177. Mulvihill, John J., Genetic repertory of human neoplasia, in *Genetics of Human Cancer*, Mulvihill, J. J., Miller, R. W., and Fraumeni, J. F., Jr., Eds., Raven Press, New York, 1977, chap. 11.

178. Lutzner, Marvin A., Nosology among the neoplastic genodermatoses in *Genetics of Human Cancer*, Mulvihill, J. J., Miller, R. W., and Fraumeni, J. F., Jr., Eds., Raven Press, New York, 1977, chap. 12.

179. Klimek, M., Formation but no excision of thymine dimers in mammalian cells after UV-irradiation, *Neoplasma*, 12, 559, 1965.

180. Regan, J. D., Tosko, J. E., and Carrier, W. L., Evidence for excision of ultraviolet-induced pyrimidine dimers from the DNA of human cells in vitro, *Biophys. J.*, 8, 318, 1968.

181. Krishnan, D. and Painter, R. B., Photoreactivation and repair replication in rat kangaroo cells, *Mutat. Res.*, 17, 213, 1973.

182. Cook, J. S. and McGrath, J. R., Photoreactivating enzyme activity in metazoa, *Proc. Natl. Acad. Sci. U.S.A.*, 58, 1359, 1967.

183. Hart, R. W. and Setlow, R. B., DNA repair and life span of mammals, in *Molecular Mechanisms for Repair of DNA*, Hanawalt, P. C. and Setlow, R. B., Eds., Plenum Press, New York, 1975, chap. 115.

184. Ben-Ishai, R. and Peleg, L., Excision-repair in primary cultures of mouse embryo cells and its decline in progressive passages and established cell lines, in *Molecular Mechanisms for Repair of DNA*, Hanawalt, P. C. and Setlow, R. B., Eds., Plenum Press, New York, 1975, chap. 85.

185. Paffenholz, Volker, Correlation between DNA repair of embryonic fibroblasts and different life span of 3 inbred mouse strains, *Mech. Aging & Dev.*, 7, 131, 1978.

186. Wheeler, K. T. and Lett, J. T., On the possibility that DNA repair is related to age in nondividing cells, *Proc. Nat. Acad. Sci. U.S.A.*, 71, 1862, 1974.

187. Craddock, V. M., Henderson, A. R., and Ansley, C. M., Repair replication of DNA in the intact animal following treatment with dimethylnitrosamine and with methylmethanesulphonate, studied by fractionation of nuclei in a zonal centrifuge, *Biochem. Biophys. Acta*, 447, 53, 1976.

188. Cox, R., Damjanov, I., Abanobi, S. E., and Sarma, D. S. R., A method for measuring DNA damage and repair in the liver in vivo, *Cancer Res.*, 33, 2114, 1973.

189. Rasmussen, R. E., unpublished experiments.

190. Swenberg, J. and Petzold, G., Detection of DNA damage and repair induced in vitro and in vivo using the alkaline elution assay, *J. Supramol. Struct.*, Suppl. 2, 46, 1978.

191. Kohn, K. W., Erickson, L. C., Regina, A. G., and Friedman, C. A., Fractionation of DNA from mammalian cells by alkaline elution, *Biochemistry*, 15(21), 4629, 1976.

192. Stich, H. F. and Kieser, D., Use of DNA repair synthesis in detecting organotropic actions of chemical carcinogens, *Proc. Soc. Exp. Biol.*, 145, 1339, 1974.

193. Sacher, G. A., Dose, dose rate, radiation quality and host factors for radiation-induced life shortening, in *Aging, Carcinogenesis and Radiation Biology. The Role of Nuceic Acid Addition Reactions*, Smith, K. C., Ed., Plenum Press, New York, 1976, 493.

194. Miller J. A., Carcinogenesis by chemicals: an overview, *Cancer Res.*, 30, 559, 1970.

195. Fishbein, L., Flamm, W. G., and Falk, H. L., *Chemical Mutagens. Environmental Effects on Biological Systems*, Academic Press, New York, 1970.

196. Gaudin, D., Guthrie, L., and Yielding, K. L., DNA repair inhibition: a new mechanism of action of steroids with possible implications for tumor therapy, *Proc. Soc. Exp. Biol. Med.*, 146, 401, 1974.

197. Tuschl, H., Klein, W., Kocsis, F., Bernat, E., and Altmann, H., Investigations into the inhibition of DNA repair processes by detergents, *Environ. Physiol. Biochem.*, 5, 84, 1975.

198. Teebor, G. W., Kuker, N. J., Ruacan, S. A., and Zachary, K. J., Inhibition of thymine dimer excision by the phorbol ester, phorbol myristate acetate, *Biochem. Biophys. Res. Commun.*, 50, 66, 1973.

199. Collins, A. R. S., Schor, S. L., and Johnson, R. T., The inhibition of repair in UV irradiated human cells, *Mutat. Res.*, 42, 413, 1977.

200. Lieberman, M. W., Sell, S., and Farber, E., Deoxyribonucleoside incorporation and the role of hydroxyurea in a model lymphocyte system for studying DNA repair in carcinogenesis, *Cancer Res.*, 31, 1307, 1971.

201. **Rasmussen, R. E.**, Inhibition of DNA replicative synthesis and DNA repair synthesis in human and mouse cells in culture by cigarette smoke condensate fractions, *Life Sci.*, 17, 767, 1975.
202. **Cleaver, J. E.**, Repair replication of mammalian cell DNA: effects of compounds that inhibit DNA synthesis or dark repair, *Radiat. Res.*, 37, 344, 1969.
203. **Cleaver, J. E. and Painter, R. B.**, Absence of specificity in inhibition of DNA repair replication by DNA-binding agents, cocarcinogens and steroids in human cells, *Cancer Res.*, 35, 1773, 1975.
204. **Poirier, M. C., DeCicco, B. T., and Lieberman, M. W.**, Nonspecific inhibition of DNA repair synthesis by tumor promoters in human diploid fibroblasts damaged with N-acetoxy-2-acetylaminofluorene, *Cancer Res.*, 35, 1392, 1975.
205. **Lavin, M. F.**, personal communication.
206. **Rasmussen, R. E.**, unpublished results.

Chapter 4

INHERITANCE OF MURINE ENDOGENOUS RNA VIRUSES

Kunjuraman, T. Nayar, Barbara O'Neill, and Richard E. Kouri

TABLE OF CONTENTS

I. INTRODUCTION

The field of viral carcinogenesis began in the early 1900s when Ellerman and Bang[1] reported that leukemia in chickens was caused by a filterable agent and Rous[2] discovered the avian sarcoma virus. Progress was then slow and hindered by disbelief and reluctance to accept the facts presented. A breakthrough finally came in 1951, when Gross[3] isolated a virus, similar in properties and morphology to the avian viruses, from AKR, an inbred strain of mice. This Gross Passage A virus, obtained from spontaneous lymphomas of AKR mice, was shown to be transmissible to another strain of mice, C3H/Bi, in which the viruses induced lymphatic leukemias. Discovery of Friend, Moloney and Rauscher murine leukemia viruses (FMR) (for review, see Gross)[4] with common serologic properties but different type-specific envelope antigens than the Gross-AKR virus was followed in the next two decades by the isolation and identification of Type C viruses in several other animal species (see Table 1) (for review, see Levy).[5]

An RNA virus whose genome is integrated in the host chromosome and whose transmission from one host to another is primarily through the germ line (vertical transmission) is defined as endogenous. Endogenous virogenes are present as an integral part of the cellular DNA in all mammalian and avian species thus far studied, even though overt expression (such as infectious virions or virus particles) is not recognized in all species. By the use of breeding experiments between specific strains of test animals that differ in their virus expression, these endogenous viruses have been shown to be genetically regulated. Spontaneous expression of virus from host cells in culture[6] and release of infectious virus from cells treated with host cell proviral DNA[7-12] are direct demonstrations of the presence of endogenous viral information in cellular DNA. Moreover, those cells which lack spontaneous virus expression, possibly due to a repressed virogene, have been shown to release infectious virus particles upon treatment with various inducing agents like 5-bromodeoxyuridine,[13-16] chemical carcinogens,[17,18] or physical agents like X-irradiation.[19] Identification of viral specific sequences in cellular DNA using molecular hybridization techniques[20-25] have further proven the endogenous nature of virogenes in all species investigated thus far.

There are two general theories that have been proposed to explain the existence of these endogenous viruses — the oncogene[26] and the provirus.[27] The oncogene theory states that the entire genome of a Type C RNA virus (virogene) is an intrinsic part of the heritable genetic material of the vertebrate cells. In other words, the oncornaviral genome is integrated into cell DNA. To this extent, the hypothesis has successfully withstood all tests. The latter half of the hypothesis states that there is a segment of the virogene called the "oncogene" which, when "switched on" by genetic regulatory mechanisms in the host genome, causes cancer.

TABLE 1

Isolation and Identification of Retroviruses From Different Animal Species

Class	Species	Source
Mammalia	Mouse (*Musmusculus*)	Endogenous virus from almost every strain of mouse so far studied
	Rat (*Rattus norvegicus*) (*Rattus rattus*)	Several endogenous viruses obtained from rat cell lines in culture and also from feral rats
	Cate (*Felis* spp.)	RD114/ccc family of endogenous viruses; FeLV, FeSV, the cat leukemia, and sarcoma viruses which are not endogenous
	Pig (*Sus scrofa*)	Endogenous virus from cells in culture
	Chinese hamster (*Cricetulus grisens*) and Syrian (or golden) hamster (*Mesocricetus auratur*)	From cells in culture and tumor extracts
	Cattle (zsBos taurus)	From lymphosarcoma tissue; Not endogenous
	Woolly monkey (Lagothrix spp.)	Simian sarcoma virus (SSV-1); Not endogenous
	Baboon (*Papio cynocephalus*)	Endogenous virus; Replicate in cells of heterologous species
	Gibbon (*Hylobates lar*)	Gibbon lymphosarcoma virus (GALV) Not endogenous
	Mink	Endogenous virus from cells in culture
	Deer	From tissues
	Horse	From tissues
Aves	Chicken, duck, pheasant, turkey, quail, partridge	Avian leukemia (ALV) and avian Sarcoma (ASV) viruses
Pisces	Fish	From cells in culture
Reptilia	Viper	From tissues

Experiments with Rous sarcoma virus which indicated that a DNA intermediate was involved in the replication of this RNA tumor virus[28] led Temin to formulate the "provirus theory".[27] It states that during the replication of RNA tumor viruses, the single-stranded RNA genome is transcribed into a DNA copy (the "provirus"), which can be integrated into the host genome. Subsequently, this DNA can be transcribed like a cellular gene, leading to the expression of viral genes and to the formation of infectious virions. The transcription of the endogenous viral RNA to DNA is catalyzed by a virion-coded enzyme, RNA-dependent DNA polymerase (RDDP) (also called the reverse transcriptase).[29,30] After cell division, all daughter cells will carry the provirus.

The origin of RNA viruses or the manner in which different types of endogenous viruses and their variants arose in different animal species was explained by Temin by his [11] "Protovirus hypothesis".[31] This is an extension of his provirus theory and states that the RNA viruses evolved along with the host organism through reverse transcription present in normal cells.

Recent reports[32] on the detection of an RDDP, unrelated to the viral enzyme, in the allantoic fluid of normal, uninfected, embryonated chicken eggs encourage speculation that this newly described enzyme may be performing some of the normal physiological functions prescribed in this protovirus hypothesis. This enzyme called "particle reverse transcriptase" shows no biological activity, such as infectivity, helper activity, or interference, and does not exhibit endogenous DNA synthesis. The presence of the enzyme activity is most noticeable during embryogenesis.

This review surveys the progress made in the study of the genetic regulation of these endogenous RNA viruses with an emphasis on Type C virus in mouse systems. First, we shall describe the properties of the viruses and then review the viral-related or host-related genes that regulate expression of these endogenous viruses. The role of this virus expression in spontaneous or chemically induced cancers will also be addressed.

II. ENDOGENOUS RNA VIRUSES

A. Classification

RNA viruses have been called oncornaviruses,[33] because of the oncogenic nature of several of these agents. The ubiquitous presence in many RNA viruses of the enzyme, RDDP, has however prompted a group of virologists to coin the term "retrovirus" for this group. This term is particularly appropriate since not all retroviruses are asociated with cancer.

Electron microscopy has revealed the existence of retroviruses that differ in morphology. Bernhard[34] was the first to propose an alphabetic nomenclature which is widely used now. Three types of RNA tumor viruses, Type A, Type B, and Type C, were described based on morphologic, antigenic, and enzymatic criteria (see Table 2). Recently a fourth, Type D, has been added.[35]

Our discussion centers on the Type C viruses. A detailed subclassification of this group, as exemplified in mice, is given in Table 3. In this case, the viruses are divided according to host-range specificity (for more descriptive reviews on the retroviruses, see References 36 to 39).

B. Structure and Composition of RNA Tumor Viruses

1. The Envelope

The envelope of the RNA type virus is derived from the host cellular membrane during the process of budding, which is their characteristic mode of release. This envelope is composed of host lipid, viral glycoprotein, and proteins. The proteins form the basis for some of their antigenic properties.

The viral envelope contains three types of antigenic determinants: type-specific, group-specific, and interspecies. The type-specific antigens help to distinguish different viruses derived from the same animal species. The group-specific antigens are common to different viruses of the same species. Interspecies antigens are defined as those that are shared by Type C viruses of different animal species. With murine leukemia viruses the envelope glycoprotein (gp) has a molecular weight of 69,000 to 71,000 daltons, abbreviated as gp69/71. Because it contains a type-specific antigen, the gp70 can be distinguished by neutralization and radioimmunoassay and provides a means of identifying specific viruses. The glycoproteins of Type C viruses from other animal species may vary in size.

2. Nucleoid or Core

The nucleoid or core of the RNA Type C viruses contains four or five structural proteins, the RDDP enzyme, and nucleic acids. The core can be exposed by disrupting the envelope through conventional methods like treatment with nonionic detergents or ether.

a. Viral Nucleic Acids

The core contains single-stranded RNA of several sizes and double-stranded DNA

TABLE 2

Properties of Retroviruses

Virus types

	A	B	C	D
Morphology (by EM)				
Size	70 nm	100nm	100 nm	60—95 nm
Nature of nucleoid in extracellular virus	Doughnut-shaped core with an electron-lucent center; density of A particles greater than Types B or C viruses	Spherical, eccentric surrounded by an intermediate layer 45 nm (dia.)	Centrally located, spherical; an electron-lucent perinucleoid space present	Centrally located electron-dense elongated nucleoid with an intermediate layer
Nucleoid at budding	Not released from cells	Complete	Incomplete	Complete
Intracytoplasmic A particles	NSI[a]	Present	Absent	Present
Intracisternal A	NSI			
Surface spikes on mature particles	NSI	Long (10 nm) sturdy spikes	Short (5 nm) or absent	Very short (?) or absent
Biochemical characteristics				
Viral genome	NSI	NSI	Single-stranded RNA 60—70S (1 × 10^7 daltons); also a 4S, 18S, and 28S species of RNA present	NSI
Buoyant density (g/ ml)				
In sucrose	NSI	1.17	1.16	1.17
In cesium chloride	NSI	1.21	1.16	1.21

TABLE 2 (continued)

Properties of Retroviruses

		Virus types		
	A	B	C	D
Enzymes				
R N A - d e p e n d e n t DNA polymerase (RDDP)	NSI	Present	Present	Present
Molecular weight of RDDP	NSI	100,000	70,000	80,000
Cofactor requirement for RDDP	NSI	Preferred divalent cation is Mg^{2+}	Preferred divalent cation is Mn^{2+}	Preferred divalent cation is Mg^{2+}

ᵃ NSI = Not sufficient information available.

TABLE 3

Classification of Endogenous Type C Viruses

	Ecotropic	Xenotropic	Amphotropic
Definition	Viruses that can infect and replicate efficiently in cells of origin	Viruses that can infect and replicate efficiently only in heterologous cells	Viruses that can infect and replicate in both the cells of their origin and cells from heterologous species
Prototype	AKR	NZB	Wild mouse from Lake Casitas in California (*Mus musculus* sp.)
Classification by preferred host-range	N-tropic — preferred growth in NIH-Swiss mouse cells B-tropic — preferred growth in BALB/c mouse cells NB-tropic — grows equally well in NIH Swiss and BALB/c mouse cells	Xe-Preferred growth in rat and rabbit cells X^p-Preferred growth in primate cells	
Examples	N-tropic-AKR-L-1 BALB: Virus-1; C58, DBA, C3H/He, A/He B-tropic-C57B1/6; WN1802, BALB/c; NB-tropic, Friend, Moloney, Murine leukemia viruses and Rauscher murine leukemia viruses	X^e-AKR, BALB/c, CBA C58, C3H X^p-NIH Swiss, C57L, NZB	Wild mice from Lake Casitas and Bouquet Canyon, California

of small size,[40] presumably of cell origin. There is a species of high molecular weight (approximately 10^7 daltons) RNA which sediments at 60 to 70S.[41] This high molecular weight RNA shifts to 35S upon treatment with heat or dimethylsulfoxide (DMSO). A reversal of 35S to a 60 to 70S has not yet been achieved. Another class of RNA, a low molecular weight RNA of 4S to 7S units, has also been identified in murine species. It has been shown that one of the 70S-associated 4S molecules serves as the major primer for reverse transcription in vitro.[42]

b. Viral Structural Proteins

The major structural proteins of the Type C RNA viruses isolated from the murine, avian, feline, and primate systems are shown in Table 4. The proteins are designated according to the prevailing nomenclature.[43] Each protein is identified by the prefix p for polypeptide, followed by the first two or three digits of its molecular weights expressed in kilodaltons. For example, p30 signifies a polypeptide of 30,000 dalton molecular weight. The genesis of these structural proteins will be discussed in Section III.A.

In brief, the existence of five major structural polypeptides in murine viruses has been reported. Four proteins are associated with the nucleoid, each with a molecular weight of approximately 30,000 (p30), 15,000 (p15), 10,000 (p10), or 12,000 (p12).[44]

TABLE 4

Major Structural Proteins of Type C Viruses[a]

Murine	Avian	Feline	Primate	Antigenic determinants
p 30	p 27	p 30	p 27	Strong group specificity and weak interspecies type specificity
p 10	p 19	p 10	p 10	A weak group specificity
p 15	p 15	p 15	p 15	Strong type specificity and weak group specificity
p 12	p 12	p 11	p 12	Strong type specificity and weak group specificity

[a] p = polypeptide; the numbers indicate molecular weights in kilodaltons.

A fifth structural polypeptide of 15,000 daltons is associated with the envelope,[45] called p15 (E).

c. RNA-Directed DNA Polymerase (RDDP)

All known retroviruses possess in their core an enzyme, RDDP, first reported in 1970.[30,31] The enzyme is coded for by the virus and is essential for its infectivity. In the ribonucleoprotein complex of the virion, the RDDP catalyzes the transcription of the endogenous RNA strand into a complementary DNA strand. The natural template for this reaction is the viral genomic RNA. The natural primer is a 4S RNA present in the 60 to 70S viral RNA complex. For reviews on RDDP, the reader is referred to several recent articles.[29,30,46-50] Some of the known properties of RDDP are enumerated in Table 5.

III. VIROGENE EXPRESSION

The different structural proteins and the envelope proteins of Type C viruses originate from precursor proteins encoded by the viral genome in all systems — murine, feline, avian, and primates alike, except for some minor variations. Biosynthesis of the viral envelope glycoproteins appears to occur independently of the structural protein in all RNA viruses. The regions of the viral genome coding for the structural proteins, RDDP and the envelope proteins, are termed *gag, pol,* and *env,* respectively. In addition to these genes, a fourth gene called *src* has been identified through studies of transformation-defective (td) deletion mutants of avian sarcoma viruses. The *src* sequences are acquired from the cellular genome and are, therefore, not required for the synthesis of infectious viral progeny.

The intrinsic cellular controls regulating the expression of viruses are still only conceptual at the present time. Depending on the genetic background of the host, different states of expression ranging from complete repression, partial expression of some viral polypeptides, to production of complete infectious viral particles can occur. These latter host factors will be discussed at length in Section IV.

The various viral precursor polypeptides are referred to in literature by an abbreviated form with a prefix Pr for precursor or gPr for glycosylated precursor, followed by the two- or three digit number indicating the molecular weight in kilodaltons. Each of the precursor polypeptides is functionally identified by the use of abbreviated superscripts. For example, the superscript *gag* represents the gene coding for the major internal virion structural proteins — p30, p15, p12, and p10. It is derived from a pre-

TABLE 5

Properties of Reverse Transcriptase in Avian and Mouse Type C Viruses

	Avian system	Murine system
Mol wt	170,000 daltons	70,000—84,000 daltons
Subunit structure	2 polypeptides 65,000 (α) mol wt 95,000 (β) mol wt	1 polypeptide
Primer to initiate DNA synthesis directed by viral RNA	Cellular tRNA^{Trp}	Cellular tRNA^{Pro}
Binding affinity of primer tRNA	Very low of (α) subunits; very high for ($\alpha\beta$) complex	Very low
Mode of action of RNAse H	Random for α subunit; processive for $\alpha\beta$ complex	Random
Immunological properties	Cross-reacts with members of the group except for Reticuloendotheliosus virus, which does not cross-react with other members of the avian group	Cross-reacts within the murine but not with avian system

cursor molecule of Pr 80^{gag} or Pr 65^{gag} depending on the molecular weight of that protein or a large precursor molecule Pr 220$^{gag-pol}$ where *pol* represents the gene responsible for the encoding of the viral RDDP. The gene that prescribes for the precursor polypeptide to make the viral envelope proteins — gp69/71, p15E, and p12E — is a 80,000 to 90,000 molecular weight protein, abbreviated as gPr 80^{env}.[51]

A. Structural Proteins (*gag* Locus)

The internal structural proteins of the murine type C viruses are derived from a common precursor polyprotein that is a translational product of the *gag* gene. The polyprotein undergoes proteolytic cleavage into the monomer forms which are then processed to the different core proteins of the virion. The precursor polyprotein is located near the 5′ end of the 35S viral RNA. In Rauscher murine leukemia virus which has been studied more thoroughly than any other murine species, this high molecular weight protein has been variously identified as a 200,000 (Pr 200$^{gag-pol}$),[52-54] 80,000 (Pr 80^{gag}), and 65,000 (Pr 65^{gag}),[54-56] dalton species. The 35S genomic viral RNA first translates the Pr 80^{gag} portion which is then rapidly cleaved to produce Pr 65^{gag}.[53,57,58] The fate of Pr 80^{gag} in the cell is unknown. It could be degraded or could exist as a functional virus-specific polypeptide. There is no evidence to date that the amino-terminal peptide sequence of PR 80^{gag} is present in virions.[59] The PR 80^{gag} portion is terminated by a terminating codon of the *gag* gene of the 35S RNA, but the latter continues to translate the remainder of the RNA containing the *pol* gene, thus producing a *gag-pol* gene product.[60] Chemical fragmentation with cyanogen bromide which has specificity for methionine residues, followed by immune precipitation with antisera specific to viral-structural proteins and tryptic peptide mapping provides evidence that Pr 80^{gag} represents a precursor polyprotein in which a long "leader" sequence is attached to Pr 65^{gag}.[59] The peptide sequence of Pr 65^{gag} has been shown to be in the order

NH_2-p15-p12-p30-p10-COOH,[60-62] the proteins lacking methionine (i.e., p15 and p10) occupying the terminal portions of the precursor. Tryptic digests of these internal proteins obtained from three principal endogenous classes of murine leukemia viruses (namely, ecotropic, xenotropic, and amphotropic) show that the major internal virion protein, p30, from each of these subgroups is strongly conserved with structural heterogeneity in only two regions.[63,64] One of these two regions is similar in all ecotropic and amphotropic viruses showing N-tropism. The peptide sequences of this particular region of the p30 among xenotropic viruses show variation within the group and these sequences are also different from those observed with eco- and amphotropic viruses. The second region of p30 protein showing heterogeneity is identical in peptide sequences in the xenotropic and amphotropic viruses and thus distinguishable from the ecotropic p30 protein at this region.[64] The differences in the murine leukemia virus p30 profiles have helped to distinguish the endogenous murine leukemia viruses from the exogenous Friend, Moloney, and Rauscher viruses. A structurally variable region of p30 has been identified that is functionally associated with *Fv*-1 tropism,[62] suggesting that p30 is the viral determinant of *Fv*-1 tropism. The p15 protein in these three classes of endogenous viruses is unique, showing the possible subgroup specificity of this protein. The p12 proteins show extensive homology among the ecotropic viruses. The NZB xenotropic virus p12 protein and the wild mouse amphotropic virus p12 are similar to each other in their peptide sequences and substantially different from the ecotropic p12 proteins. The partial immunological cross-reactivity between xenotropic and amphotropic viruses not shared by ecotropic viruses could be attributed to this shared homology in the p12 protein.[64] The structural proteins, especially the major structural protein p30, may prove a useful tool in determining the nature of the novel biochemical or biological properties of unique virus types that arise through phenotypic mixing or genetic recombination.

B. RNA-Directed DNA Polymerase (RDDP) (*pol* Locus)

RDDP is located in the core of the virus as a complex with the viral RNA. This enzyme catalyzes in vivo the synthesis of DNA complementary to the RNA of tumor viruses. This enzyme requires a template to direct DNA synthesis. The natural template is the viral genomic RNA. The enzyme cannot initiate a new DNA chain. It can only help in elongation of the DNA chain at the 3′ OH end of an already existing primer strand, hydrogen bonded to the template. Therefore, the direction of synthesis of the enzyme is from 5′ to 3′. The natural primer is the 4S RNA present in the 60 to 70S RNA complex. The 4S RNA of the murine type C viruses has been identified as a proline tRNA.[65]

The RDDP is encoded by a gene called *pol* identified in the virogene as closer to the *gag* gene. In the Rauscher murine leukemia virus, the precursor polypeptide responsible for the formation of RDDP has been identified as a 200,000 molecular weight protein (Pr 200$^{gag-pol}$).[66,67] This large precursor protein contains both p30 and RDDP information (see Section III.A). The Pr 200$^{gag-pol}$ through proteolytic cleavage produces intermediate RDDP related precursors of 145,000 (Pr 145^{pol}), 135,000 (Pr 135^{pol}), 125,000 (Pr 125^{pol}), and 80,000 (Pr 80^{pol}) molecular weight proteins in that order.[67] The last three precursor proteins are relatively stable. The Rauscher leukemia virus RDDP has a molecular weight of 80,000 daltons. It remains to be determined whether or not Pr 80^{pol} is further processed to virion p80^{pol}.

C. Envelope (*env* Locus)

The envelope (*env*) precursor in the murine system is a glycosylated protein, gPr 80^{env}. This precursor protein is synthesized and processed in cellular membranes by proteolysis and carbohydrate alteration to the finished envelope gene products gp70 and p15 (E).[51,68-72] The gp70 through further proteolysis gives rise to a smaller glyco-protein gp45, which has recently been shown to share similar amino-terminal amino acid sequences.[73] The p15(E) is a 15,000 molecular weight protein located in the viral envelope.[74,75] This further cleaves to produce p12(E).[52] The p15(E) protein species possesses strong group-specific antigenic reactivity and is different from the structural protein, p15. Both gp70 and p15(E) are derived from the same precursor polyprotein. The gp70-p15(E) complex may play a role in the proper assembly of the virion surface components and in determining the surface morphology of mature virions.

D. Sarcoma-Specific Gene (*src* Gene)

The oncogene theory[26] which suggests the presence of an "oncogene" within or close to the virogene and perhaps under the host gene regulatory mechanism has been identified in the avian system as a single viral gene called *src*. This gene has been mapped near the 3' terminus of the avian sarcoma virus RNA.[76] The interesting observation that nucleotide sequences related to *src* are present in the DNA of the chickens[77] led several investigators to believe that *src* or the product(s) of the *src* gene may be present in all the mammalian species as well. The product of the avian sarcoma virus *src* gene has been identified as a phosphoprotein of 60,000 daltons, pp60^{src}. The pp60^{src} acts as a protein kinase.[78-80] Recently, uninfected cells from a variety of vertebrate species were found to possess a highly conserved phosphoprotein that has antigenic, chemical, and functional homology with pp60^{src}.[81] As yet, a *src* gene has not been identified in the murine system. The closest to identifying a *src* gene in the murine system is the observation that the DNA of uninfected mouse cells contain specific sequences of the Moloney murine sarcoma virus-genome as a single copy per haploid genome.[82-84] The most likely interpretation of this observation is that the Moloney murine sarcoma virus-specific sequence is a normal cell sequence which was incorporated into the Moloney murine sarcoma virus genome by a rare combination event between Moloney murine leukemia virus and cell RNAs or between proviral DNA and cell DNA. A correlation between the amount of Moloney murine sarcoma virus-specific RNA in the cytoplasm of certain clones of NIH 3T3 cells and the degree of transformation has also been shown.[85]

The dual-tropic viruses[86-87] — that is, viruses which arose as genetic recombinants between ecotropic viruses and endogenous viral sequences coding for envelope glyco-protein determinants[88] — may provide insight into factors influencing the oncogenic potential and the possibility of recognizing a *src* or *leuk* gene in mice. The dual-tropic oncogenic virus isolates obtained from AKR and C3H have been found to possess in them common envelope glycoprotein determinants of a unique type not shared by the nononcogenic ecotropic viruses from which they were derived[89,90] and which are presumably required, but not necessarily sufficient, for oncogenicity.

E. Retrovirus Assembly and Maturation

The previous section has described the different viral components that are independently synthesized within the cellular machinery. Through biosynthesis and proteolytic cleavage, these viral precursor polypeptides undergo morphogenesis, culminating in the characteristic Type C virion substructures that result in the formation of infectious virion particles. However, the precise site in the cell where the precursor polypeptide cleavage takes place is not known with certainty. The sequence of events leading to the virus assembly at the cell surface prior to budding and the containment of the viral core with the cell membrane is also poorly understood. One of the prerequisities of virus assembly is the specific recognition and association of structural components during the budding process. Temperature-sensitive (*ts*) replication mutants of the Rauscher-murine leukemia virus (conditional lethal mutants), defective in post-translational processing of the *gag* gene coded precursor (Pr 65^{gag}), provided evidence that the cleavage of the Rauscher murine leukemia virus *gag* gene polypeptide precursor occurs at the cell surface at the time of the virus assembly.[91,92] One proposed mechanism of virus assembly[93] suggests that the interior portion of the transmembrane protein serves as a recognition site for the amino-terminal polypeptide of the *gag* precursor during virus formation. The type-specific internal protein, p12, which is at the amino-terminal, would thus be a likely candidate to specifically recognize the viral envelope constituents. The observation of a distinct pool of structural antigens (p30, p15, and p10) in the form of precursor polypeptide (Pr 65^{gag}) below the cell membrane in cells infected with *ts* mutants of Rauscher murine leukemia viruses at the nonpermissive temperature as seen through immunofluorescence and electron microscopy studies[92,94] gives credence to the recognition site suggested for the *gag* precursor protein during maturation of the virus particle. Further substantiating evidence is obtained through the rapidity with which virus assembly takes place; the virus assembly and the release of mature virions are completed within 2 to 4 min.[92] Virus assembly is unlikely in the absence of virus glycoprotein, which is required for packaging the virion to an infectious particle. More research of the sequential steps in assembly and the release of virus from the cell surface is needed to answer questions such as the nature of the cleavage enzymes responsible for processing the *gag* and *env* precursors or the viral glycoprotein complex.

IV. GENETIC CONTROL OF VIRUS EXPRESSION

A. Host-Genes Regulating Virus Expression

The foregoing discussion pertained to the various steps that take place at the molecular level for the formation of an infectious virion particle. However, these sequences are not expressed in all cells at all times. It seems quite likely that the level or degree of expression is somehow regulated by the host cell. These regulatory gene sequences can be mapped on specific chromosomes using standard procedures of genetic linkage analysis. This section will describe those genes in the mouse that regulate the expression of murine leukemia virus. There are examples of similar regulatory mechanisms in other animal systems.

Table 6 lists the genes that have been identified as controlling the expression of murine leukemia virus. The genes are divided into those controlling spontaneous virus production and those which respond to inducing agents and express murine leukemia virus. A brief description of each follows.

1. Murine Ecotropic Viruses
a. Spontaneous Expression

By the use of mating experiments between high virus-yielding AKR and the low virus-yielding NIH-Swiss strains, two genes, *Akv*-1 and *Akv*-2, which seem to control independently the production of infectious endogenous leukemia virus in AKR mice, have been described.[95] These two genes were shown to be segregating in a Mendelian fashion, thus providing proof that these genes are integrated DNA proviruses of endogenous murine leukemia virus.[96,97] One of these two genes, the *Akv*-1, has been mapped on chromosome 7, linkage group I.[98,99] The *Akv*-2 has not yet been mapped. The viruses regulated by these two genetic loci have been found to be indistinguishable by biological criteria, as well as through fingerprint analysis using RNase T-1 resistant

TABLE 6

Host Genes that Regulate Expression of Viruses

Murine Ecotropic Viruses

Locus	Host in which gene identified	Chromosome no.	Linkage data	Genetic function	Virus regulated	Ref.
Spontaneous expression						
Akv-1	AKR	7	c-Gpi-1, Akv-1	Spontaneous and induced expression of infectious virus	AKR-MuLV	98
Akv-2	AKR	NR	NR	Same as Akv-1	AKR-MuLV	99
A single gene	AKR	NR	NR	NR	AKR-MuLV	101
A single gene	C3H	NR	Unlinked to G-6PD es-1, or 3-Hbb-H2 or c, and to C57BL/6 MuLV gene	Expression of infectious virus	AKR-type MuLV	103
A single gene	C57BL/6	NR	Unlinked to the gene described above in C3H for MuLV production	Expression of infectious virus	AKR-type MULV	100
2 genes	C57BL/6 × DBA/2	NR	NR	Group-specific (p30) antigen expression	Ecotropic MuLV	104
2 dominant genes	C57BL/6 × AKR and AKR × B10	NR	NR	Group-specific (p30) antigen expression	Ecotropic MuLV	105
1 semidominant gene; 2 dominant genes	AKR × C57L	NR	NR	Group-specific (p30) antigen expression	Ecotropic MuLV	106
Induced expression						
Ind	BALB/c	NR	Nonlinked to Fv-1	Induced expression of N-tropic MuLV (BALB: Virus-1)	AKR-type MuLV	110
A single gene	BALB/c	NR	NR	Induced expression of B-tropic MuLV	AKR-type MuLV	111

TABLE 6 (continued)

Host Genes that Regulate Expression of Viruses

Locus	Host in which gene identified	Chromosome no.	Linkage data	Genetic function	Virus regulated	Ref.
Murine Ecotropic Viruses						
Multiple loci (more than 2 genes)	C58	NR	NR	Induced expression	AKR-type MuLV	112
Murine Xenotropic Viruses						
Spontaneous expression						
Nzv-1	NZB	NR	NR	Regulation of high titers either by acting alone or with Nzv-2	NZB xenotropic virus	115
$ Nzv-2	NZB	NR	NR	Regulation of low titers of infectious virus	Same as Nzv-1	115
A single gene	NZB	NR	NR	Regulation of infectious NZB xenotropic virus	NZB xenotropic virus	114
Induced expression						
A single gene	BALB/c	1	Linked to Dip-1; nonallelic to Bxv-1	Induced virus expression	BALB: Virus-2	118
Bxv-1	C57BL/10 and B10.Br/Sgli (congenic strain)	1	Linked Dip-1	Inducible virus expression	Xenotropic virus	119

oligonucleotides generated by enzymatic cleavage of ^{32}P-labeled viral RNA and through two-dimensional gel electrophoresis.[100] The inherent disadvantage in RNA fingerprinting is that only a small percentage of the viral RNA is taken into account for the analysis. Thus, it is quite conceivable that the difference in sequence between the viruses formed by the Akv-1 gene and Akv-2 gene might go unnoticed. Perhaps these two genetic loci may have been the result of two integrations of the same viral genetic material or these two loci are the result of independent exogenous infection by two closely related viruses.

A third viral locus which regulates the expression of infectious AKR murine leukemia virus in AKR mice has recently been identified.[101] This locus is not detectable through focus-forming assay with tail extracts from various crosses over FG-10 indicator cells. In backcrosses of NIH × (NIH × AKR), three main phenotypes emerged: viremic mice without any free antibody against murine leukemia virus, nonviremic mice with high titers of antibody, and nonviremic mice without any detectable antibody. These three categories were present in proportions conforming to Mendelian segregation for three independently segregating genetic loci and were further confirmed through backcrosses with other inbred strains such as BALB/c and C57BL/6 mice.

The AKR-type ecotropic murine leukemia virus is also present in other inbred strains of mice such as C3H and C57BL/6. The C3H phenotype is characteristically associated with the early appearance of high titers of antibody, whereas the C57BL/6 has a late phenotype in which antibodies occur later in life, are transient, and are at lower titers. This immune response has been shown to be correlated to virus expression in vivo and has been used to follow virus expression in vivo through appropriate genetic crosses.[102] The genetics of expression of the endogenous C3H AKR-type murine leukemia virus has been followed utilizing crosses between C3H and NIH Swiss mice as well as C57BL/6 and NIH/Swiss, their F_1 and F_2, and backcross progeny. Virus expression was followed logically using radioimmuneprecipitation assay, and the segregation of proviral DNA was studied using DNA-DNA hybridization. In both C3H and C57BL/6, the endogenous AKR-type murine leukemia virus expression has been shown to be regulated by a single gene. The single gene in C3H has been shown to be nonallelic and unlinked to the single gene in C57BL/6 by appropriate genetic crosses between C3H and C57BL/6 strains.[103]

Host-gene regulated expression of the group-specific (p30) antigen in crosses between C57BL/6 and DBA/2 strains of mice has indicated that at least two genes influence endogenous virus expression in this cross.[104] Detection of viral antigen from splenic tissues from C57BL/6 and DBA/2, their F_1s and backcross progeny were studied. Whereas all the DBA/2 strain examined are positive for group-specific (p30) antigen, only a low percentage (7%) of mice from the other parental strain, C57BL/6, showed the presence of viral antigen. The percentage of mice that show the viral antigen expression in the F_1 hybrids, F_2, and the backcross progeny segregated conforming to the Mendelian ratio for two genes. These results are similar to those reported using high leukemic strains such as AKR and C58, crossed to low leukemic strains C57BL/6 and B-10.[105] In this latter study, group-specific viral antigen expression was studied through an immunofluorescence absorption test and a test based on disappearance rate of antimurine leukemia virus antibody. The results indicate that the genetic control of murine leukemia virus group-specific (p30) antigen expression in crosses between high and low leukemic strains is in concordance with the "two dominant genes-one semidominant gene" model, the influence of the semidominant host gene depending on the Fv-1 allele of the strains used, (i.e., Fv-1^n or Fv-1^b allele (see next section for details).

In crosses between low leukemic C57BL and AKR, two dominant genes controlling

the group-specific antigen (p30) have been reported.[106] Both these strains possess the
Fv-1" allele and hence the influence of Fv-1 gene cannot be detected from these crosses.

b. Induced Expression

In cells which lack spontaneous expression of endogenous type C viruses, two groups
of chemicals, halogenated pyrimidines and inhibitors of protein synthesis, have been
shown to be highly efficient inducers of these viruses.[15,107,108] Following this, several
studies have shown the presence of genetic loci for virus induction in cells of many
inbred strains of mice.[96,99,109]

BALB/c strain has a low incidence of endogenous virus expression but these viruses
can be induced following treatment with 5-iododeoxyuridine. In order to determine
the number of genes involved in the inducibility of endogenous virus in BALB/c mice,
cell lines derived from crosses between inducible BALB/c and the noninducible NIH/
Swiss mice were used in a study in which a single locus, tentatively designated as *Ind*,
was identified.[110] This gene controls the expression of a virus that grows preferentially
in NIH Swiss mouse cells and hence are N-tropic in host range. This virus is called the
BALB:virus 1. A gene known to affect cell susceptibility to exogenous infection by
many strains of murine leukemia virus, the Fv-1 gene, has been shown to be genetically
unlinked to the *Ind* locus.[110] Recently, another gene controlling the induction of an
ecotropic murine leukemia virus preferentially growing in BALB/c cells (B-tropic) has
been identified.[111]

The virus inducibility loci represent viral structural rather than regulatory information. This can be demonstrated by showing that all virus isolates induced from the
same locus are identical and yet distinct from those activated at some other locus.
Studying inducibility and biological properties of virus isolates from genetic backcrosses is one of the ways in which the nature of the loci (structural or regulatory) can
be determined.

In the high leukemic incidence C58 strain of mice, the induction of murine leukemia
virus has been shown to be under the control of multiple (more than two genes) genetic
loci.[112] Using genetic crosses involving C58 and NIH Swiss mice, the existence of more
than one genetic loci was determined, thereby raising the possibility of finding additional alleles representing viruses in other inbred strains of mice.

2. Murine Xenotropic Viruses

a. Spontaneous Expression

The NZB strain of mice spontaneously releases high levels of infectious xenotropic
virus and has been the model for studying the genetics of xenotropic virus expression.
Genetic studies using embryonic cells derived from NZB and NIH Swiss (a strain which
does not spontaneously release xenotropic virus) provided evidence for a single dominant-like autosomal gene responsible for virus production in the NZB strain.[113] Genetic
studies in our laboratory using NZB/B1NJ and 129/J (another inbred strain which
lacks spontaneous production of infectious xenotropic virus) also indicate that a single,
autosomal, dominant-like gene is responsible for the spontaneous release of infectious
xenotropic virus from the NZB/B1NJ strain.[114] All the F_1 hybrids and the backcross
progeny derived from (NZB/129) × NZB show spontaneous xenotropic virus production. Progeny obtained from crosses involving (NZB × 129)F_1 to 129/J strain and its
reciprocal backcrosses provided evidence of spontaneous infectious xenotropic virus
in 52% of their progeny. This data along with the data obtained from (NZB/129)F_2
progeny where 77% were virus-positive and 23% virus-negative mice are consistent
with the Mendelian segregation for a single gene (Table 7). This was confirmed by
examining the second backcross generation. The virus-positive (NZB/129)F_1 × 129

TABLE 7

Expression of Infectious Xenotropic Virus in Genetic
Crosses of NZB/B1NJ and 129/J Mice[a]

Strain	+/Tested[b]
NZB/B1NJ	42/42
129/J	0/51
(NZB × 129)F$_1$	32/32
(129 × NZB)F$_1$	4/4
(NZB/129)F$_1$ × NZB	4/4
NZB × (NZB/129)F$_1$	14/14
(NZB/129)F$_1$ × 129	26/50
129 × (NZB/129)F$_1$	4/5
((NZB/129)F$_1$ × (NZB/129)F$_1$)F$_2$	37/48

[a] In all crosses, the female is listed first. Infectious
virus production was measured by cocultivation with
human foreskin cells, as described in text.

[b] Number of animals positive for X-tropic virus per
the total number of animals examined.

mice (Bc-1) mated to the virus-negative strain 129/J resulted in progeny animals that
differed in virus production; that is, 47% of the progeny (17/36) were virus positive.
Virus-negative (NZB/129)F$_1$ × 129 mated to 129/J mice yielded only virus-negative
progeny (0/34) (Table 8).

In contradistinction to the aforementioned studies, Datta and Schwartz[115,116] found
two independently segregating autosomal dominant genes, Nzv-1 and Nzv-2, regulating the level of spontaneous production of infectious xenotropic virus. These two genes
are not linked to H-2 type, coat color, or sex. Their genetic studies used two inbred
strains of mice, NZB and SWR. From the analyses of F$_1$, F$_2$, and progeny derived
from backcross to either parent, these investigators concluded that the expression of
high virus titer is controlled by Nzv-1 alone or in association with Nzv-2. When present
alone, low virus titer is under genetic control of Nzv-2.

The information on the number of genes involved in spontaneous xenotropic virus
production in studies using NZB and NFS (an inbred strain derived from random bred
NIH Swiss mice) is confusing. A single, autosomal semidominant gene as well as two
genes are reported in the spontaneous virus expression in NZB[117] depending on the
methods of detection for virus expression.

The conflicting data on the number of genes that determine the spontaneous production of infectious xenotropic virus in NZB need to be resolved by further studies.
The difference could be attributed to the influence of modifier genes contributed by
the particular mouse strain used or, perhaps, the virus detected show preferential
expression in certain heterologous host cells (For more details, see Reference 117.)

An important approach to understanding the expression of xenotropic virus regulation in NZB would be the derivation of a congenic strain — congenic for xenotropic
virus expression. A congenic mouse strain is an inbred strain which has been derived
so that it differs from an established inbred strain in only one particular character.
Congenic strains can be produced for any gene that exhibits genetic variation and for
which a screening method of any kind is available. The simplest mating system leading
to establishment of a congenic strain consists of repeated backcrossing. The genetic
crossing starts with the two strains of mice. One of them provides the genetic background for the congenic line and is therefore called the background strain. This strain
must be inbred. The second strain donates the locus at which the congenic lines will

TABLE 8

Xenotropic Virus Expression in Second-back-
cross Progeny of NZB and 129/J Mice

Family	Parental strain[a]	+ / Tested[b]
1	$129 \times (F_1 \times 129)^+$	6/12
2	$(F_1 \times 129)^+ \times 129$	7/16
3	$(F_1 \times 129)^+ \times 129$	4/8
4	$129 \times (F_1 \times 129)^-$	0/22
5	$129 \times (F_1 \times 129)^-$	0/7
6	$(F_1 \times 129)^- \times 129$	0/5

[a] + = mouse whose spleen showed presence
of infectious virus.
 − = mouse whose spleen showed no infectious virus.

[b] Number of animals positive for X-tropic virus per total number of animals examined.

differ (donor strain)., The locus at which the congenic line differs from its background
strain is called the differntial locus and its allele is called the differential allele. Derivation of such a strain would greatly minimize the interaction of modifying genes and
thus provide an excellent model which could be utilized not only for genetics, but also
6for studies related to cancers in mice. The derivation of a strain of mouse that is
congenic to the 129/J strain for virus expression (i.e., carrying the gene from the NZB
strain that determines virus expression) is now being generated in our laboratory.

b. Induced Expression

The genetics of induction of xenotropic virus has been studied in cell cultures derived
from specific strains of mice and using such inducers as halogenated pyrimidines or
protein synthesis inhibitors. Detailed description of the various inducing agents used
for release of xenotropic viruses from different cell lines and the proposed mechanisms
involved are beyond the scope of this chapter and the reader is directed to a recent
review of these principles.[117] Table 6 shows the two genetic loci recently identified.
Utilizing embryo cell lines derived from genetic crosses between BALB/c and NIH
Swiss mice, an endogenous xenotropic virus was induced by treatment of cells with 5-
iododeoxyuridine.[118] This virus is called BALB:virus-2. This virus, like the NZB-mu-
rine leukemia virus, transmits to and replicates in normal rat kidney cells. BALB:virus-
2 is unable to infect NIH Swiss or BALB/c mouse embryo cells. The genetic locus
governing the BALB:virus-2 inducibility segregates independently of the locus regulating the ecotropic BALB:virus-1. The gene has not yet been named, nor has its precise
location in the mouse genome been identified.

An inducibility locus has been identified in C57BL/10 mice and is named *Bxv*-1.
Virus inducibility is linked to the enzyme dipeptidase-1 (*Dip*-1) on chromosome-1,[119]
Bxv-1 is nonallelic to the locus controlling the BALB:virus-2.[119]

B. Host-Genes Regulating Infectivity to Viruses

Strains of mice differ in their susceptibility to exogenous retrovirus infection. Most
factors that regulate retrovirus replication and expression could operate at different
levels of virus-host interactions. For example, control can be exercised at the level of
viral adsorption onto cells, viral integration, or maturation. Biological activities associated with virus infection can also be regulated by the host immune system (Table 9).

TABLE 9

Host Genes Affecting Infectivity to Viruses

Gene	Chromosome #	Dominant allele	Linkage group	Mechanism	Ref.
Fv-1	4	Resistance to infection of exogenous MuLV	VIII Linked to *Gpd*-1	Replication according to the NB tropism of the helper	128, 129
Rev	5	NR	Syntenic with *Pgm*-1	Regulation of MuLV adsorption	121, 122
Srv	NR	Affects the sensitivity of virus infection	NR	Regulates both insensitivity and hitness (infectivity) along with *Fv*-1 gene	150
Fv-2	9	Sensitivity to infection of exogenous MuLV	II, Linked to "dilute" (*d*)	Interaction of SFFV with erythropoietic precursors	142
Fv-4	NR	Resistance to replication of NB-tropic	Unlinked to "dilute" (*d*)	*In vivo* resistance is independent of *Fv*-1 and *Fv*-2 and epistatic to both	146, 148
Fv-3	NR	NR	NR	Influence on murine lymphocytes to respond to mitogens	154
Rgv-1	17	Resistance	IX, Linked to H2	Control of the antivirus (Gross virus) or antitumor immune response	157, 158
Rgv-2	NR	Resistance	Not linked to H2	Not known; may be identical to action of *Fv*-1	161
Rgv-3	NR	Resistance	NR	NR	161
Av-1	NR	Sensitivity	NR	Susceptibility to lymphoma genesis to MuLV-A strain	162
Av-2	NR	Sensitivity	NR	Same as above	162

The current picture of susceptibility is one of complex control with a number of genes involved. Hence, discussion in this section will be limited to only the important and well-recognized genes in the murine system. One other system which is well studied in the avian group, but a discussion of this group is beyond the scope of this chapter.

1. Genes Involved at the Level of Virus Adsorption

Virus adsorption onto cells is affected as a result of specific interactions between the viral envelope and the receptor molecule on the cell surface. The viral envelope glycoprotein specifically recognizes the cell surface receptors. It is these cell surface receptors that restrict certain types of cells to exogenous infection of retroviruses. The receptor-viral glycoprotein complex formation has been studied using purified gp70 in a cell-free system by gel filtration through Sepharose-CL6B[120] or through somatic cell hybrids using murine × Chinese hamster cells.[121,122] Tissue specificity in the expression of viral receptors in vitro has been observed in certain cases of murine leukemia viruses.[123] In the plasma membranes of Kirsten murine sarcoma virus-transformed A31 clone of BALB/c-3T3 (KA 31) cells, a receptor has been identified for the binding of Rauscher murine leukemia virus. This receptor has been characterized as a lipoprotein.[120] In experiments on mouse × Chinese hamster cells that segregate murine chromosomes, the gene responsible for ecotropic murine leukemia virus has been identified and designated *Rev* and assigned to mouse chromosome 5.[121-124]

Multiple viral receptors have been identified in the wild mouse, *Mus cervicolor*. A minimum of two unlinked genes for ecotropic receptors as well as a third independently segregating receptor gene for xenotropic virus have been reported.[124]

The mechanism of mouse cell resistance to xenotropic virus has been studied using human × mouse cell hybrids. The xenotropic virus, AT-124, was only infectious for hybrid cells containing a complete complement of human chromosomes and very few mouse chromosomes.[125] The restriction of xenotropic viruses by mouse cells is presumed to be at the level of virus adsorption. Presumably, this is caused by glycoproteins coded for by endogenous viral genomes in the mouse cells and expressed on the surface of the cell hybrids.[126] The mechanism of the mouse cell surface restriction to xenotropic viruses is still not completely understood..

2. Genes Acting at the Intracellular Level

A thoroughly studied gene that regulates exogenous infection of mouse cells by naturally occurring murine leukemia virus is $Fv\text{-}1$.[127] This locus mapped on mouse chromosome 4[128,129] has two alleles — $Fv\text{-}1^n$ and $Fv\text{-}1^b$. Each represents a dominant resistance to virus of a certain tropism. $Fv\text{-}1^{nn}$ cells are susceptible to N-tropic (viruses that propagate better in cells of NIH Swiss mice) virus, whereas $Fv\text{-}1^{bb}$ cells replicate B-tropic (those viruses propagating best in BALB/c cells) viruses efficiently. NB-tropic viruses can grow in either type of cell.[96,130-132] Crosses of $Fv\text{-}1^{nn}$ and $Fv\text{-}1^{bb}$ cells lead to heterozygotes $Fv\text{-}1^{nb}$ cells with resistance to N- and B-tropic virus. Recently, RF, 129, NZB, and NZW mouse strains previously characterized as N-type have been reported to be more resistant to N-tropic murine leukemia virus than to other N-type cells, and a third allele, $Fv\text{-}1^{nr}$ (r for resistance), has been defined.[133]

Studies on the molecular basis of this $Fv\text{-}1$ restriction suggest that the host-cell control is at a step between viral DNA synthesis and its integration into the host genome.[134-140] Through Sendai virus-induced fusion of permissive and nonpermissive cells, virus expressions were studied by simultaneous autoradiography and fluorescent antibody assays which permitted the detection of virus-induced proteins.[141] These heterokaryons were found to dominantly restrict both N- and B-tropic virus but not NB-tropic virus. This restriction is, however, not at the level of virus adsorption, but at some post-penetration step extending to at least 6 hr after infection. Thus, it appears that Fv-1 restriction functions at some step in the virus replication cycle which follows adsorption but precedes the provirus stage.[141]

The gene Fv-2, segregating independantly of the Fv-1 gene and imparting susceptibility of mouse cells to spleen focus-forming virus (SFFV) of the Friend virus complex, has been described. This gene is linked to the gene for coat color dilute (d) on linkage Group II (Chromosome 9).[142] The spleen focus-forming virus is a defective virus in that it can no longer carry out its entire infectious cycle or induce erythroleukemia in mice in the absence of a helper virus like the lymphatic leukemia virus (a Friend virus which is under the regulation of the Fv-1 gene). The resistance of Fv-2 is absolute. The genetic influence of the Fv-1 and Fv-2 genes in viral leukemogenesis is discussed exhaustively in several reviews.[143-145]

A gene called Fv-4, imparting resistance to viral-induced leukemia in an inbred strain of mice, the G strain (derived from a noninbred ddY mouse colony in Japan), has recently been identified.[146] Fv-4 acts independently of Fv-1 and Fv-2 renes. Fv-4 controlled resistance to leukemia and is believed to result from a complete repression of the growth of ecotropic murine leukemia virus of N-, B-, or NB-tropism.[146,147] The dominant allele of the Fv-4 gene is Fv-4^n.[146,148] Recently, G mouse cells were shown to be fully permissive to amphotropic murine leukemia virus and to focus formation by amphotropic murine sarcoma virus.[149] The resistance to murine leukemia virus by G cells is unstable and tends to be lost during culture due to a selective loss of sensitive cells.[149]

Another gene, whose mechanism of action is not known but seems to regulate susceptibility to the radiation-leukemia virus (RadLV) at an intracellular level, is Srv. The action of this gene specifically influences susceptibility to this B-tropic murine leukemia virus. The action of this gene on other viruses is not yet known.[150]

3. Control of Virus Infectivity by Host Immune Systems

Several oncogenic viruses are profoundly immunosuppressive in vivo.[151] This immunosuppression has been reported on both humoral antibody synthesis[152] as well as on cell-mediated immunity.[153] The relevance of the immunosuppressive effects of viruses to their oncogenicity is still not clear. The Friend murine leukemia virus, which causes erythroleukemia in different strains of mice, has been a useful model to study the mechanism of immunosuppression by this virus on susceptible mouse cells. Immunosuppression by this virus in vivo is under host genetic control.

Susceptibility to immunosuppression by Friend murine leukemia virus, studied using a lymphocyte-mitogenesis assay in vitro, has provided evidence that suppression of lymphocyte-mitogenesis is under the control of a single, autosomal, dominant gene, Fv-3.[154] This gene is distinct from the Fv-2 gene described earlier and not linked to H-2 locus. Through genetic analyses between susceptible DBA/2 and resistant B10 D2/n strains, their F_1, intercross, and backcross progeny, it was shown that susceptibility to immunosuppression in vivo is also regulated by Fv-3 or a closely linked gene.[155] The role of this gene in leukemogenesis or the relevance of this gene in regulating the host's ability to mount an immune response against viral antigens is still unclear. If the latter case is true, then one could expect the gene to influence the recovery and survival of mice from Friend erythroleukemia.

The observation of a common histocompatibility allele H-2K in strains of mice that have a high leukemia, or are highly sensitive to the leukemia induced by exogenous retroviruses, led to the identification of the Rgv-1 gene (resistance to Gross virus, Passage A). This gene controls Gross virus-induced leukemia and resistance is dominant.[156-158] The Rgv-1 appears to control the immunological response against antigens associated with virus infection. The existence of *Rgv*-1 and an immune response gene (*Ir*-1) in the same subregion of H-2 is very suggestive of a strong influence of these two genes on the fate of viral disease by eliciting antibodies to the virus itself or the surface antigens of the leukemic cells.[159-160] The *Rgv*-1 gene is on Linkage Group IX of the mouse.

The existence of two more genes, segregating independently of the H-2 and therefore of *Rgv*-1, was known through analyses of F_1, F_2, and backcross progeny derived from crosses between two strains sensitive to Gross virus-induced leukemia, B10.BR and C3H.[161] These two genes are called *Rgv*-2 and *Rgv*-3.[161] Resistance is dominant for both these genes. These two genes are not yet mapped in the mouse chromosome.

A variant of Moloney leukemia virus isolated from a nonthymic lymphoma of a BALB/c mouse, termed Abelson murine leukemia virus, has been shown to cause a malignant disease of a B-lymphocytes-plasmacytomas. Recombinant inbred lines derived from (BALB/c × C57BL/6) have shown that susceptibility to Abelson murine leukemia virus lymphomagenesis is controlled by two genes designated as *Av*-1 and *Av*-2.[162] Susceptibility to lymphomagenesis is dominant at both these loci for the prototype, sensitive strain BALB/c. The mechanism of action of these genes in vivo is still not understood.

V. GENETICS OF VIRAL EXPRESSION AND DISEASE STATES

A. Viral-Chemical Interactions

Viruses can cause leukemia and lymphoma in mice, cats, and chickens. Yet certain cofactors are also known to play an important role in the development of clinically apparent disease. In these studies, the viral-chemical interaction on the host cell has been tested by monitoring the susceptibility of various clones of cells to chemicals and viruses alone and to the two agents together.

1. In Vitro Models

Table 10 summarizes the lines of evidence linking chemicals and viruses to neoplasia. Freeman and his co-workers[18,163] were among the first to study virus-chemical interactions in tissue culture. They showed that both diethylnitrosamine and Rauscher leukemia virus were required for transformation of Fischer and Osborne-Mendel secondary rat embryo cell cultures. However, the order in which the cells were treated was very important. Virus added after chemical treatment did not lead to cell transformation. They suggested that virus must be present and actively replicating at the time of chemical treatment.[18] Similar results were reported[164] using benzo(a)pyrene. Using high and low passage (P <60) Fischer rat embryo cells pretreated with 5-bromodeoxyuridine followed by treatment with the potent chemical carcinogen 3-methylcholanthrene,[165,166] Freeman and his group found transformation only when virus expression was observed. It is postulated that partial expression of Type C RNA virus in the cells is sufficient to act as a cocarcinogen with 3-methylcholanthrene. Rat cells are transformed by either 3-methylcholanthrene or 7,12- dimethylbenz(a)anthracene only with prior infection with an exogenous virus or with prior treatment with 5-bromodeoxyuridine.[167]

Transformation of rat embryo cells by 4-nitroquinoline-*N*-oxide or 3-methylcholanthrene occurs only in the presence of xenotropic virus.[168] No transformation occurred when the xenotropic virus was suppressed in these cells by a type-specific antibody.[168] These results suggest that the xenotropic viruses provide the necessary conditions for transformation by chemicals.

AKR-2B is a clone of AKR mouse embryo cells which does not produce infectious

TABLE 10

Transformation of Mammalian Cells by Combined Action of Chemicals and Viruses

System	Chemicals tested (concentration)	Transformation		Virus studied	Ref.
		In the presence of virus	In the absence of virus		
Rat systems					
Rat embryo cells from Fischer, Osborne-Mendel and Wistar strains	Diethylnitrosamine (0.1 mM)	+	—	RLV	18, 163
	Benzo(a)pyrene (10—25 µg/ml)	+	—	RLV	164
	3-Methylcholanthrene (0.01—10 µg/ml)	+	—	RLV	165, 166
	7,12-Dimethylbenz(a)-anthracene (0.01—0.1 µg/ml)	+	—	RLV	167
	Nitroquinoline-oxide	+	—	X-tropic AT-124 and H-5031	168
	3-Methylcholanthrene	+	—		
Mouse system					
AKR Mouse embryo cells Clone AKR-2B cells.	Benzo(a)pyrene, 5,6 dibenzathracene, 7,12 dimethylbenzanthracene 3-Methylcholanthrene	+	—	AKR-MuLV	170
NIH Swiss Mouse embryo cells.	3-Methylcholanthrene (0.1—1.0 µg/ml)	+	—	AKR-MuLV	171
	Benzo(a)pyrene (1.0—5.0 µg/ml)	+	—	AKR-MuLV	171
	7,12-Dimethylbenzanthracene (0.01—0.1 µg/ml)	+	—	AKR-MuLV	171
C3H10T¹ᐟ²	3-Methylcholanthrene (various doses)	+	+	C3H-MuLV	172

viruses, but which can be induced by halogenated pyrimidines to produce AKR murine leukemia virus.[169] Using AKR-2B cells as the control, two sets of these clonal cells — namely AKR-2B cells in which endogenous Type C virus was previously activated by 5-iododeoxyuridine were treated with four different carcinogenic polycyclic hydrocarbons — 3-methylcholanthrene, benzo(a)pyrene, 5,6-dibenzanthracene, and 7,12-dimethylbenzanthracene.[170] Similar experiments also used NIH-Swiss mouse embryo cells exogenously infected with AKR-murine leukemia virus in the presence of carcinogenic hydrocarbons: 3-methylcholanthrene, benzo(a)pyrene, and 7,12-dimethylbenzanthracene.[171] Cell transformation was enhanced when virus was expressed and the results suggest that both virus production and chemical treatment are required for cell transformation. Neither spontaneous endogenous virus production, exogenous virus infection of cells, nor treatment by chemical alone was sufficient for transformation.

The murine system utilizing the C3H 10T½ cells seems not to require the involvement of virus expression for chemical transformation.[172] Normal and chemically transformed cells express the same degree of viral activity.

2. In Vivo Models
a. Background

The foregoing discussion on the viral chemical cocarcinogenesis in vitro has been extended by several investigators to in vivo systems. Although the naturally occurring incidence of cancer among inbred strains of mice parallels the naturally occurring level of ecotropic virus expression,[106] susceptibility to chemically induced tumors usually does not parallel this virus expression. Correlation between virus expression and chemical carcinogenesis using 3-methylcholanthrene and 7,12-dimethylbenzanthracene subcutaneously on several inbred strains of mice shows that endogenous virus expression is independent of susceptibility to chemically induced tumors.[173,174] Some of the studies relating the degree of virus expression to susceptibility to chemically induced tumors are described in the following sections.

b. Ecotropic Virus and Chemical Carcinogenesis

The role of ecotropic viruses in chemically induced cancers has been studied using the subcutaneous model system. In this system, chemical carcinogens are inoculated once in the interscapular region, and fibrosarcomas at the site of inoculation are monitored. In genetic crosses between C57BL/6 and DBA/2, *gs* antigen expression segregates independently of 3-methylcholanthrene-induced fibrosarcomas.[104] Similar results are reported using two other strains of mice — AKR/J and C3H/HeJ.[105] AKR/J strain produces high levels of endogenous murine leukemia virus. Virus production in this strain is under the genetic regulation of two independently segregating host genes, *Akv*-1 and *Akv*-2 (for details see Section IV.A). The AKR strain is resistant to 3-methylcholanthrene-induced sarcomagenesis. C3H/HeJ lacks detectable virus and is susceptible to 3-methylcholanthrene-induced sarcoma. In genetic crosses between these two strains, susceptibility to 3-methylcholanthrene-induced sarcoma is independent of virus expression,[175] indicating that overt production of infectious virus does not play any role in determining susceptibility of the mice to chemical carcinogenesis.

The role of virus expression in chemically induced leukemia has been studied in strains that differ in their level of endogenous virus expression following 7,12-dimethylbenz(a)anthracene treatment.[176] 7,12-Dimethylbenz(a)anthracene treatment had little effect on p30 expression in C3H and BALB/c mice, which are less sensitive to 7,12-dimethylbenz(a)anthracene-induced leukemogenesis. The chemical, however, did result in increased p30 expression in the leukemia-sensitive strains, ST and DBA/2. The

TABLE 11

Susceptibility to 3 MC-Induced Fibrosarcomas In NZB/B1NJ, 129/J The F_1s, and Backcross to NZB[a,b]

Strain[c]	Total # on test	Total # tumors	% Mice with tumors	Avg latency period (days)	CI[d]
NZB/B1NJ	26	12	46	171	27
129/J	40	14	35	183	19
(NZB/129) F_1	33	21	64	167	38
(NZB/129)NZB Bc1	26	17	65	159	41

[a] Mice treated with 500 μg/0.05 ml of 3 MC in trioctanoin, subcutaneously.
[b] Susceptibility based on a 10-month test period.
[c] Mice 9 to 10 weeks old.
[d] CI = carcinogenic index:

$$\frac{\% \text{ Tumors}}{\text{Average Latency Period}} \times 100$$

results indicate an association of C-type viral activation with chemical induction of leukemia but do not necessarily imply an etiological role of the virus of the disease.

c. Xenotropic Virus and Chemical Carcinogenesis

A role of xenotropic virus in chemical carcinogenesis has been studied in our laboratory for the past 3 years. The high xenotropic virus-yielding NZB/B1NJ and nonvirus-yielding 129/J strains, the F_1 hybrids, the backcross progeny to either parents, and the second backcross progeny were treated with 3-methylcholanthrene subcutaneously, and the mice were monitored for tumors over a 10-month period.[177] The data obtained are presented in Tables 11 and 12. After treatment with the chemical carcinogen 3-methylcholanthrene, the parental strain NZB developed fibrosarcomas in 43% of the total mice tested with a carcinogenic index (a parameter equating latency period to tumor incidence and, therefore, indicating the degree of susceptibility) of 27 which is slightly higher than susceptibility to the chemical shown by the other parental strain, 129/J (Table 11). The F_1 hybrids and the backcross progeny derived from the F_1s mated to the NZB parent are all positive for xenotropic virus expression.[114] The degree of susceptibility to carcinogen-induced fibrosarcomas in the F_1s and (NZB × 129) × NZB backcross progeny was very much identical, both in terms of percent mice that developed tumors and the carcinogenic index (Table 11).

To study the correlation between xenotropic virus expression and susceptibility to chemical carcinogenesis, the virus-segregating populations from the progeny derived from the backcross F_1 × 129 and the F_2, as well as the second backcross (F_1 × 129) × 129, were inoculated with 3-methylcholanthrene and monitored for the appearance of fibrosarcomas at the site of inoculation (Table 12). In the backcross progeny derived from the F_1 × 129 genetic crosses, 50% of the mice were positive for virus expression.

Among the F_2s, the virus segregated on a 3:1 ratio of virus-positive to virus-negative mice. Among the second backcross progeny a 1:1 ratio of virus-positive to virus-negative mice was observed.[114]

Susceptibility to 3-methylcholanthrene-induced tumors in the virus-positive and virus-negative F_2 populations was identical with a carcinogenic index of 31 and 33, respectively. This, along with the data obtained from the second backcross families, confirmed that the virus-positive mice are no more susceptible to chemically induced cancers than the virus-negative mice (Table 12). These experiments showed that no correlation exists between xenotropic virus expression and 3-methylcholanthrene-induced fibrosarcomas.

TABLE 12

Susceptibility to 3 MC-Induced Fibrosarcomas in Progeny where Xenotropic Virus is Segregating[a,b]

Strain[c]	XTV status	Total # tested	Total # tumors	% of mice with tumors	Average latency period (days)	CI[d]
(NZB/219) × 129/J Bcl	+	12	5	42	202	21
	−	9	2	22	137	16
(NZB/129) F₂	+	31	16	51	166	31
	−	9	5	56	169	33
129/J × [(F₁) 129⁺] Bc2	+	6	3	50	189	26
	−	6	5	83	155	53
[(F₁) 129⁺] × 129/J	+	7	4	57	152	37
	−	9	6	67	212	31
[(F₁) 129⁺] × 129/J Bc2	+	4	2	50	188	26
	−	4	3	75	119	63

[a] Mice treated with 500 μg/0.05 mℓ of 3 MC in trioctanoin, subcutaneously.
[b] Susceptibility based on a 10-month test period.
[c] Mice 9 to 10 weeks old.
[d] CI = carcinogenic index:

$$\frac{\% \text{ Tumors}}{\text{Average Latency Period}} \times 100$$

B. Autoimmunity

It has been postulated that the endogenous viruses stimulate autoantibodies. An example would be antinuclear antibodies produced in mice that are immunologically hyperresponsive to nucleic acid antigens.[178]

The NZB strain is an excellent model system to study possible links between autoimmunity, malignancy, and virus infection. Through reciprocal matings between NZB and BALB/c strain, and progeny from three generations of this cross, and the backcross, the full course of autoimmune hemolytic disease was monitored throughout the life span of the mice.[179] The appearance of the disease in the hybrids was found to be relatively weak and much delayed (about 20 months) compared to the normal latency period of 12 months in the parental NZB strain. Electron microscopy studies confirmed evidence of viral segregation in the NZB × BALB/c F₁ hybrids. More viral particles in the hybrid tissues were noticed in comparison to the tissues of the parental strain BALB/c. The virus transmitted vertically in these hybrids was found to be different from the virus described in the NZB[180,181] in its host range and was found to be infective for newborn BALB/c, NZB, or F₁ hybrid recipients.

No correlation between the NZB xenotropic virus and autoimmunity has been observed in crosses between NZB mice and SWR, C57BL/6, and B10.A mice despite high titers of xenotropic virus in all of the F₁ hybrids tested at an early age. Whether the autoimmune disease is time dependent is not known at present.[116] In other studies, Datta et al.[182,183] concluded that the segregation of NZB xenotropic virus is independent of autoimmune syndrome in these animals through examination of both the infectious xenotropic virus expression and levels of serum gp70.

The cellular basis and the specific immunoregulatory events underlying the autoimmune hemolytic anemia are still not completely understood. Further work is required in order to understand the role of Type C RNA viruses in this autoimmune phenomenon.

VI. SEARCH FOR VIRAL FOOTPRINTS IN MAN

Attempts to isolate infectious RNA Type C viruses from human neoplasia have not yet been successful. However, the possibility of the presence of noninfectious endogenous RNA tumor viral genomes in human cells cannot be ruled out. Identification of nucleic acid sequences homologous to Type C viruses or RDDP activities similar to mammalian Type C viruses has been reported from a wide variety of human neoplasms including leukemias,[184] lymphomas,[185] sarcomas,[186] and brain tumors.[187] Sarngadharan et al.[188] isolated an enzyme with biochemical properties similar to those of the RDDP of mammalian Type C viruses from leukemic peripheral blood leukocytes. The presence of proviral sequences has been reported in DNA of a patient with acute myelogenous leukemia through viral RNA-cell DNA hybridization. Two types of infectious viruses have been identified, one type closely related to Simian sarcoma-leukemia virus and another type closely related to the baboon endogenous virus (see References 189 and 190). The most consistent evidence for a virus particle from human tissue is that of budding atypical virus-like particles from the base of syncitiotrophoblast layer of human not primate placentas found by several investigators.[191-196]

Several teams have reported the presence of viral nucleotide sequences in human leukemia cells.[197-202] In all these investigations, polynucleotide probes of murine and primate origin were used in the absence of a clearly defined human leukemia virus. Analyses of human cellular DNA indicate that none of these viral groups is genetically endogenous to human cells.

More research is needed in probing for a causal virus in various human malignancies. One cannot rule out the possibility of the presence of an endogenous xenotropic virus in the human cell DNA, strictly under some genetic regulation or probably not being able to be detected under the present assay methods. A possible association between Type C viruses and human neoplastic disease is still unproven. Levy[202,203] suggests a role for this endogenous viral information in normal cellular development as positive regulators for normal life processes such as embryogenesis, differentiation, autoimmunity, and cancer. The endogenous xenotropic viruses seem the most likely candidates for the variety of roles suggested in cells during all stages of their development.

VII. RECAPITULATION

One of the most important concepts to emerge in cancer research during the past two decades is that of genetic transmission of information regulating oncogenic virus expression in mice. As yet, a viral origin (RNA tumor virus) for cancer has not been demonstrated in man. However, one cannot ignore the many clinical, pathologic, and epidemiologic similarities between some human tumors and those of lower animals which have been shown to be caused by viruses. A priori, the genotypic change presumed to underlie the cellular transformation to malignancy could be ascribed to the insertion of RNA viral information into the cellular genome, thereby dictating the cellular machinery to copy the viral RNA, and alter the normal phenotype of the cells.

Significant progress has been made in the study of RNA tumor viruses in mammalian species. We know that these viruses, when expressed as infectious particles, can be transmitted horizontally from animal to animal, congenitally through the mother and vertically through either parent in whose genome the viral information is integrated. But what is not known with certainty is the nature or function of those endogenous virogenes that remain repressed in the cellular DNA of many species throughout their life span. Evidence that these endogenous virogenes are preserved over a long period of species evolution prompted many investigators to suggest some function in embryogenesis and differentiation.[204] Oncogenicity, then, could very well be the result of a breakdown in the equilibrium of the host-viral steady-state, leading the virus on its hostile path. For example, those species of *Felis* which acquired primate Type C viral genes from baboons millions of years ago have been shown to be resistant to infection by the endogenous baboon viruses, while those *Felis* species that lack the viral information are susceptible to baboon viral infection.[205] Type C viruses may provide an important mechanism by which interspecies genetic information can be transmitted. In their course of vertical transmission the viral genes almost always "carry" some cellular genes along with it. Thus, these viruses can recombine with cellular gene sequences including transforming genes and transmit these to distantly related species.[206,207] The observations[208,209] that transformed cells in culture, whether transformed spontaneously, by chemical carcinogens, or by other viruses, release their endogenous Type C viruses more readily than do their normal, untransformed counterparts have led to the suggestions that the released virus may have some role in alerting the host immune system by way of altering the cell membrane. The detection in the allantoic fluid of normal uninfected, embryonated chicken eggs of the enzyme "particle reverse transcriptase"[32] which lacks biological activity such as infectivity, helper activity, or interference and no endogenous DNA synthesis is significant. This enzyme is coded by a'gene different from the one that regulates the viral RDDP and is expressed at least sometime during embryogenesis. The presence of the activity of this enzyme during embryogenesis makes it a candidate for such functions as mutations, recombination, and translocation of genetic information envisaged by Temin[27] in his "provirus theory".

Identification of RDDP activity similar in biochemical and immunological properties to that of known Type C viral reverse transcriptase as well as particles resembling RNA tumor viruses in various human malignancies (see Reference 117) should be viewed as further evidence of a possible link of a putative human virus to the viral agents associated with similar neoplasia in the mouse and monkey models. The presence of endogenous viral information in all mammalian species studied including the few reports from normal human cells further augments the variety of roles these viruses may play in normal cell function.

In summary, we are only a few steps further in unraveling the nature of genetic regulations of viruses in host cells. Also, host cells can selectively express certain virogene products. The key to understanding this complex regulatory mechanism of virus expression probably lies in the determination of, and understanding the nature of, those genes controlling for virus assembly and expression. This genetic approach should yield the necessary information for a realistic determination of the role of virus expression in such processes as cancer, autoimmunity, or developmental biology.

ACKNOWLEDGMENT

The authors thank Dr. J. A. Levy, Cancer Research Center, University of San Francisco, California, for useful discussions and critical and constructive review of the chapter and The Council for Tobacco Research — U.S.A., Inc., New York, who funded much of the work from our laboratory described in this chapter. Thanks are also due to Dr. P. Reddy for many helpful discussions. The technical assistance of Miss P. Moody is gratefully acknowledged. Thanks are also extended to Ms. A. Ventura, Ms. J. Williams, and Miss C. Dwyer for clerical assistance.

REFERENCES

1. **Ellerman, V. and Bang, O.**, Experimentelle Leukamie bei Huhnern *Zentralbl. Bakteriol. Parasitenkd. Infektionskr. Abt. 1*, 46, 596, 1908.
2. **Rous, P.**, A sarcoma of the fowl transmissible by an agent separable from the tumor cells, *J. Exp. Med.*, 13, 397, 1911.
3. **Gross, L.**, Pathogenic properties and "vertical" transmission of the mouse leukemia agent, *Proc. Soc. Expr. Biol. Med.*, 78, 342, 1951.
4. **Gross, L.**, Oncogenic Viruses, 2nd ed., Pergamon Press, New York, 1970, 286.
5. **Levy, J. A.**, Endogenous C-type viruses in normal and "abnormal" cell development, *Cancer Res.*, 37, 2957, 1977.
6. **Aaronson, S. A., Hartley, J. W., and Todaro, G. J.**, Mouse leukemia virus: "spontaneous" release by mouse embryo cells after long-term *in vitro* cultivation, *Proc. Natl. Acad. Sci. U.S.A.*, 64, 87, 1969.
7. **Hill, M. and Hillova, J.**, Virus recovery in chicken cells tested with Rous sarcoma cell DNA, *Nature (New Biol.)*, 237, 35, 1972.
8. **Cooper, G. M. and Temin, H. M.**, Infectious DNA from cells infected with Rous sarcoma virus, reticuloendotheliosis virus or Rous associate virus-O, *Cold Spring Harbor Symp. Quant. Biol.*, 39, 1027, 1974.
9. **Levy, J. A., Kazan, P. M., and Varmus, H. E.**, The importance of DNA size for successful transfection of chicken embryo fibroblasts, *Virology*, 61, 297, 1974.
10. **McAllister, R. M., Gardner, M. B., Nicolson, M. O., Gilden, R. V., and Davidson, N.**, RD-114 virus: characterization and identification, *Prog. Exp. Tumor Res.*, 21, 196, 1978.
11. **McAllister, R. M., Nicolson, M. O., Heberling, R., Charman, H., Rice, N., and Gilden, R. V.**, Infectivity of endogenous baboon type-C virus related genes, in *Proc. 8th Int. Symp. Comp. Leukemia Res.*, Bentvelzen, P., Hilgers, J., and Yohn, D. S., Eds., Elsevier North Holland, New York, 1977, 135.
12. **Nicolson, M. O., McAllister, R. M., Okabe, H., and Gilden, R. V.**, Transfection with endogenous RD-114 provirus of cat cells, in *Proc. 8th Int. Symp. Comp. Leukemia Res.*, Bentvelzen, P., Hilgers, J., and Yohn, D. S., Eds., Elsvier-North Holand, New York, 1977, 139.
13. **Teich, N., Lowy, D. R., Hartley, J. W., and Rowe, W. P.**, Studies on the mechanism of induction of infectious murine leukemia virus from AKR mouse embryo cell lines by 5-iododeoxyuridine and 5-bromodeoxyuridine, *Virology*, 51, 163, 1973.
14. **Schwartz, S. A., Horio, D., and Kirsten, W. H.**, Non-random incorporation of 5-bromodeoxyuridine in rat cell DNA, *Biochem. Biophys. Res. Commun.*, 61, 927, 1974.
15. **Aaronson, S. A., Todaro, G. J., and Scolnick, E. N.**, Induction of murine C-type viruses from clonal lines of virus-free BALB/3T3 cells, *Science*, 174, 157, 1971.
16. **Klement, V., Nicolson, M. O., and Huebner, R. J.**, Rescue of the genome of focus forming virus from rat non-productive lines by 5-bromodeoxyuridine, *Nature (New Biol.)*, 234, 12, 1971.
17. **Rhim, J. S., Duh, F. G., Cho, H. Y., Elder, E., and Vernon, M. L.**, Brief communication: activation of a type-C RNA virus from tumors induced by rat kidney cells transformed by a chemical carcinogen, *J. Natl. Cancer Inst.*, 50, 155, 1973.
18. **Freeman, A. E., Price, P. J., Igel, H. J., Young, J. C., Maryak, J. M., and Huebner, R. J.**, Morphological transformation of rat embryo cells induced by diethylnitrosamine and murine leukemia viruses, *J. Natl. Cancer Inst.*, 44, 65, 1970.
19. **Decleve, A., Niwa, O., Gelmen, E. and Kaplan, H. S.**, Radiation activation of endogenous leukemia viruses in cell culture: acute X-irradiation, in *Biology of Radiation Carcinogenesis*, Yuhas, J. M., Tennant, R. W., and Regan, J. D., Eds., Raven Press, New York, 1976, 217.
20. **Varmus, H. E., Weiss, R. A., Friis, R. R., Levinson, W., and Bishop, J. M.**, Detection of avian tumor virus-specific nucleotide sequences in avian cell-DNAs, *Proc. Natl. Acad. Sci. U.S.A.*, 69, 20, 1972.
21. **Gelb, L. D., Milstein, J. B., Martin, M. A., and Aaronson, S. A.**, Characterization of murine leukemia virus-specific DNA present in normal mouse cells, *Nature (New Biol.)*, 244, 76, 1973.
22. **Rowe, W. P.**, Genetic factors in the natural history of murine leukemia virus infection: G.H.A. Clowes Memorial Lecture, *Cancer Res.*, 33, 3061, 1973.
23. **Benveniste, R. E., Lieber, M. M., Livingson, D. M., Sherr, C. J., Todaro, G. J., and Kalter, S. S.**, Infectious C-type virus isolated from a baboon placenta, *Nature (London)*, 248, 17, 1974.
24. **Chattopadhyay, S. K., Rowe, W. P., and Levine, A. S.**, Quantitative studies of integration of murine leukemia virus after exogenous infection, *Proc. Natl. Acad. Sci. U.S.A.*, 73, 4905, 1976.
25. **Varmus, H. E., Bishop, J. M., Nowinski, R. C., and Sarkar, N. H.**, Mammary tumor virus specific nucleotide sequences in mouse DNA, *Nature (New Biol.)* 9, 189, 1972.

26. **Huebner, R. J. and Todaro, G. J.**, Oncogenes of RNA tumor viruses as determinants of cancer, *Proc. Natl. Acad. Sci. U.S.A.*, 64, 1087, 1969.
27. **Temin, H. M.**, Nature of the provirus of Rous sarcoma, *Natl. Cancer Inst. Monogr.*, 17, 557, 1964.
28. **Temin, H. M.**, The participation of DNA in Rous sarcoma virus production, *Virology*, 23, 486, 1964.
29. **Temin, H. M. and Mizutani, S.**, RNA-dependent DNA polymerase in virions of Rous sarcoma virus, *Nature (London)*, 226, 1211, 1970.
30. **Baltimore, D.**, Viral RNA-dependent DNA polymerase, *Nature (London)*, 226, 1209, 1970.
31. **Temin, H. M.**, The protovirus hypothesis: speculations on the significance of RNA-directed DNA synthesis for normal development and for carcinogenesis, *J. Natl. Cancer Inst.*, 46, 3, 1971.
32. **Bauer, G.**, RNA-dependent DNA polymerase (reverse transcriptase), *Blut*, 35, 3, 1977.
33. **Nowinski, R. C., Old, L. J., Sarkar, N. H., and Moore, D. H.**, Common properties of the oncogenic RNA viruses (oncornaviruses), *Virology*, 42, 1152, 1970.
34. **Bernhard, W.**, The detection and study of tumor viruses with the electron microscope, *Cancer Res.*, 20, 712, 1960.
35. **Dalton, A. J., Melnick, J. L., Bauer, H., Beaudreau, G., Bentvelzen, P., Bolognesi, D., Gallo, R. C., Graffi, A., Haguenau, F., Heston, W., Huebner, R. J., Todaro, G. J., and Heine, U. I.**, The case for a family of reverse transcriptase viruses: Retroviridae. *Intervirology*, 4, 201, 1974.
36. **Temin, H. M.**, Mechanism of cell transformation by RNA tumor viruses, *Annu. Rev. Microbiol.*, 25, 609, 1971.
37. **Schidlovsky, G.**, Structure of RNA tumor viruses, in *Recent Advances in Cancer Research: Cell Biology Molecular Biology and Tumor Virology*, Vol. I, Gallo, R. C., Ed., CRC Press, Boca Raton, Fla., 1977, 189.
38. **Fine, D. and Schochetman, G.**, Type D primate retroviruses: a review, *Cancer Res.*, 38, 3123, 1978.
39. **Vogt, P. K.**, The genetics of RNA tumor viruses, in *Comprehensive Virology*, Fraenkel-Conrat, H. and Wagner, R., Eds., Plenum Press, New York, 1977, 341.
40. **Levinson, W., Bishop, J. M., Quintrell, N., Jackson, J.**, Presence of DNA in the Rous sarcoma virus, *Nature (London)*, 227, 1023, 1970.
41. **Duesberg, P. H. and Robinson, W. S.**, Nucleic acid and proteins isolated from Rauscher mouse leukemia virus, *Proc. Natl. Acad. Sci. U.S.A.*, 55, 219, 1966.
42. **Peters, G., Harada, F., Dahlberg, J. E., Panet, A., Haseltin, W. A., and Baltimore, D.**, Low molecular weight RNAs of Moloney murine leukemia virus: identification of the primer for RNA-directed DNA Synthesis, *J. Virol.*, 21, 1031, 1977.
43. **August, J. T., Bolognesi, D. P., Fleissner, E., Gilden, R. V., and Nowinski, R. C.**, A proposed nomenclature for the virion proteins of oncogenic RNA viruses, *Virology*, 60, 595, 1974.
44. **Bolognesi, D. P., Luftig, R., and Shaper, J. H.**, Localization of RNA tumor virus polypeptides. I. Isolation of further virus substructures, *Virology*, 56, 549, 1973.
45. **Ikeda, H., Hardy, W., Jr., Tress, E., and Fleissner, E.**, Chromatographic separation and antigenic analysis of proteins of the oncornaviruses. V. Identification of a new murine viral protein, p15(E), *J. Virol.*, 16, 53, 1975.
46. **Sarin, P. S. and Gallo, R. C.**, RNA directed DNA polymerases, in *Nucleic Acids, International Review of Science Series in Biochemistry*, Vol. VI Burton, K., Ed., Butterworth and Medical and Technical Publishing, Oxford, 1974, 219.
47. **Green, M. and Gerard, G. F.**, RNA — directed DNA polymerase — properties and functions in oncogenic RNA viruses and cells, *Prog. Nucl. Acid. Res. Mol. Biol.*, 14, 187, 1974.
48. **Sarngadharan, M. G., Allaudeen, H. S., and Gallo, R. C.**, Reverse transcriptase of RNA tumor viruses and animal cells, *Methods Cancer Res.*, 12, 3, 1976.
49. **Sarngadharan, M. G., Robert-Guroff, M., and Gallo, R. C.**, DNA polymerases of normal and neoplastic mammalian cells, *Biochim. Biophys. Acta*, 516, 419, 1978.
50. **Verma, I. M.**, The reverse transcriptase, *Biochim. Biophys. Acta*, 473, 1, 1977.
51. **Famulari, N. G., Buchhagen, D. L., Klenk, H. D., and Fleissner, E.**, Presence of murine leukemia virus envelope proteins gp70 and p15(E) in a common polyprotein of infected cells, *J. Virol.*, 20, 501, 1976.
52. **Arcement, L. J., Karshin, W. L., Naso, R. B., Jamjoom, G., and Arlinghaus, R. B.**, Biosynthesis of Rauscher leukemia viral proteins: presence of p30 and envelope p15 sequences in precursor polypeptides, *Virology*, 69, 763, 1976.
53. **Jamjoom, G. A., Nasu, R. B., and Arlinghaus, R. B.**, Further characterization of intracellular precursor polyproteins of Rauscher leukemia virus, *Virology*, 78, 11, 1977.
54. **Arcement, L. J., Karshin, W. L., Naso, R. B., and Arlinghaus, R. B.**, "gag" polyprotein precursors of Rauscher murine leukemia virus, *Virology*, 81, 284, 1977.
55. **Naso, R. B., Arcement, L. J., and Arlinghaus, R. B.**, Biosynthesis of Rauscher leukemia viral proteins, *Cell*, 4, 31, 1975.

56. Arlinghaus, R. B., Naso, R. B., Jamjoom, G. A., Arcement, L. J., and Karshin, W. L., Biosynthesis and processing of Rauscher leukemia viral precursor polyproteins, in *Animal Virology: ICN-UCLA Symposia on Molecular and Cellular Biology,* Vol. IV, Baltimore, D., Huang, A. S., and Fox, C. F., Eds., Academic Press, New York, 1976, 689.

57. Van Zaane, D., Gielkens, A. L. J., Dekker-Mecheslsen, M. J. A., and Bloemers, H. P. J., Virus-specific precursor polypeptides in cells infected with Rauscher leukemia virus, *Virology,* 67, 544, 1975.

58. Murphy, E. C., Jr., Kopchick, J. J., Watson, K. F., and Arlinghaus, R. B., Cell-free synthesis of a precursor polyprotein containing both *gag* and *pol* gene products by Rauscher murine leukemia virus 35S RNA, *Cell,* 13, 359, 1978.

59. Schultz, A. M. and Oroszlan, S., Murine leukemia virus *gag* polyproteins, The peptide chain unique to Pr80 is located at the amino terminus, *Virology,* 91, 481, 1978.

60. Murphy, E. C., Jr. and Arlinghaus, R. B., Tryptic peptide analyses of polypeptides generated by premature termination of cell-free protein synthesis allow a determination of the Rauscher leukemia virus *gag* gene order, *J. Virol.,* 28, 929, 1978.

61. Barbacid, M., Stephenson, J. R., and Aaronson, S. A., *Gag* gene of mammalian type-C RNA tumor viruses, *Nature (London),* 262, 554, 1976.

62. Reynolds, R. K. and Stephenson, J. R., Intracistronic mapping of the murine type C viral *gag* gene by use of conditional lethal replication mutants, *Virology,* 81, 328, 1977.

63. Gautsch, J. W., Elder, J. H., Schindler, J., Jensen, F. C., and Lerner, R. A., Structural markers on core protein p30 of murine leukemia virus: functional correlation with *Fv-1* tropism, *Proc. Natl. Acad. Sci. U.S.A.,* 75, 4170, 1978.

64. Albino, A., Korngold, L., and Mellors, R. C., Tryptic peptide analysis of *gag* gene proteins of endogenous mouse type C viruses, *J. Virol.,* 29, 102, 1979.

65. Waters, L. C., Transfer RNAs associated with the 70s RNA of AKR murine leukemia virus, *Biochem. Biophys. Res. Commun.,* 65, 1130, 1975.

66. Jamjoom, G. A., Karshin, W. L., and Naso, R. B., Proteins of Rauscher murine leukemia virus: resoltuion of a 70,000-dalton, nonglycosylated polypeptide containing p30 peptide sequences, *Virology,* 68, 135, 1975.

67. Kopchick, J. J., Jamjoom, G. A., Watson, K. F., and Arlinghaus, R. B., Biosynthesis of reverse transcriptase from Rauscher murine leukemia virus by synthesis and cleavage of a *gag-pol* read-through viral precursor polyprotein, *Proc. Natl. Acad. Sci. U.S.A.,* 75, 2016, 1978.

68. Naso, R. B., Arcement, L. J., Karshin, W. L., Jamjoom, G. A., and Arlinghaus, R. B., Fucose-deficient glycoprotein precursor to Rauscher leukemia virus gp69-71, *Proc. Natl. Acad. Sci. U.S.A.,* 73, 2325, 1976.

69. VanZaane, D. and Bloemers, H. P. J., Identification of Rauscher leukemia virus precursor polypeptides by chymotryptic peptide analysis, *Virology,* 75, 113, 1976.

70. Shapiro, S. Z., Strand, M., and August, J. T., High molecular weight precursor polypeptides to structural proteins of Rauscher murine leukemia virus, *J. Mol. Biol.,* 107, 459, 1976.

71. Pinter, A. and Fleissner, E., The presence of disulfide-linked gp70-p15(E) complexes in AKR murine leukemia viruses, *Virology,* 83, 417, 1977.

72. Witte, O. N., Tsukamoto-Adey, A., and Weissman, I. L., Cellular maturation of oncornavirus glycoproteins: topological arrangement of precursor and product forms in cellular membranes, *Virology,* 76, 539, 1977.

73. Henderson, L. E., Copeland, T. D., Smythers, G. W., Marquardt, H., and Oroszlan, S., Amino-terminal amino acid sequence and carboxyl-terminal analysis of Rauscher murine leukemia virus glycoproteins, *Virology,* 85, 319, 1978.

74. Ikeda, H., Hardy, W., Tress, E., and Fleissner, E., Chromatographic separation and antigenic analysis of proteins of the oncornaviruses. V. Identification of a new murine viral protein, p15(E), *J. Virol.,* 16, 53, 1975.

75. Ihle, J., Hanna, M., Schafer, W., Hunsmann, G., Bolognesi, D. P., and Huper, G., Polypeptides of mammalian oncornaviruses. III. Localization of p15 and reactivity with natural antibody, *Virology,* 63, 60, 1975.

76. Stehelin, D., Varmus, H. E., Bishop, J. M., and Vogt, P. K., DNA related to the transforming gene(s) of avian sarcoma viruses is present in normal avian cells, *Nature (London),* 260, 170, 1976.

77. Duesberg, P. H., Wang, L. H., Mellon, P., Mason, W. S., and Vogt, P. K., Towards a complete genetic map of Rous Sarcoma Virus, in *ICN-UCLA Symp. Molecular and Cellular Biology,* Vol. IV, Baltimore, D., Huang, A. S., and Fox, C. F., Eds., Academic Press, New York, 1976, 107.

78. Brugge, J. S. and Erikson, R. L., Identification of a transformation-specific antigen induced by an avian sarcoma virus, *Nature (London),* 269, 346, 1977.

79. Collett, M. S. and Erikson, R. L., Protein kinase activity associated with the avian sarcoma virus *src* gene prduct, *Proc. Natl. Acad. Sci. U.S.A.,* 75, 2021, 1978.

80. Purchio, A. F., Erikson, E., Brugge, J. S., and Erikson, R. L., Identification of a polypeptide encoded by the avian sarcoma virus *src* gene, *Proc. Natl. Acad. Sci. U.S.A.*, 76, 1979.

81. Oppermann, H., Levinson, A. D., Varmus, H. E., Levintow, L. and Bishop, M., Uninfected vertebrate cells contain a protein that is closely related to the product of the avian sarcoma transforming gene *(src)*, *Proc. Natl. Acad. Sci. U.S.A.*, 76, 1804, 1979.

82. Frankel, A. E. and Fischinger, P. J., Nucleotide sequences in mouse DNA and RNA specific for Moloney sarcoma virus, *Proc. Natl. Acad. Sci. U.S.A.*, 73, 3705, 1976.

83. Frankel, A. E. and Fischinger, P. J., Rate of divergence of cellular sequences homologous to segments of Moloney sarcoma virus, *J. Virol.*, 21, 153, 1977.

84. Frankel, A. E., Gilbert, J. H., and Fischinger, P. J., Effect of Helper virus on the number of murine sarcoma virus DNA copies in infected mammalian cells, *J. Virol.*, 23, 492, 1977.

85. Bondurant, M., Ramabhadran, R., Green, M., and Wold, W. S. M., "*Sarc*" sequence transcription in Moloney sarcoma virus transformed non-producer cell lines, *J. Virol.*, 29, 76, 1979.

86. Hartley, J. W., Wolford, N. K., Old, L. J., and Rowe, W. P., A new class of murine leukemia virus associated with development of spontaneous lympomas, *Proc. Natl. Acad. Sci. U.S.A.*, 74, 789, 1977.

87. Rapp, U. R. and Todaro, G. J., Generation of oncogenic Type-C viruses: Rapid leukemia viruses from C3H mouse cells derived *in vivo* and *in vitro*, *Proc. Natl. Acad. Sci. U.S.A.*, 75, 2468, 1978.

88. Elder, J. H., Gautsch, J. W., Jensen F. C., Lerner, R. A., Hartley, J. W., and Rowe, W. P., Biochemical evidence that MCF murine leukemia viruses are enveloped *(env)* gene recombinants, *Proc. Natl. Acad. Sci. U..A.*, 74, 4676, 1977.

89. Devare, S. G., Rapp, U. R., Todaro, G. J., and Stephenson, J. R., Acquisition of oncogenicity of endogenous mouse Type-C viruses: Effects of variations in *env* and *gag* genes, *J. Virol.*, 28, 457, 1978.

90. Rommelaere, J., Faller, D. V., and Hopkins, N., Characterization and mapping of RNase T-1 resistant oligonucleotides derived from the genomes of *Akv* and MCF murine leukemia viruses, *Proc. Natl. Acad. Sci. U.S.A.*, 75, 495, 1978.

91. Yeger, H., Kalnins, V. J., and Stephenson, J. R., Electron microscopy of mammalian Type-C RNA viruses: use of conditional lethal mutants in studies of virion maturation and assembly, *Virology*, 74, 459, 1976.

92. Yeger, H., Kalnins, V. J., and Stephenson, J. R., Type-C retrovirus maturation and assembly: post-translational cleavage of the *gag* coded precursor polypeptide occurs at the cell membrane, *Virology*, 89, 34, 1978.

93. Bolognesi, D. P., Montelaro, R. C., Sullivan, S. J., Frank, H., and Schafer, W., A model for assembly of Type-C oncornaviruses, *Med. Microbiol. Immunol.*, 164, 97, 1977.

94. Yoshinaka, Y. and Luftig, R. B., Murine leukemia virus morphogenesis: cleavage of p70 *in vitro* can be accompanied by a shift from a concentrically coiled internal strand ("immature") to a collapsed ("mature") form of the virus core, *Proc. Natl. Acad. Sci. U.S.A.*, 74, 3446, 1977.

95. Rowe, W. P. and Hartley, J. W., Studies of genetic transmission of murine leukemia virus by AKR mice. II. Crosses with *Fv-1ᵇ* strains of mice, *J. Exp. Med.*, 136, 1286, 1972.

96. Chattopadhyay, S. K., Lowy, D. R., Teich, N. M., Levine, A. S., and Rowe, W. P., Qualitative and quantitative studies of AKR type murine leukemia virus sequences in mouse DNA, *Cold Spring Harbor Symp. Quant. Biol.*, 39, 1805, 1974.

97. Chattopadhyay, S. K., Rowe, W. P., Teich, N. M., and Lowy, D. R., Definitive evidence that the murine C-Type virus inducing locus *Akv-1* is viral genetic material, *Proc. Natl. Acad. Sci. U.S.A.*, 72, 906, 1975.

98. Rowe, W. P., Hartley, J. W., and Bremner, T., Genetic mapping of a murine leukemia virus-inducing locus of AKR mice, *Science*, 178, 860, 1972.

99. Rowe, W. P., Studies of genetic transmission of murine leukemia virus by AKR mice. I. Crosses with *Fv-1ⁿ* strains of mice, *J. Exp.Med.*, 136, 1272, 1972.

100. Rommelaere, J., Faller, D. V., and Hopkins, N., RNase T1-resistant oligonucleotides of *Akv-1* and *Akv-2* Type-C of AKR mice, *J. Virol.*, 24, 690, 1970.

101. Ihle, J. N. and Joseph, D. R., Serological and virological analysis of NIH(NIH × AKR) mice: evidence for three AKR murine leukemia virus loci, *Virology*, 87, 287, 1978.

102. Ihle, J. N., Domotor, J. J., Jr., and Bengali, K. M., Strain-dependent development of an autogenous immune response in mice to endogenous C-Type viruses, *Bibl. Hematol.*, 43, 177, 1976.

103. Ihle, J. N. and Joseph, D. R., Genetic analysis of the endogenous C3H murine leukemia virus genome: evidence for one locus unlinked to the endogenous murine leukemia virus genome of C57BL/6 mice, *Virology*, 87, 298, 1978.

104. Kouri, R. E., Ratrie, H., and Whitmire, C. E., Genetic control of susceptibility to 3-methylcholanthrene-induced subcutaneous sarcomas, *Int. J. Cancer*, 13, 714, 1974.

105. Hilgers, J. and Galesloot, J., Genetic control of MuLV-gs expression in crosses between high and low leukemia incidence strains, Int. J. Cancer, 11, 780, 1973.

106. Taylor, B. A., Meier, H., and Myers, D. D., Host-gene control of C-Type RNA tumor virus expression and tumorigenesis: inheritance of the group-specific antigen(s) of murine leukemia virus, Proc. Natl. Acad. Sci. U.S.A., 68, 3190, 1971.

107. Aaronson, S. A. and Dunn, C. Y., High frequency C-Type virus induction by inhibitors of protein synthesis, Science, 183, 422, 1974.

108. Lowy, D. R., Rowe, W. P., Teich, N., and Hartley, J. W., Murine leukemia virus: high frequency activation in vitro by 5'-iododeoyuridine and 5'-bromodeoxyuridine, Science, 174, 155, 1971.

109. Stephenson, J. R. and Aaronson, S. A., Genetic factors influencing C-Type RNA virus induction, J. Exp. Med., 136, 175, 1972.

110. Stephenson, J. R. and Aaronson, S. A., A genetic locus for inducibility of C-Type virus in BALB/c cells: the effect of a non-linked regulatory gene on detection of virus after chemical activation, Proc. Natl. Acad. Sci. U.S.A., 69, 2798, 1972.

111. Robbins, K. C., Cabradilla, C. D., Stephenson, J. R., and Aaronson, S. A., Segregation of genetic information for a B-tropic leukemia virus with the structural locus for BALB: virus 1, Proc. Natl. Acad. Sci. U.S.A., 74, 2953, 1977.

112. Stephenson, J. R. and Aaronson, S. A., Segregation of loci for C-Type virus induction in strains of mice with high and low incidence of leukemia, Science, 180, 865, 1973.

113. Stephenson, J. R. and Aaronson, S. A., Demonstration of genetic factor influencing spontaneous release of a xenotropic virus of mouse cells, Proc. Natl. Acad. Sci. U.S.A., 71, 4925, 1974.

114. Levy, J. A., Joyner, J., Nayar, K., and Kouri, R. E., Genetics of xenotropic virus expression in mice. I. Evidence for a single locus regulating spontaneous production of infectious virus in crosses involving NZB/BlNJ and 129/J strains, J. Virol., in press.

115. Datta, S. K. and Schwartz, R. S., Genetics of expression of xenotropic virus and autoimmunity in NZB mice, Nature (London), 263, 412, 1976.

116. Datta, S. K. and Schwartz, R. S., Mendelian segregation of loci controlling xenotropic virus production in NZB crosses, Virology, 83, 449, 1977.

117. Levy, J. A., Xenotropic Type-C viruses, Curr. Top. Microbiol., Imunol., 79, 113, 1978.

118. Aaronson, S. A. and Stephenson, J. R., Independent segregation of loci for activations of biologically distinguishable RNA C-Type viruses in mouse cells, Proc. Natl. Acad. Sci. U.S.A., 70, 2055, 1973.

119. Kozak, C. and Rowe, W. P., Genetic mapping of xenotropic leukemia virus-inducing loci in two mouse strains, Science, 199, 1448, 1978.

120. Kalyanaraman, V. S., Sarngadharan, M. G., and Gallo, R. C., Characterizations of Rauscher murine leukemia virus envelope glycoprotein receptor in membranes from murine fibroblasts, J. Virol., 28, 688, 1978.

121. Gazdar, A. F., Oie, H., Lalley, P., Moss, W., Minna, J. D., and Francke, U., Identification of mouse chromosomes required for murine leukemia virus replication, Cell, 11, 949, 1977.

122. Ruddle, N. H., Conta, B. S., Leinwand, L., Kozak, C., Ruddle, F., Besmer, P., and Baltimore, D., Assignment of the receptor for ecotropic murine leukemia virus to mouse chromosome 5, J. Exp. Med., 148, 451, 1978.

123. DeLarco, J. E., Rapp, U. R., and Todaro, G. J., Cell surface receptors for ecotropic MuLV: detection and tissue distribution of free receptors in vitro, Int. J. Cancer, 21, 356, 1978.

124. Marshall, T. H. and Rapp, U. R., Genes controlling receptors for ecotropic and xenotropic Type C virus in Mus cervicolor and Mus musculus, J. Virol., 29, 501, 1979.

125. Gazdar, A. F., Russell, E. K., and Minna, J. D., Replication of mouse-tropic and xenotropic strains of murine leukemia virus in human × mouse hybrid cells, Proc. Natl. Acad. Sci. U.S.A., 71, 2642, 1974.

126. Besmer, P. and Baltimore, D., Mechanism of restriction of ecotropic and xenotropic murine leukemia viruses and formation of pseudotypes between the two viruses, J. Virol., 21, 965, 1977.

127. Lilly, F., Susceptibility in two strains of Friend leukemia virus in mice, Science, 155, 461, 1967.

128. Rowe, W. P. and Sato, H., Genetic mapping of the Fv-1 locus of the mouse, Science, 180, 640, 1973.

129. Rowe, W. P., Humphrey, J. B., and Lilly, F., A major genetic locus affecting resistance to infection with murine leukemia viruses. III. Assignment of the Fv-1 locus to linkage group VIII of the mouse, J. Exp. Med., 137, 850, 1973.

130. Klement, V., Rowe, W. P., Hartley, J. W., and Pugh, W. E., Mixed culture cytopathogenicity: a new test for growth of murine leukemia viruses in tissue culture, Proc. Natl. Acad. Sci. U.S.A., 63, 753, 1969.

131. Pincus, T., Hartley, J. W., and Rowe, W. P., A major genetic loci affecting resistance to infection with murine leukemia viruses. I. Tissue culture studies of naturally occurring viruses, J. Exp. Med., 133, 1219, 1971.

132. **Pincus, T., Rowe, W. P., and Lilly, F.**, A major genetic locus affecting resistance to infection with murine leukemia viruses. II. Apparent identity to a major locus described for resistance to Friend murine leukemia virus, *J. Exp. Med.*, 133, 1234, 1971.
133. **Steeves, R. and Lilly, F.**, Interactions between host and viral genomes in mouse leukemia, *Annu. Rev. Genet.*, 11, 277, 1977.
134. **Rein, A., Kashmiri, S. V. S., Bassin, R. H., Gerwin, B. I., and Duran-Troise, G.**, Phenotypic mixing between N- and B-tropic murine leukemia viruses: infectious particles with dual sensitivity to *Fv-1* restriction, *Cell*, 7, 373, 1976.
135. **Sveda, M. M., Fields, B. N., and Soeiro, R.**, Host restriction of Friend leukemia virus: fate of input virion RNA, *Cell*, 2, 271, 1974.
136. **Jolicoeur, P. and Baltimore, D.**, Effect of *Fv-1* gene on synthesis of N-Tropic and B-Tropic murine leukemia viral RNA, *Cell*, 7, 33, 1976.
137. **Jolicoeur, P. and Baltimore, D.**, Effect of *Fv-1* gene product on proviral DNA formation and integration in cells infected with murine leukemia viruses, *Proc. Natl. Acad. Sci. U.S.A.*, 73, 2236, 1976.
138. **Sveda, M. M. and Soeiro, R.**, Host restriction of Friend leukemia virus: synthesis and integration of the provirus, *Proc. Natl. Acad. Sci., U.S.A.*, 73, 2356, 1976.
139. **Tennant, R. W., Schluter, B., Yang, W. K., and Brown, A.**, Reciprocal inhibition of mouse leukemia infection by *Fv-1* allele cell extracts, *Proc. Natl. Acad. Sci. U.S.A.*, 71, 4241, 1974.
140. **Tennant, R. W., Schluter, B., Myer, F. V., Olten, J. A., Yang, W. K., and Brown, A.**, Genetic evidence for a product of the *Fv-1* locus that transfers resistance to mouse leukemia viruses, *J. Virol.*, 20, 589, 1976.
141. **Tennant, R. W., Myer, F. E., and McGrath, L.**, Effect of the *Fv-1* gene on leukemia virus in mouse cell heterokaryons, *Int. J. Cancer*, 14, 504, 1974.
142. **Lilly, F.**, Identification and location of a second gene governing the spleen focus response to Friend leukemia virus in mice, *J. Natl. Cancer Inst.*, 45, 163, 1970.
143. **Lilly, F.**, Mouse leukemia: a model of a multiple-gene disease, *J. Natl. Cancer Inst.*, 49, 927, 1972.
144. **Gisselbrecht, S. and Levy, J. P.**, The genetic control of leukemogenesis. II. Genetic systems involved in the control of leukemogenesis as they are detected *in vivo*, *Biomedicine*, 20, 170, 1974.
145. **Meredith, R. F. and Okunewich, J. P.**, Genetic influence in murine viral leukemogenesis, *Biomedicine*, 24, 374, 1976.
146. **Suzuki, S.**, *Fv-4*: A new gene affecting the splenomegaly induction by Friend Leukemia virus, *Jpn. J. Exp. Med.*, 45, 473, 1975.
147. **Kai, K., Ikeda, H., Yussa, Y., Suzuki, S., and Odalea, T.**, Mouse strain resistant to N-, B-, and NB-tropic murine leukemia viruses, *J. Virol.*, 20, 436, 1976.
148. **Odaka, T., Ikeda, H., Moriwaki, K., Matsuzawa, A., and Mizuno, M.**, Genetic resistance in Japanese wild mice (*Mus musculus molossinus*) to and NB-Tropic Friend murine virus, *J. Natl. Cancer Inst.*, 61, 1301, 1978.
149. **Yoshikura, H., Naito, Y., and Moriwaki, K.**, Unstable resistance of G mouse fibroblasts to ecotropic murine leukemia virus infection, *J. Virol.*, 29, 1078, 1979.
150. **Decleve, A., Niwa, O., Kojola, J., and Kaplan, H. S.**, New gene locus modifying susceptibility to certain B-tropic murine leukemia viruses, *Proc. Natl. Acad. Sci. U.S.A.*, 73, 2, 1976.
151. **Dent, P. B.**, Immunodepression by oncogenic viruses, *Prog. Med. Virol.*, 14, 1, 1972.
152. **Bennett, M. and Steeves, R. A.**, Immunocompetent cell functions in mice infected with Friend leukemia virus, *J. Natl. Cancer Inst.*, 44, 1107, 1970.
153. **Mortensen, R. F., Geglowski, W. S., and Friedmen, H.**, Leukemia virus-induced immunosuppression. X. Depression of T-cell mediated cytotoxicity after infection of mice with Friend leukemia virus, *J. Immunol.*, 112, 2077, 1974.
154. **Kumar, V., Goldschmidt, L., Eastcott, J. W., and Bennett, M.**, Mechanism of genetic resistance to Friend virus leukemia in mice. IV. Identification of a gene (*Fv-3*) regulating immunosuppression *in vitro* and its distinction from *Fv-2* and genes regulating marrow allograft reactivity, *J. Exp. Med.*, 147, 422, 1978.
155. **Kumar, V., Resnick, P., Eastcott, J. W., and Bennett, M.**, Mechanism of genetic resistance to Friend virus leukemia in mice. V. Relevance of *Fv-3* gene in the regulation of *in vivo* immunosuppression, *J. Natl. Cancer Inst.*, 61, 1117, 1978.
156. **Lilly, F., Boyse, E. A., and Old, L. J.**, Genetic basis of susceptibility to viral leukemogenesis, *Lancet*, 2, 1207, 1964.
157. **Lilly, F.**, The histocompatibility 2 locus and susceptibility to tumor induction, *Natl. Cancer Inst. Mongr.*, 22, 631, 1966.
158. **Lilly, F.**, The inheritance of susceptibility to the Gross leukemia virus, *Genetics*, 53, 529, 1966.
159. **Aoki, T., Boyse, E. A., and Old, L. J.**, Occurrence of natural antibody to the G (Gross) leukemia antigen in mice, *Cancer Res.*, 26, 1415, 1966.

160. Aoki, T., Boyse, E. A., and Old, L. J., Wild type Gross leukemia virus. II. Influence of immunogenetic factors on natural transmission and on the consequence of infection, *J. Natl. Cancer Inst.*, 41, 97, 1968.

161. Lilly, F., The influence of H-2 type on Gross virus leukemogenesis in mice, *Transplant. Proc.*, 3, 1239, 1971.

162. Risser, R., Potter, M., and Rowe, W. P., Abelson virus-induced lymphomagenesis in mice, *J. Exp. Med.*, 148, 714, 1978.

163. Freeman, A. E., Price, P. J., Zimmerman, E. M., Kelloff, G. J., and Huebner, R. J., RNA tumor virus genomes as determinants of chemically-induced transformation *in vitro*, *Bibl. Haematol (Basel)*, 39, 617, 1973.

164. Freeman, A. E., Price, P. J., Poryan, R. J., Gordon, R. J., Gilden, R. V., Kelloff, G. J., and Huebner, R. J., Transformation of rat and hamster embryo cells by extracts of city-smog., *Proc. Natl. Acad. Sci. U.S.A.*, 68, 445, 1971.

165. Freeman, A. E., Gilden, R. V., Vernon, M. L., Wolford, R. G., Hugunin, P. E., and Huebner, R. J., 5-Bromo-2′ deoxyuridine potentiation of transformation of rat embryo cells induced *in vitro* by 3-methylcholanthrene: induction of rat leukemia virus *gs* antigen in transformed cells, *Proc. Natl. Acad. Sci. U.S.A.*, 70, 2415, 1973.

166. Price, P. J., Freeman, A. E., Lane, W. T., and Huebner, R. J., Morphological transformation of rat embryo cells by the combined action of 3-methylcholanthrene and Rauscher-leukemia virus, *Nature (New Biol.)*, 230, 144, 1971.

167. Rhim, J. S., Vass, W., Cho, H. Y., and Huebner, R. J., Malignant transformation induced by 7,12, dimethylbenz(a)anthracene in rat embryo cells infected with Rauscher leukemia virus, *Int. J. Cancer*, 7, 65, 1971.

168. Price, P. J., Suk, W. A., Peters, R. L., Gilden, R. V., and Huebner, R. J., Chemical transformation of rat cells infected with xenotropic Type-C RNA virus and its suppression by virus-specific antiserum, *Proc. Natl. Acad Sci. U.S.A.*, 74, 579, 1977.

169. Lowy, D. R., Rowe, W. P., Teich, N., and Hartley, J. W., Murine leukemia virus: high frequency activation *in vitro* by 5′ iododeoxyuridine and 5′-bromodeoxyuridine, *Science*, 174, 155, 1971.

170. Reiman, H. M., Branum, E. L., and Moses, H. L., Effects of chemical carcinogens and C-Type RNA viruses on transformation of mouse embryo cells, *J. Cell Biol. Abstr.*, 67, 358, 1975.

171. Rhim, J. S., Creasy, B., and Huebner, R. J., Production of altered cell foci by 3-methylcholanthrene in mouse cells infected with AKR leukemia virus, *Proc. Natl. Acad. Sci. U.S.A.*, 68, 2212, 1971.

172. Rapp, U. R., Nowinski, R. C., Reznikoff, C. A., and Heidelberger, C., Endogenous oncornaviruses in chemically-induced transformation. I. Transformation independent of virus production, *Virology*, 65, 392, 1975.

173. Meier, H. and Myers, D. D., Chemical co-carcinogenesis: differential action of various compounds, derepression of endogenous C-type RNA genomes, and influence of different genotypes of mice, *Bibl. Haematol. (Basel)*, 39, 551, 1973.

174. Whitmire, C. E., Salerno, R. A., Rabstein, L. S., and Huebner, R. J., RNA tumor virus antigen expression in chemically-induced tumors — significance of specific chemical carcinogens to the C-Type RNA virogene and oncogene expressions, *Bibl. Haematol. (Basel)*, 39, 574, 1973.

175. Nowinski, R. C. and Miller, E. C., Endogenous oncornaviruses in chemically-induced transformation. II. Effect of virus production *in vivo*, *J. Natl. Cancer Inst.*, 57, 1347, 1976.

176. Nexo, B. A. and Ulrich, K., Activation of C-type virus during chemically-induced leukemogenesis in mice, *Cancer Res.*, 38, 729, 1978.

177. Nayar, K. T., Levy, J. A., and Kouri, R. E., Xenotropic virus expression and susceptibility to chemically-induced cancer, *Abstr. Ann. Meet. Am. Soc. Microbiol.*, 272, 1978.

178. Tonietti, G., Oldstone, M. B. A., and Dixon, F. J., The effect of induced chronic viral infections on the immunologic disease of New Zealand mice, *J Exp. Med.*, 132, 89, 1970.

179. East, J., Harvey, J. J., and Tilly, R. J., Transmission of auto-immune hemolytic anemia and murine leukemia virus in NZB-BALB/c hybrid mice, *Clin. Exp. Immunol.*, 24, 196, 1976.

180. Levy, J. A., Xenotropic viruses: murine leukemia viruses associated with NIH Swiss, NZB, and other mouse strains, *Science*, 182, 1151, 1973.

181. Levy, J. A. and Pincus, T., Demonstration of biological activity of a murine leukemia virus of New Zealand Black mice, *Science*, 170, 326, 1970.

182. Datta, S. K., Manny, N., Andrzejewski, C., Andre-Schwartz, J., and Schwartz, R. S., Genetic studies on autoimmunity and retrovirus expression in crosses of New Zealand Black mice, I. Xenotropic virus, *J. Exp. Med.*, 147, 854, 1978.

183. Datta, S. K., McConahey, P. J., Manny, N., Theofilopoulos, A. N., Dixon, F. J., and Schwartz, R. S., Genetic studies of autoimmunity and retrovirus expression in crosses of New Zealand Black mice. II. The viral envelope glycoprotein gp70, *J. Exp. Med.*, 147, 872, 1978.

184. Hehlmann, R., Kufe, D., and Spiegelman, S., RNA in human leukemia cells related to the RNA of a mouse leukemia virus, *Proc. Natl. Acad. Sci. U.S.A.,* 69, 435, 1972.

185. Hehlmann, R., Kufe, D., and Spiegelman, S., Viral-related RNA in Hodgin's disease and other human lymphomas, *Proc. Natl. Acad. Sci. U.S.A.,* 69, 1727, 1972.

186. Kufe, D., Hehlmann, R., and Spiegelman, S., Human sarcomas contain RNA related to the RNA of a mouse leukemia virus, *Science,* 175, 182, 1972.

187. Cuatico, W., Cho, R., and Spiegelman, S., Particles with RNA of high molecular weight and RNA-directed DNA polymerase in human brain tumors, *Proc. Natl. Acad. Sci. U.S.A.,* 70, 2789, 1973.

188. Sarngadharan, M. G., Sarin, P., Reitz, M., and Gallo, R. C., Reverse transcriptase activity of human acute leukemic cells: purification of the enzyme response to AMV 70S RNA, and characterization of the DNA product, *Nature (New Biol.)* 240, 67, 1972.

189. Gillespie, D., Use of molecular hybridization in detecting viral genetic information in DNA of human cancer cells, in *Recent Advances in Cancer Research: Cell Biology, Molecular Biology and Tumor Virology,* Vol. I, Gallo, R. C., Eds., CRC Press, Boca Raton, Fla., 1977, 139.

190. Gardner, M. B., Rasheed, S., Shimizu, S., Rongey, R. W., Henderson, B. E., McAllister, R. M., Klement, V., Charman, H. P., Gilden, R. V., Heberling, R. L., and Huebner, R. J., Search for RNA tumor virus in human, in *Origins of Human Cancer,* Book B., Hiatt, H. H., Watson, J. D., and Winsten, J. A., Eds., Cold Spring Harbor Laboratory, Cold Spring Harbor, N.Y., 1977, 1235.

191. Kalter, S. S., Helmke, R. J., Heberling, R. L., Panigel, M., Fowler, A. K., Strickland, J. E., and Hellman, A., C-Type particles in normal human placentas, *J. Natl. Cancer Inst.,* 50, 1081, 1973.

192. Schidlovsky, G. and Ahmed, M., C-type virus particles in placentas and fetal tissues of rhesus monkeys, *J. Natl. Cancer Inst.,* 51, 225, 1973.

193. Dalton, A. J., Hellman, A., Kalter, S. S., and Helmke, R. J., Ultrastructural comparison of placental virus with several Type-C oncogenic viruses, *J. Natl. Cancer Inst.,* 52, 1379, 1974.

194. Vernon, M. L., McMahon, J. M., and Hadgett, J. J., Additional evidence of Type-C particles in human placentas, *J. Natl. Cancer Inst.,* 52, 987, 1974.

195. Dirksen, E. R. and Levy, J. A., Type C virus-like particles in placentas from normal individuals and patients with lupus erythematosus, *J. Natl. Cancer Inst.,* 59, 1187, 1977.

196. Aulakh, G. and Gallo, R. C., Rauscher leukemia virus related sequences in human DNA: presence in some tissues of some patients with hematopoietic neoplasias and absence in DNA from other tissues, *Proc. Natl. Acad. Sci. U.S.A.,* 74, 3531, 1977.

197. Baxt, W. G. and Spiegelman, S., Human leukemic cells contain reverse transcriptase associated with a high molecular weight virus-related RNA, *Nature (New Biol.),* 244, 72, 1972.

198. Gallo, R. C., Gallagher, R. E., Miller, N. R., Mondal, H., Saxinger, W., Mayer, R. J., Smith, R. G., and Gillespie, D. H., Relationships between components in primate RNA tumor viruses and in the cytoplasm of human leukemic cells: implications to leukemogenesis, *Cold Spring Harbor Symp. Quant. Biol.,* 39, 933, 1974.

199. Gallagher, R. E., Todaro, G. J., Smith, R. G., Livingston, D. M., and Gallo, R. C., Relationship between reverse transcriptase from human acute leukemic blood cells and primate Type-C viruses, *Proc. Natl. Acad. Sci. U.S.A.,* 71, 1309, 1974.

200. Larsen, C. J., Marty, M., Hamelin, R., Peries, J., Boiron, M., and Tavitian, A., Search for nucleic acid sequences complementary to a murine oncornaviral genome in poly(A)-rich RNA of human leukemic cells, *Proc. Natl. Acad. Sci. U.S.A.,* 72, 4900, 1975.

201. Tavitian, A., Hamelin, R., Larsen, C. J., Marty, M., Peries, J., and Boiron, M., Characterization of the viral-type nucleotide sequences detected in the RNA of human leukemic cells by probes of murine and simian origins, *Bull. Cancer,* 65(1), 25, 1978.

202. Levy, J. A., Endogenous C-type viruses: double-agents in natural life processes, *Biomedicine,* 24, 84, 1976.

203. Levy, J. A., C-Type RNA viruses and autoimmune disease, in *Autoimmunity,* Talal, N., Ed., Academic Press, New York, 1977, 404.

204. Todaro, G. J., Evidence for the interspecies transmission of tumor virus genes, in *Recent Advances in Cancer Research: Cell Biology, Molecular Biology and Tumor Virology,* Vol. II, Gallo, R. C., Ed., CRC Press, Boca Raton, Fla., 1977, 51.

205. Benveniste, R. E. and Todaro, G. J., Evolution of C-Type viral genes: inheritance of exogenously acquired viral genes, *Nature (London),* 252, 456, 1974.

206. Scolnick, E. M., Rands, E., Williams, D., and Parks, W. P., Studies on the nucleic acid sequences of Kirsten sarcoma virus, *J. Virol.,* 12, 458, 1973.

207. Weiss, R. A., Mason, W. S., and Vogt, P. K., Genetic recombinants and heterozygotes derived from endogenous and exogenous avian RNA tumor viruses, *Virology,* 52, 535, 1973.

208. Todaro, G. J., Spontaneous release of Type-C viruses from clonal lines of "spontaneously" transformed BALB/3T3 cells, *Nature (New Biol.),* 240, 157, 1972.

209. Lieber, M. M. and Todaro, G. J., Spontaneous and induced production of endogenous Type-C RNA virus from a clonal line of spontaneously transformed BALB/3T3, *Int. J. Cancer,* 11, 616, 1973.

Chapter 5

TWO STAGE CARCINOGENESIS: POSSIBLE ROLE OF PROMOTERS

Sukdeb Mondal

TABLE OF CONTENTS

I. INTRODUCTION AND HISTORICAL BACKGROUND

The overall conclusion from modern epidemiology is that 90% of all human cancers are environmentally related.[1] Boyland[2] claims that this percentage is due to chemicals and attributes the remaining 10% of cancer incidence to genetic, viral, and radiation factors. Chemicals were first suggested in 1761, by John Hill, a British physician, to cause cancer.[3] He observed a high incidence of nasal polypus among snuff users, from which he suggested the possibility of snuff being the real cause of that ailment, or that it acted as an irritant to the parts that already had the "mischief" and hastened the process of polypus formation (promotion!). In 1775 another British surgeon, Percival Pott, associated soot as the cause for the high incidence of scrotal skin cancer among the chimney sweeps in London.[4] Long after that, in 1915, two Japanese investigators, Yamagiwa and Ichikawa, first demonstrated the production of cancer in rabbits ears by painting coal tar.[5] Thus, the foundation for chemical carcinogenesis research was laid. Since then, the list of cancer causing chemicals for humans is ever increasing.

It is now generally agreed that the carcinogenic process is usually a multistep one, and that various and diverse factors influence the likelihood that a normal cell exposed to a cancer causing agent will progress through the subsequent steps required for its transformation into a cancer cell and start a malignant tumor. In 1927 Deelman[6] reported that wounding mouse skin that had been pretreated with coal tar led to the appearance of tumors. In the experimental production of tumors in rabbit skin, it was often found that the induced papillomas tended to regress completely, but could be made to reappear at the identical sites by means of nonspecific stimuli, e.g., punching holes or by application of substances such as turpentine and chloroform.[7,8] Thus, by studying the role of wounding and irritation that resulted in stimulation of rapid cell division during the process of tumor formation, Rous and his co-workers[9] identified two stages in the formation of skin tumors in rabbits: (1) initiation — formation of "latent tumor cells" in the epidermis as a result of previous treatment with carcinogenic compound (tar), and (2) promotion — when those latent tumor cells would be revealed as tumors by subsequent treatment of the same area with a nonspecific stimuli, such as wounding or application of an irritant. These two stages depended on different kinds of stimuli, and Rous et al.[9] suggested, therefore, the involvement of two independent mechanisms. Thus the terms "Initiation" and "Promotion" in two stage carcinogenesis were coined by Rous and his co-workers. However, at present initiation does not mean the formation of "latent tumor cells", but rather causes an alteration of cells such that subsequent specific treatment transforms the initiated cells to dormant tumor cells. In 1941 Berenblum published his development of a two stage carcinogenesis regimen on mouse skin.[10] In his experiments he found that croton oil applied alternately with a subeffective dose of benzo[a]pyrene (BP) to mouse skin had a remarkable ability to cause tumors. Later Mottram[11] showed that BP needed to be applied only once in subeffective doses to initiate the process, so that subsequent multiple application of croton oil was able to elicit tumors. In recent years Berenblum et al.[12,13] have proposed that such a two stage process also occured in the production of mammary tumors and leukemias in female Wistar rats, and of liver and lung tumors in AKR mice. Peraino et al.[14] have also produced evidence that the chemical induction of rat hepatomas is a two stage process. Since the original work, many investigators have studied the two stage process of carcinogenesis, and the subject has been reviewed periodically.[15-21]

Rabbit and mouse skin, however, are not ideal tissues for the study of the cellular events that occur during initiation and promotion, because of the difficulty in obtaining a homogenous population of target cells. For the study of carcinogenesis in a well-controlled uniform environment, various quantitative systems for obtaining chemical carcinogenesis in cell culture have been developed, and important mechanistic information has been obtained. These have also provided systems with the potential for rapid and economical preliminary screening of chemical carcinogens. The subject has been reviewed by Heidelberger[22,23] and Casto and DiPaolo.[24] Lasne et al.[25,26] reported experiments suggesting a promoting effect of phorbol ester, 12-0-tetradecanoyl-phorbol-13-acetate (TPA) in the oncogenic transformation of rat embryo cells in culture initiated with BP. Sivak and van Duuren[27,28] and Sivak[29] demonstrated some effects of phorbol esters on cultured 3T3 cells suggesting tumor promoting action of TPA. Recently Mondal and his co-workers have definitely established the two stage carcinogenesis phenomenon in cultures of C3H/10T1/2 mouse embryo cells with polycyclic aromatic hydrocarbons,[30] UV radiation,[31] and X-irradiation[32] as initiating agents, and TPA as promoter. This system has now provided the unique opportunity of studying the mechanism of action of promoters as well as a potentially rapid and economical tool for the primary screening of environmental pollutants for their carcinogenic, initiating, and/or promoting activities.

II. SOME BIOLOGICAL ASPECTS OF INITIATION AND PROMOTION

All carcinogens are found to be initiators. Many of the carcinogens at sufficiently high doses are found to act both as initiator and promoter. Urethane is a unique compound in the sense that it is a complete carcinogen for lung and other tissues,[33,34,35] an initiator for mouse skin,[36,37] and a promoter in radiation leukemogenesis.[36] Noncarcinogens in general were found to have no initiating effect. The initiation is accompolished by subcarcinogenic concentrations of carcinogen, usually applied only once. In the C3H/10T1/2 cell culture system it was found that 0.1 μg/ml of 3-methylcholanthrene (MCA), BP, and 7, 12-Dimethylbenz[a]anthracene (DMBA) produced essentially no transformation of the cells, but when the same nontoxic concentration of TPA was added to the culture 5 days after the carcinogen treatment there was a high frequency of transformation.[30] By contrast, in cultures that received TPA 5 days after treatment with the three hydrocarbons at an effective transforming concentration of 0.25 μg/ml, there was no significant effect on the frequency of transformation. This showed, in analogy with the mouse skin model, that when the concentration of carcinogen is adequate by itself there was no need for promotion (Table 1). When ultraviolet (UV) light was used as initiator there was no transformation of cells at any dose from 10 to 200 ergs/mm^2. However, when the irradiated cells were cultured in medium containing 0.1 μg/ml of TPA, starting immediately after or 120 hr after the irradiation, a high frequency of transformation was produced (Table 2). In case of X-ray transformation it was found that when cells were exposed to minimally transforming doses (100 rd) followed by TPA treatment beginning either immediately or 96 hr afterwards, there was a marked increase in the transformation frequencies (see Reference 32).

We have seen if we treated the cells immediately after a subthreshold concentration of a chemical carcinogen that there was no transformation, but this was not true in the case of UV and X-ray initiation. The cause of this difference is still to be discovered. Cells need not show any morphological changes at initiation although some carcinogens such as β-propiolactone cause cytotoxicity and gross damage at initiating dose.[39] Whatever changes the initiator produces in the cells have been regarded as irreversible and long lasting. This has been tested in the two stage process of skin carcinogenesis by applying the promoting agents at varying intervals after the application of initiating treatment.[17,21,40-42] There was no significant diminution in tumor yield, in most cases, by lengthening the interval between initiation and promotion from

TABLE 1

Transformation of C3H/10T1/2 Cells Produced by Hydrocarbon and TPA Treatment

Treatment schedule	Plating efficiency (%)	Number of dishes with Type III foci/total number of dishes
0.5% acetone	20	0/89
0.5% acetone, 1 day; TPA (0.1)[a]	20	1/84
0.5% acetone, 5 days; TPA (0.1)	20	0/72
MCA (0.1)	19	1/89
MCA (0.1), 1 day; TPA (0.1)	20	1/49
MCA (0.1), 5 days; TPA (0.1)	20	11/40
MCA (0.25)	19	27/57
MCA (0.25), 1 day TPA (0.1)	19	3/19
MCA (0.25), 5 days TPA (0.1)	19	13/19
BP (0.1)	19	0/23
BP (0.1), 1 day TPA (0.1)	18	0/12
BP (0.1), 5 days TPA (0.1)	17	3/10
BP (0.25)	17	20/49
BP (0.25), 1 day; TPA (0.1)	16	6/20
BP (0.25), 5 days; TPA (0.1)	18	10/12
DMBA (0.1)	18	4/31
DMBA (0.1), 1 day, TPA (0.1)	17	1/18
DMBA (0.1), 5 days; TPA (0.1)	18	2/10
DMBA (0.25)	18	16/25
DMBA (0.25), 1 day; TPA (0.1)	19	5/22
DMBA (0.25), 5 days; TPA (0.1)	19	12/20
Anthracene (1.0)	16	0/11
Anthracene (1.0), 5 days; TPA (0.1)	19	0/10
Phenanthrene (1.0)	18	0/10
Phenanthrene (1.0), 5 days; TPA (0.1)	18	0/8
MCA-11, 12-oxide (1.0)	17	0/11
MCA-11,12-oxide (1.0), 5 days; TPA (0.1)	19	0/9

[a] Numbers in parenthesis, concentration (μg/mℓ).

7 to 112 days. The action of the initiator can also be additive in that very low doses of carcinogen can be applied repeatedly to have an additive effect. There is no evidence of a threshold dose below which the initiating effect is completely lost.[17] In this two stage process the promoting action operates only on initiated cells, because, i.e., if promoters are applied before the initiating agents there is no tumor production.[43,44] This is the essential characteristic of the promoters. Berenblum classifies a promoter as an incomplete carcinogen, since it is able to accomplish only one stage of the carcinogenic process.[45]

On the other hand, most complete chemical carcinogens at an optimal dose act both as initiator and promoter. Most carcinogens either generate or are converted metabolically to electrophilic reactants that bind covalently at the nucleophilic sites of cellular DNA, RNA, proteins, and other components. Binding with DNA may be the decisive

TABLE 2

Toxicity and % Dishes of C3H/10Tl/2 Cells with Transformed
Type 111 Foci at Doses of Light and Light + TPA

Treatment schedule	Plating effi- ciency %	Number of dishes with Type 111 foci/total num- ber of dishes
Acetone—0.5%	19	0/35
TPA (0.1 μg/ml)	20	0/36
10 ergsdimm²	19	0/24
+ TPA—0 hr	19	3/10
+ TPA—24 hr	19	2/11
+ TPA—48 hr	19	2/12
+ TPA—96 hr	19	4/12
+ TPA—120 hr	19	3/12
25 ergs/mm²	18	0/39
+ TPA—0 hr	18	6/36
+ TPA—24 hr	18	7/23
+ TPA—48 hr	18	13/24
+ TPA—76 hr	18	15/23
+ TPA—96 hr	18	14/22
+ TPA—120 hr	18	15/24
50 ergs/mm²	8	0/38
+ TPA—0 hr	8	1/11
+ TPA—24 hr	18	4/24
+ TPA—48 hr	8	8/12
+ TPA—72 hr	8	10/24
+ TPA—96 hr	8	7/12
+ TPA—120 hr	8	5/11
100 ergs/mm²	1	0/35
+ TPA—0 hr	1	1/10
+ TPA—24 hr	1	7/22
+ TPA—48 hr	1	6/15
+ TPA—72 hr	1	8/19
+ TPA—96 hr	1	3/12
+ TPA—120 hr	1	3/11
150 ergs/mm²	0.6	0/20
+ TPA—0 hr	0.6	2/10
+ TPA—24 hr	0.6	2/10
200 ergs/mm²	0.3	0/25
+ TPA—0 hr	0.3	0/12
+ TPA—24 hr	0.3	1/11

step in initiation, since most of the carcinogens or their activated forms are mutagenic, and since cancer is also considered to be a result of somatic mutation (to be discussed later). In contrast to one single treatment with initiators, promoters require multiple treatments for a prolonged period. Their action is reversible and not necessarily additive. Their effect is cumulative only when given in sufficient amounts at each application and not at too long intervals.[17,21] Promoters per se have no or little carcinogenic activity. Boutwell has divided the promotion phase into two separate stages.[17] He initiated the skin of mice with DMBA and followed by croton oil painting for 5 weeks and thereafter by painting with turpentine for another 5 weeks. In this case the tumor yield was significantly higher than when turpentine was painted first, after DMBA initiation followed by croton oil painting. Turpentine stimulates cell growth in mouse skin but has little promoting action. He interpreted these experiments that the first painting with croton oil converted the initiated cells to dormant tumor cells and then turpentine caused the dormant tumor cells to multiply and form the visible tumors. Thus Boutwell postulated that a promoter is capable of two functions: conversion of the initiated cells to dormant tumor cells (conversion) and propagation of the dormant tumor cells by cell division to visible tumor formation (propagation). In contrast to carcinogens the phorbol esters do not bind covalently with DNA and RNA. However, they bind at low level with proteins, but it is doubtful that this binding is essential for tumor promotion.[18] It appears that the total tumor incidence is determined by the potency of the initiating stimulus while the latent period depends on the efficiency and persistence of the action of the promoting agent. By proper manipulation of this latter phase the tumor incidence can be reduced or even abolished.[17,46,47]

In the early studies by Berenblum and co-workers, the promoting agent used in the mouse skin experiments was the irritant croton oil, a crude extract of the seeds of the plant *croteus tiglium*. E. Hecker in Germany isolated, characterized, and determined the structures of a number of phorbol diesters with specific fatty acid chains in particular positions in the phorbol molecule.[19,48] The most active derivative is TPA, now widely being used in various laboratories as a promoting agent. In addition to phorbol esters, there are many other chemicals that have been shown to possess significant promoting activity. Among them are certain detergents, e.g., Tween and Span,[49,50] iodoacetic acid and chloroacetophenone,[51] phenol,[52] anthranil (1,8,9-trihydroxyan-thracene),[53] n-dodecane,[54] canthridine,[55] some alkanes and 1-alkanols,[56] citrus oil,[57] Euphorbia lattices, the active constituent of which are related to those of croton oil,[58] and cigarette smoke condensates.[59-62] From the study of Hecker and his co-workers[63] it seems possible that many active principles of various plants all over the world have some promoting action. Of particular interest is recent epidemiologic evidence suggesting that the use of a tea made from *Croteus flavus* may be associated with a higher incidence of esophageal cancer in Curacao.[63] This should be considered seriously in future epidemiological studies of human cancer.

iII. ANALYSIS OF BIOLOGICAL AND BIOCHEMICAL EFFECTS — DNA, RNA, AND PROTEIN SYNTHESIS

The initiation phase of carcinogenesis, the first step in neoplastic transformation, is of very short duration and most probably involves changes in the genetic apparatus of the cells. The facts now available suggest that the initiation process does not cause the formation of cancer cells in dormant condition. None of the data so far available relates to the speed of initiation with chemical carcinogens, but if we consider X-ray and UV light as initiators,[31,32] it takes only seconds. In the case of chemical carcinogens it may take some hours.[16] Initiation may also result from incorporation of genetic material of viral nucleic acid into the host cell.[64] Furthermore, the irreversible nature of the initiation of skin carcinogenesis implies changes hereditably transmissible to daughter cells. A widely discussed concept is that carcinogenesis brings about an irreversible change in the hereditary nucleic acid (DNA) of the cell leading to its transformation into malignancy.[65]

It is possible to increase the initiating effect by pretreating the skin either with croton oil or any nonspecific skin irritant for one or two days before the initiating stimulus.[66,67] This pretreatment stimulated the cell division. This led to the belief that initiation takes place during a mitotic cycle. There is, however, no general agreement about the exact phase of the cell cycle when the initiation takes place. Working with synchronous cell·Marquardt[68] and Jones et al.[69,70] showed the maximum frequency of transformation by treating the cells at "S" phase, whereas Bertram and Heidelberger[71] found evidence that the G_1-S boundary was the phase for maximum transformation frequency with chemical carcinogens. Berenblum and Armuth[72] suggested the "M" phase as being the probable time for initiation. The cause of this difference is not known; each one of them used different chemical carcinogens, and it might be that different chemical carcinogens preferentially acted on different phases of growth.

All these suggest a possible interaction of the initiating agents with DNA of the cell resulting in a heritable defect in the genome compatible with the concept of a somatic mutation. Bruce Ames has shown a good correlation between mutagenic and carcinogenic activity with his test on a selected strain of *Salmonella*.[73] He concluded that carcinogenesis is a mutational process. The covalent binding of carcinogens to mouse skin DNA has been studied extensively by several groups of investigators.[74-76]

There seems to be a fairly good correlation between the amount bound to DNA and the carcinogenic activity of the hydrocarbons. In addition to the interaction with DNA, the active form of a carcinogen binds covalently with RNA, protein, and other components of the cell. Kuroki and Heidelberger[77] studied the binding of several polycyclic hydrocarbons to DNA, RNA, and total protein of transformable hamster embryo and prostate cells. The hydrocarbons were firmly bound to the DNA, RNA, and proteins of both cells; binding of DMBA was found highest to the nucleic acids but relatively low to proteins; BP was bound to proteins to the highest extent. The weakly carcinogenic dibenz[a,c]anthracene was bound to all constituents of the cells to a greater extent than its more carcinogenic isomer, dibenz[a,h]anthracene. There was much less (5 to 10 times) macromolecular binding in chemically and spontaneously transformed clones. With azo dyes and AAF, the covalent binding to proteins has been known for a long time.[78] Abell and Heidelberger[79] showed with polycyclic hydrocarbons that there was a direct relation between the covalent binding to a certain soluble protein fraction of mouse skin and their carcinogenic activity. Later on this h-protein was partially purified by Tasseron et al.,[80] and the binding of polycyclic hydrocarbons to this protein in cultured transformable but not transformed cells has been demonstrated in the same laboratory.[81]

From all these findings of carcinogen binding to DNA, RNA, and proteins of target cells, it is assumed that one or more of those interactions is responsible for the initiation of carcinogenesis. Now the question is, which of these interactions is most significant. Pitot and Heidelberger[82] postulated that the binding of a carcinogen to a specific protein (possibly a repressor) could give rise to a perpetuated change, based on the theory of Jacob and Monod for the genetic control of gene expression.s;8[3] The Millers showed the loss of a particular protein from the liver cells of rats fed with p-dimethylaminoazobenzene was associated with hepatocarcinogenesis.[84] But this was from continuous and longstanding feeding of the compound to the rats. This is more applicable to the promoting phase. The working hypothesis at present is that initiation results in the formation of a permanent and heritable change in the genetic structure of the cell and promotion causes the phenotypic expression of the changes as malignancy.

Promoting action is very slow, which accounts of the long latent period of tumor formation. It can be stopped or reversed by discontinuing the promoter treatment,[85] or by administration of anticarcinogenic agents.[86,87] Effects of promoters on cells have been studied for a long time. Epidermal hyperplasia has always been documented with the application of promoters,[18] thus one of the functions of promoters was considered to increase cell division as has been shown by many workers.[6,7,8,17,55] It is also true that many agents such as turpentine, acridine, castor oil, etc., which are skin irritants and cause hyperplasia of epidermal cells, are devoid of promoting action for mouse skin.[20,88] In the C3H/10T1/2 cell culture system, Mondal et al.[30] showed very clearly

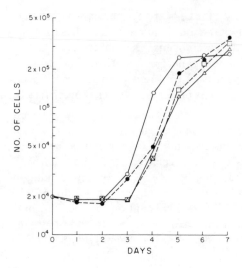

FIGURE 1. Growth of C3H/10T1/2 cells in
different media: 0, medium with 0.5% Acetone,
●, medium with 0.1 µg/m*l* of TPA; △, medium
with 0.1 µg/m*l* MCA; □, medium with 0.1 µg/
m*l* of MCA + 0.1 µg/m*l* of TPA.

that cellular multiplication was necessary for promotion; however, it needed some additional factors supplied by the promoting agent. In their experiment TPA was found not to increase saturation density; thus it did not alter the contact inhibition of the cells. If continuous cell division were the sole factor in promotion, in cell culture systems where multiplication of cells is obvious, promoting agents were not necessary or phase of promotion could not have been shown. In systemic promotion experiments, cellular hyperplasia has not been shown to be associated with promotion.[12-14]

From the hyperplastic effect of TPA on mouse epidermis it was logical to study DNA synthesis by the cells after TPA application. It was found in mouse skin that tumor promoters depressed the incorporation of tritiated thymidine into cellular DNA for the first 6 to 12 hr, but by 18 to 24 hr there was a strong stimulation (four to five fold) of incorporation.[89-93] In the work with C3H/10T1/2 cell cultures, Peterson et al.[93] showed that treatment during the log phase of growth with TPA, phorbol-12-13-didecanoate, and 4 α-phorbol-12-13-didecanoate caused an inhibition of (³H)TdR incorporation with the maximum at 12 hr after treatment. This resulted in a temporary delay of growth followed by a recovery of the normal cell doubling time. Because of this delay the treated cells reached confluency one day later than the control untreated cells whose DNA synthesis was at that time minimum. Therefore at that time the DNA synthesis in the treated cells was three to four fold higher than in the control (Figures 1 and 2). Thus there was no stimulation of DNA synthesis in the treated cells. They concluded[93] that inhibition of DNA synthesis is more related to promoting action, because phorbol, which was a nonpromoter in their system, did not have such an inhibitory action.

Bertsch and Marks[94] showed that tumor promoting phorbol esters did not stimulate DNA synthesis by epidermal cells of newborn mice. The responsiveness of epidermal DNA synthesis to the stimulatory effect of the above tumor promoting agents was age dependent. That may be the reason why Peterson et al.[93] did not find any stimulation of DNA synthesis by those agents using mouse embryo fibroblasts. Misrepair of the damage in the DNA caused by the carcinogens is presumed to be related to malignant

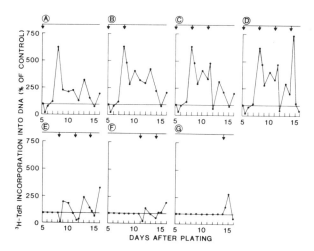

FIGURE 2. The effects of multiple treatments with 0.1 μg TPA/ml on ³H-TdR incorporation in C3H/10Tl/2 cells. 2000 cells were seeded in 60 mm plastic petri dishes, treated after 24 hr with 0.1 μg MCA/ml for 24 hr, and on 5, 8, 11 and 14 days with TPA as shown by the arrows. At 6 and 24 hr intervals after the cells received TPA, they were incubated for 30 min with ³H-TdR (2 μCi/ml, 2 Ci.mM), and the radioactivity in the cold acid precipitable material was determined by scintillation counting.

transformation of the cells.[95] Tumor promoters were found at very high doses to inhibit both semiconservative and repair DNA synthesis[96-99] and it was proposed that the inhibition of DNA repair was the general mechanism of action of promotion. There are some objections to this generalization. Promoters were found to be effective long (even a year) after carcinogen treatment, and it is difficult to believe that the DNA of the carcinogen treated cells remained damaged or unrepaired for such a long time. In C3H/10T1/2 cell cultures it was found also that promoters were effective after 10 days from carcinogen treatment, and moreover the concentration of TPA used in cell culture experiment was very much lower than that reported to inhibit DNA repair.[30] Krieg et al.[100] found that TPA is effective in disturbing the chalone mechanism which is thought to control cell multiplication in mouse epidermis. After treatment with TPA or phorbol dibenzoate, the inhibitory effect of pigskin extracts (which contain an epidermis-specific inhibitor of DNA synthesis — G_1 Chalone) was transiently diminished or completely abolished.

Marks and Relevian[101] suggested that epidermal chalone plus adrenalin exert their inhibiting action on cell mitosis by stimulating the epidermal adenylcyclase, which means that cyclic adenosine-3′,5′-monophosphate (cAMP) is the ultimate inhibitor of epidermal mitosis. The role of cAMP in controlling epidermal mitosis was also suggested by other workers;[102] Marks et al.[103] prevented completely the elevation of cAMP levels following adrenalin administration. Bellman and Troll inhibited the tumor promoting and mitogenic action of TPA in mouse skin by treatment with cAMP and theophyllin, and there was a marked decrease in cAMP levels in mouse skin after TPA treatment.[46] In cell culture the mitogenic effect of TPA on 3T3 cells was shown to be inhibited by dibutyryl cAMP.[104] Cyclic GMP level in 3T3 cells was found to have increased to about 25 times following TPA treatment, which is followed by increased ³H-TdR uptake and cell division.[105]

RNA synthesis was also found to be increased after treatment with tumor promoters in mouse epidermis[91,106-108] and also in cell culture.[109] Unlike the effect on DNA synthesis, there was no early inhibition in RNA synthesis, which increased over control 3 hr after croton oil application on mouse skin and was maximum 6 hr afterwards; by 6 days it had returned to normal. Looking at the species of RNA, Baird et al.[108] found that by 3 hr after treatment with effective tumor promoters, there was a large stimulation of incorporation of tritiated cytidine into 32S RNA, γRNA and 4 to 5 S RNA. The effect on 32S RNA was observed as early as 30 min after promoter application. In our laboratory[166] the increase in RNA synthesis was detected as early as 1 hr after treating C3H/10T1/2 mouse fibroblast cells with TPA. The increased synthesis was maintained up to 8 days. Phorbol, a nontumor promoter, had no such effect.

Protein synthesis was also found to increase in mouse epidermal cells following the application of croton oil or TPA.[91,106,110] The stimulus to protein synthesis was noticed 3 hr after promoter treatment, was maximum at 18 hr, and returned to normal by 6 days. Scribner and Boutwell reported induction of selective protein synthesis in mouse skin epidermis by TPA treatment.[111] By gel electrophoresis of mouse skin soluble proteins, they found near the top of the gels two bands that were lacking or only faintly present among the soluble proteins from untreated skin. Their appearance correlated with the tumor-promoting activity of three phorbol esters. The highly potent tumor promoter TPA binds with skin protein. Berenblum maintains that binding of the promoters with cellular protein is responsible for their promoting action.[112] A similar suggestion has also been put forward by Scribner and Boutwell.[111] These studies may suggest that the long continued binding of a protein with a promoter may lead to elimination of that protein from the cell. When genome (DNA) of the cell is damaged or changed by an initiating carcinogen, this protein loss would be irreversible leading to derepression of a particular gene responsible for uninhibited cell division, a characteristic of malignant transformation. The inflammation-producing compounds which produce hyperplasia of cells do not bind with skin protein.[111,113] Traut et al.[113] found that 4 α PDD, which was a nonpromoter in mouse skin, also bound with skin protein. It was a strange anomaly to them but in cell culture system Mondal et al.[30] found 4 α PDD was a weak promoter.

IV. POSSIBILITY OF GENE ACTIVATION AND GENETIC SUSCEPTIBILITY IN PROMOTION PHASE

The increase or decrease in protein synthesis by the cells following TPA treatment may bring about the altered enzyme levels in the cells, which has been associated for a long time with cancer.[114,115] The alteration in enzyme levels may be caused by the appearance of a new and unique protein or alteration in the concentration of preexisting enzymes. One of such enzymes is ornithine decarboxylase, a key enzyme in the biosynthesis of polyamines. The level of ornithinine decarboxylase in mouse skin is increased many fold 3 to 6 hr following treatment with TPA.[116] The same stimulatory effect was noticed after topical application of other tumor promoting phorbol esters, iodoacetic acid, anthralin, and tween 60. The hyperplastic agents, acetic acid, cantharidine, and ethylphenylpropiolate had little such effect. Such stimulatory effects were also noticed when 7,12-dimethylbenz[a]anthracene (DMBA) was applied in a completely carcinogenic dose but not with an initiating dose. Epidermal tumors produced by a two stage procedure showed consistently high levels of this enzyme. From these results, Boutwell and co-workers suggested that the induction of ornithine decarboxylase and subsequent accumulation of polyamines may be involved in tumor promotion. According to them, an initiated cell has a genetic or epigenetic change in the regulatory gene(s) controlling the level of ornithine decarboxylase resulting to maintain the very high enzyme levels reached after promoter treatment, while in normal cells only a transient spike of activity occurs; after a critical number of promoter applications, a permanently elevated level of this enzyme results leading to accumulation of polyamine, responsible for the selective growth advantage of the initiated cells. In a preliminary study with C3H/10T1/2 mouse embryo cell culture, in collaboration with Dr. Boutwell, we have also found that TPA increased the level of ornithine decarboxylase.[166]

Another enzyme which has been frequently associated with malignant transformation is a protease, plasminogen activator.[117-120] It has been shown that cells transformed by chemicals and viruses express a high level of plasminogen activator; but this was not found to be a universal association.[121-123] An interesting development in this aspect was the finding of Troll et al.,[124] who detected trypsin-like proteinase activity in the mouse ear as early as 30 min after topical application of TPA. To test the hypothesis that this proteinase activity was intimately associated with tumor promotion, a variety of proteinase inhibitors were applied to the mouse skin ear in conjunction with TPA. Those proteinase inhibitors (tosyl lysine chloromethyl ketone, tosyl phenylalanine chloromethyl ketone, tosyl arginine methyl ester) applied in small amounts with TPA after initiating the skin of the ear of mice with DMBA, suppressed tumor formation for 200 days and reduced the number of tumor-bearing mice to 50% of the control. This was also confirmed from another laboratory using the protease inhibitor, leupeptin, to inhibit the promoting action of croton oil.[125]

Sex hormones have been considered possible promoters in the malignant transformation of hormone target organs, such as uterus, breast, and prostate.[18,126] Troll et al. found the localization of trypsin-like protease in the nucleus and 12,000 g granules in the uterus following administration of sex hormones to the ovarectomized rats.[126] They suggested those proteins were synthesized in the cytosol, packaged in 12,000 g granules and transferred to the nucleus, where they caused the derepression of the genome by histone modification, permitting increased transcription. Cortical steroid hormones which protect the integrity of lysosomes, which were suggested to liberate protease by the lytic action of the promoters,[127] inhibit tumor promotion.[46,47]

In cell cultures, Wigler and Weinstein[128] demonstrated the induction of plasminogen activator in chick embryo fibroblasts, mouse cells, and HeLa cells by treatment with TPA and related compounds. Very low concentrations of TPA, 30 ng/mℓ, led to a marked induction of plasminogen activator which began within 3 hr and reached a maximum at about 24 hr in chick embryo fibroblasts. They found that TPA not only induced the synthesis of plasminogen activator in normal cells but it also markedly increased the synthesis of this protease in malignant cells. Actinomyin D completely blocked the induction, suggesting that RNA synthesis is required. The nontumor promoter, phorbol, did not induce the synthesis. Dexamethasone inhibited the production of plasminogen activator in certain tumor cell cultures[129] and in normal activated macrophages[130] as it did in in vivo experiments.[46] This may be another reason for glucocorticoid inhibition of tumor promotion as shown by Slaga and Scribner.[47] Testosterone or estradiol did not inhibit its production.[129] It was suggested that the glucocorticoid inhibition of plasminogen activator synthesis was not due to a direct inhibition of the transcription of plasminogen activator mRNA; rather it induces the synthesis, at the level of transcription, of a substance that inhibits the translation of plasminogen activator mRNA.[129]

Recently Levine and Hassid reported that two tumor promoting phorbol esters, TPA and phorbol-12,13-decanoate, at a very low concentration, stimulated prostaglandin production by dog kidney (MDCK) cells in culture. The nontumor promoting phorbol esters, at a dose higher than above, had no effect.[131] From the same laboratory it was shown that MDCK cells could be stimulated to produce prostaglandins by carcinogenic aromatic hydrocarbons and the potent carcinogen aflatoxin B_1, but not by noncarcinogenic compounds.[132] Anti-inflammatory glucocorticoids inhibited the serum-stimulated prostaglandin synthesis by methylcholanthrene-transformed mouse fibroblasts.[133] They suggested that inhibition of the phospolipase activation by the steroids affected the synthesis of a regulator for the phospholipase activity. Tumor promoters caused increased deacylation of the phospholipase, which may be one of the causes for the stimulation of prostaglandin synthesis.[131] TPA also stimulates increased phospholipid turnover, as measured by incorporation of choline[134] and ^{32}P[135] into phospholipids.

There are many reports suggesting that a TPA-membrane interaction could be the initial event in the mechanism of action of TPA. Demonstrable morphological and biochemical changes have been shown to be produced by tumor promoters. In chicken embryo fibroblasts (CEF) and mouse embryo fibroblast culture tumor promoting phorbol ester produced morphological changes[136,137] making the cells smaller and longer with extended processes. Weinstein et al. showed with CEF that TPA potentiates the changes in the cell surface glycopeptides characteristic of RSV transformed cells.[138] Cultures of normal CEF exposed to TPA, 30 ng/mℓ, for 18 hr synthesized more of the earlier eluting glucose-labeled glycopeptides than the control cultures. Blumberg et al.[139] reported that TPA at nM concentrations caused a striking decrease in LETS (large external transformation sensitive) protein in CEF. Similar changes were seen in CEF transformed by RSV. Transport of nutrients through the cell surface has been studied by measuring the 2-deoxy-D-glucose uptake by the cells exposed to tumor promoters[136,140] using CEF and C3H/10T1/2 mouse embryo cells. Both cell lines showed a concentration dependent deoxyglucose uptake; at lower concentrations the uptake of glucose by the cells was increased, at a concentration (0.1 μg/mℓ) used in promotion experiment in cell culture glucose uptake was inhibited.[140] It is known that chemically and virally transformed cells show a marked increase in the uptake of 2-deoxy-D-glucose compared to their nontransformed counterparts.[141,142] Lillehaug et al.[140] found, with 10T1/2 cells, that transformed cells in log phase had a lower glucose uptake than their normal counterpart. Mondal et al.[137] showed that TPA treated cells can grow in a medium with 1% fetal calf serum, as do the transformed cells, whereas, untreated normal cells could not grow at this serum concentration. All these experiments indicate that TPA induces a number of changes in the phenotype of normal cells, which tend to mimic those found in malignant cells. In other words it can be said that TPA induces a change in the program of gene expression of the normal cells mimicking the malignant cells.

Increased phosphorylation of histones, as well as a change in the rate of synthesis of individual histone fractions, have been associated with gene activation; a correlation between histone phosphorylation and DNA, and RNA synthesis was demonstrated by Ord and Stocken[143] in regenerating liver. It was postulated that the phosphorylation affects DNA-histone interaction, causing an increase in template activity and increased RNA and protein synthesis. Raineri et al.[144] found a positive correlation between the increased phosphorylation of histones, together with increased synthesis of certain histone fractions, caused by different phorbol esters and their tumor promoting activities in mouse skin. Their observance of two peaks of phosphorylation at roughly the same times as peaks in RNA and DNA synthesis lead them to suggest a gene activation to the phenomenon of promotion. Balmain et al.[145] found a similar increased phosphorylation of H1 and H2A histone of mouse epidermis following a low dose of TPA, and they considered increased phosphorylation to be directly related to the stimulation of DNA replication and mitotic activity, rather than to a gene activation phenomenon. H1 histone has been implicated with the maturation or differentiation of the cells.[146,147]

Balmain et al.[145] did not find any significant difference of histone fractions obtained from the epidermis at different times after treatment with TPA. The inhibition of differentiation was demonstrated by TPA treatment in cell cultures by several authors. TPA inhibited chicken embryo myoblasts undergoing myogenesis,[148] Friend erythroleukemia cells undergoing either spontaneous or induced erythroid differentiation,[149,150] and differentiations of 3T3 cells to lipocytes.[151] The mechanism by which TPA inhibits differentiation is not known. Yamasaki et al.[150] found an association between inhibition of differentiation of mouse erythroleukemic cells by TPA and a decrease in globin mRNA. This may reflect an altered transcription blocking the steps involved in terminal differentiation. This again points out the possibility of gene activation as mechanisms of action for the tumor promoters.

The pleiotypic response, i.e., the sequence of molecular events that occur when a more or less quiescent cell population is triggered to undergo cell division, is considered to be following the triggering of a mechanism located in the outer cell membrane.[152] The biochemical reactions such as synthesis of DNA, RNA, and protein, stimulation of phospholipid metabolism, alteration in membrane permeability, phosphorylation of nuclear protein, etc., seen after treatment of epidermis with phorbol esters, are also pleiotypic responses so it may be assumed that TPA acts on the cellular membrane for its tumor promoting activity and there are experiments in favor of it.[104,127,135,153-155] This led to the search of a receptor site for TPA, but so far it has not yet been found.

All cells do not act in the same way to a particular tumor promoter treatment. Susceptibility to the tumor promoting action of different agents varies from organ to organ and also from species to species. Phorbol, which is quite ineffective in skin, is a good promoter in liver, lung in AKR mice,[12] and for mammary carcinomas and leukemia in Wistar rats.[13] There might be some metabolic esterification of phorbol when used systemically for its promoting action. Shubik found that in rabbits, scarring (wound healing) was a good promoter but croton oil was not, while wound healing had no promoting activity in mice.[88] Croton oil was also found by the same author to be ineffective as a tumor promoter in rats and Guinea pigs for the production of skin tumor. In cell cultures of rat embryo fibro blasts, TPA was found to have a promoting effect.[25,26] Boutwell, by selective breeding, showed that it is possible to breed mice for susceptibility and resistance to two stage carcinogenesis.[17] Using same amounts of DMBA followed by the same number of croton oil treatment in two separate strains of mice which he developed by selective breeding, 100% of the susceptible strain developed tumors at an average of 12 tumors per mouse, whereas in resistant strains less than 20% of the animals at average of 0.24 tumors per animal developed tumors. Thus there is a genetic susceptibility for tumor promotion as is found in the induction of tumor by a chemical carcinogen (this is being dealt with in other chapters of this book).

One of the important causes behind the difference of susceptibility in chemical carcinogenesis is the presence or absence of some enzymes related to the metabolism of cancer producing agents as many chemical compounds need to be metabolically activated to form the ultimate carcinogen. In tumor promotion the most widely studied compound is TPA, which does not require metabolic activation for its action,[18] but this does not suggest that the other tumor promoters do not need to be metabolically activated for their action. TPA is metabolized by L cells and newborn mouse skin cells but not by HeLa cells.[156] Nobody knows whether TPA can act as a promoter in human cells; so far the results are negative in our laboratory,[166] although TPA has a growth stimulating property in human fibroblast cultures.[157] Segal et al. found a metabolite of phorbol myristate acetate in mouse skin.[158] Their preliminary results suggested that the metabolite, phorbolol myristate acetate, was approximately equivalent to its parent compound in its potency to induce mitosis and to enhance thymidine incorporation in the interfollicular epidermal basal cell layer. Sivak has shown that phorbolol myristate acetate had one fiftieth of the potency for the induction of cell division in stationary cultures of BALB/c-3T3 cells and in a mixed cell culture assay, which he devised for detection of tumor-promoting agents, it showed only a small fraction of the activity compared to the unmetabolized parent compound.[29] Metabolism of TPA may be related to some genetic factor, but its action may not be dependent on its metabolism; thus the difference of its promoting activity in different species may be related to the presence or absence of some receptor sites which is also genetically determined. Unfortunately no such receptor site has so far been identified.

V. DISCUSSION WITH PERSPECTIVES

The foregoing parts of this chapter may be considered as an overview rather than a complete review of the large number of experimental data emerging with ever increasing rapidity in the field of two stage chemical carcinogenesis. At the present moment we cannot differentiate between obligatory molecular changes and the broad spectrum of unrelated effects produced by carcinogens and promoters. We are currently at a loss to define the key molecular events produced by these agents. The most exciting and provocative theory of promotion is by gene activation, which has been supported by many experiments mentioned before. In many respects the action of promoters resembles that of hormones; they include the extremely low concentrations at which they are effective, pleiotropic effects that they induce in the exposed cells, and the variation in the details of the response manifest in different target cells. Many hormones act by gene activation, and it is quite tempting to explain the high frequency of cancer of hormone dependent organs by the promoting action of hormones through this pathway on some initiated cells that originated from the low exposure to some other carcinogen. Most of the work on the role of promoters in carcinogenesis has been done in mouse skin as the model system. From the work of Armuth and Berenblum,[12,13] of Peraino and others,[14] and from other epidemiological studies,[63,160] it is quite clear that promotion is an important factor in the course of development of many malignancies. From our work on cell culture models with different chemical and physical carcinogens as initiators[30,31,32] and that of Dr. Weinstein and his co-workers with oncogenic virus as initiator,[161] and TPA as promoter, it may be assumed that promotion could be a general phenomenon in the causation of cancer. Reports are now available that promoters also play a role as enhancing factors in the frequency of mutation.[159,160]

In the effective cancer control program, the value of the search for etiology of cancer is undisputed. As etiologic factors both carcinogens (initiators) and promoters may play equally important roles. Identification and elimination of these factors from the human environment form the key of the cancer prevention program. The knowledge of their chemical structure and physical characteristics may help us in better understanding their mechanism of action, which could lead to the formulation of a cancer cure. We need a rapid, inexpensive, and highly predictable assay system to screen the cancer related agents which include carcinogens, procarcinogens, co-carcinogens, promoters and other modifying agents. They are innumerable in numbers. It is prohibitably expensive and also in some respect impossible to test them on whole animals and follow those animals throughout the length of their life time. The recent developments in the field of malignant transformation in cell culture with chemicals, viruses, and also with two stage procedures is quite promising. Beside screening compounds rapidly and economically the cell culture systems provide the unique opportunity of studying the mechanism of carcinogenesis at the cellular and molecular levels at different stages, e.g., initiation and promotion.

In practical consideration, avoidance of carcinogenic (initiators) agents to reduce the incidence of cancer may not be altogether possible. In addition to large numbers of naturally occuring carcinogens (including sunlight), synthetic chemical carcinogens are daily being added to the environment in ever increasing numbers. Thus, one is led to the feeling that we are all immersed in an uncontrollable sea of carcinogens. If very low noncarcinogenic concentrations of a carcinogen can initiate the cells in the process of malignancy, then it may be presumed that each one of us has one or more initiated cells in our body. Then the determining factor for the development of cancer is the effects of promoters on those cells. Individual hormonal status and genetic background can act as a promoting or modifying factor. There are also many chemicals, seemingly harmless, which can act as promoters. Like carcinogens, they are also widely distributed in human environment; they may be in diet, drink, drugs, cosmetics, and also associated with personal habits, i.e., smoking, and drinking. Relation of nutrition to cancer has drawn attention of many investigators[162] and we believe that besides a specific carcinogenic role the diet plays a major role as a modifying factor in the development of cancer. Diet fat and tobacco smoke are known to have promoting effects.[163-165] It has been shown that tumor incidence can be reduced or even abolished by stopping the application of promoters or by modifying their action.[17,46,47] We know that personal lifestyle plays an important role in the development of cancer and it is possible for an individual to limit significantly his own risk by appropriately altering his lifestyle.

ACKNOWLEDGMENTS

I wish to express my sincere thanks to Professor Charles Heidelberger, Director of Basic Research, LAC/USC Cancer Research Center, Los Angeles, for his kind help in preparing the manuscript.

REFERENCES

1. **Higginson, J.**, Present trends in cancer epidemiology, *Proc. Can. Cancer Res. Conf.*, 8, 40, 1969.
2. **Boyland, E.**, The correlation of experimental carcinogenesis and cancer in man, *Prog. Exp. Tumor Res.*, 11, 222, 1967.
3. **Hill, J.**, Cautions Against the Immoderate Use of Snuff, etc., 2nd ed., R. Baldwin, London, 1971; **Redmond, D. E., Jr.**, Tobacco and cancer: the first clinical report, 1761, *N. Engl. J. Med.*, 282, 1823, 1970.
4. **Pott, P.**, in *Chirurgical Observation*, London, Hawkes, Clarke and Collins, 1775, 63.
5. **Yamagiwa, K. and Ichikawa, K.**, Experimentelle Studies uber die pathogenese der Epithelialgeschwulste, *Mitt. Med. Fak. K. Jpn. Univ.*, 15, 295, 1915.
6. **Deelman, H. T.**, The part played by injury and repair in the development of cancer, *Br. Med. J.*, 1, 872, 1927.
7. **Rous, P. and Kidd, J. G.**, Conditional neoplasms and subthreshold neoplastic states. A study of tar tumors in rabbits, *J. Exp. Med.*, 73, 365, 1941.
8. **MacKenzie, I. and Rous, P.**, The environmental disclosure of latent neoplastic changes in tarred skin, *J. Exp. Med.*, 73, 391, 1941.
9. **Friedwald, W. F. and Rous, P.**, The initiating and promoting elements in tumor production, *J. Exp. Med.*, 80, 101, 1944.

10. **Berenblum, I.**, The co-carcinogenic action of croton resin, *Cancer Res.,* 1, 44, 1941.
11. **Mottram, J. C.**, A developing factor in experimental blastogenesis, *J. Pathol. Bacteriol.,* 56, 181, 1944.
12. **Armuth, V. and Berenblum, I.**, Systemic promoting action of phorbol in liver and lung carcinogenesis in AKR mice, *Cancer Res.,* 32, 2259, 1972.
13. **Armuth, V. and Berenblum, I.**, Promotion of mammary carcinogenesis and leukemogenic action by phorbol in virgin female Wistar rats, *Cancer Res.,* 34, 2704, 1974.
14. **Peraino, C., Fry, R. J. M., Staffeldt, E., and Christopher, J. P.**, Comparative enhancing effects of phenobarbital, aminobarbital, diphenylhydantoin and dichlorodiphenyltrichloroethane on 2-Acetylaminofluorene-induced hepatic tumorigenesis in the rat, *Cancer Res.,* 35, 2884, 1975.
15. **Berenblum, I.**, A speculative review: the probable nature of promoting action and its significance in the understanding of the mechanism of carcinogenesis, *Cancer Res.,* 14, 471, 1954.
16. **Berenblum, I.**, *Sequential aspects of Chemical Carcinogenesis: Skin, Cancer,* Vol. 1, Becker, F. F., Ed., Plenum Press, New York, 1975, 323.
17. **Boutwell, R. K.**, Some biological aspects of skin carcinogenesis, *Prog. Exp. Tumor Res.,* 4, 207, 1964.
18. **Boutwell, R. K.**, The function and mechanism of promoters of carcinogenesis, *CRC Crit. Rev. Toxicol.,* 2, 419, 1974.
19. **Hecker, E.**, Isolation and characterisation of the co-carcinogenic principles from croton oil, *Methods in Cancer Research,* Vol. 6, Busch, H., Ed., Academic Press, New York, 1971, 439.
20. **Saffiotti, U. and Shubik, P.**, Studies on promoting action in skin carcinogenesis, *Nat. Cancer Inst. Monogr.,* 10, 489, 1963.
21. **Van Duuren, B. L.**, Tumor promoting agents in two-stage carcinogenesis, *Prog. Exp. Tumor Res.,* 11, 31, 1969.
22. **Heidelberger, C.**, Chemical oncogenesis in culture, *Adv. Cancer Res.,* 18, 317, 1974.
23. **Heidelberger, C.**, Chemical carcinogenesis, *Ann. Rev. Biochem.,* 44, 79, 1975.
24. **Casto, B. C. and DiPaolo, J. A.**, Virus, chemicals and cancer, *Prog. Med. Virol.,* 16, 1, 1973.
25. **Lasne, C., Gentil, A., and Chouroulinkov, I.**, Two stage malignant transformation of rat fibroblasts in tissue culture, *Nature,* 247, 490, 1974.
26. **Lasne, C., Gentil, A., and Chouroulinkov, I.**, Two stage carcinogenesis with rat embryo cells in tissue culture, *Br. J. Cancer,* 35, 722, 1977.
27. **Sivak, A. and Van Duuren, B. L.**, Phenotypic expression of transformation induction in cell culture by phorbol esters, *Science,* 157, 1443, 1967.
28. **Sivak, A. and Van Duuren, B. L.**, A cell culture system for the assessment of tumor promoting activity, *J. Nat. Cancer Inst.,* 44, 1091, 1970.
29. **Sivak, A.**, Comparison of the biological activity of the tumor promoter phorbol myristate acetate and a metabolite phorbolol myristate acetate in the cell culture, *Cancer Lett.,* 2, 285, 1977.
30. **Mondal, S., Brankow, D. W., and Heidelberger, C.**, Two-stage chemical oncogenesis in cultures of C3H/10T1/2 cells, *Cancer Res.,* 36, 2254, 1976.
31. **Mondal, S. and Heidelberger, C.**, Transformation of C3H/10T1/2 C18 mouse embryo fibroblasts by UV radiation and a phorbol ester, *Nature,* 260, 710, 1976.
32. **Kennedy, A., Mondal, S., Heidelberger, C., and Little, J. B.**, Enhancement of X-ray transformation of 12-0-Tetradecanoyl-phorbol-12-acetate in a cloned line of C_3H mouse embryo cells, *Cancer Res.,* 38, 439, 1978.
33. **Nettleship, A., Henshaw, P. S., and Meyer, H. L.**, Induction of pulmonary tumors in mice with ethylcarbamate (urethan), *J. Nat. Cancer Inst.,* 4, 309, 1943.
34. **Mirvish, S. S.**, The carcinogenic action and metabolism of urethan and N-hydroxyurethan, *Adv. Cancer Res.,* 11, 1, 1968.
35. **Tannenbaum, A. and Silverstone, H.**, Urethane (ethylcarbamate) as a multipotential carcinogen, *Cancer Res.,* 18, 1225, 1958.
36. **Salaman, M. H. and Roe, F. J. C.**, Incomplete carcinogens: ethyl carbamate (urethan) as an initiator of skin tumor formation in the mouse, *Br. J. Cancer,* 7, 472, 1953.
37. **Haran, N. and Berenblum, I.**, The induction of the initiating phase of carcinogenesis in the mouse by oral administration of urethan (ethylcarbamate), *Br. J. Cancer,* 10, 57, 1956.
38. **Berenblum, I. and Trainin, N.**, Possible two stage mechanism in experimental leukemogenesis, *Science,* 132, 40, 1960.
39. **Colburn, N. H. and Boutwell, R. K.**, The binding of β-propiolactone to mouse DNA in vivo; its correlation with tumor initiating activity, *Cancer Res.,* 26, 1701, 1966.
40. **Berenblum, I. and Shubik, P.**, The persistance of latent tumor cells induced in the mouse's skin by a single application of 9,10-dimethyl-1,2-benzanthracene, *Br. J. Cancer,* 3, 384, 1949.
41. **Roe, F. J. C. and Salaman, M. H.**, A quantitative study of the power and persistence of the tumor-initiating effect of ethyl carbamate (urethan) on mouse skin, *Br. J. Cancer,* 8, 666, 1954.

42. Salaman, M. J. and Gwynn, R. H., The histology of co-carcinogenesis in mouse skin, *Br. J. Cancer*, 5, 252, 1951.
43. Berenblum, I. and Haran, N., The significance of the sequence of initiating and promoting actions in the process of skin carcinogenesis in the mouse, *Br. J. Cancer*, 9, 268, 1955.
44. Roe, F. J. C., The effect of applying croton oil before a single application of 9,10-dimethyl-1,2-benzanthracene (DMBA), *Br. J. Cancer*, 13, 87, 1959.
45. Berenblum, I., A re-evaluation of the concepts of co-carcinogenesis, *Prog Exp. Tumor Res.*, 11, 21, 1969.
46. Bellman, S. and Troll, W., The effect of 12-0-tetradecanoyl-phorbol-13-acetate on cyclic AMP levels in mouse skin, *Proc. Am. Assoc. Cancer Res.*, 14, 21, 1973.
47. Slaga, T. J. and Scribner, J. D., Inhibition of tumor initiation and promotion by anti-inflammatory agents, *J. Nat. Cancer Inst.*, 51, 1723, 1973.
48. Hecker, E., Co-carcinogenic principles from the seed oil of croton tiglium and other euphorbiacae, *Cancer Res.*, 28, 2338, 1968.
49. Setälä, K., Progress in carcinogenesis, tumor enhancing factors: a bio-assay of skin tumor formation, *Prog. Exp. Tumor Res.*, 1, 225, 1960.
50. Setälä, K., Setala, H., and Holsti, P., A new physiochemically well-defined group of tumor promoting (co-carcinogenic) agents for mouse skin, *Science*, 120, 1075, 1954.
51. Gwynn, R. H. and Salaman, M. H., Studies on co-carcinogenesis: SH-reactors and other substances tested for co-carcinogenic action in mouse skin, *Br. J. Cancer*, 7, 482, 1953.
52. Rusch, H. P., Bosch, D., and Boutwell, R. K., The influence of irritants on mitotic activity and tumor formation in mouse epidermis, *Acta Unio Int. Contra Cancrum*, 11, 699, 1955.
53. Bock, F. C. and Burns, R., Tumor promoting properties of anthratriol (1,8,9-anthratriol), *J. Natl. Cancer Inst.*, 30, 393, 1963.
54. Saffiotti, U. and Shubik, P., The effects of low concentrations in epidermal carcinogenesis: a comparison with promoting agents, *J. Nat. Cancer Inst.*, 16, 961, 1956.
55. Hennings, H. and Boutwell, R. K., Studies on the mechanism of skin tumor promotion, *Cancer Res.*, 30, 312, 1970.
56. Sicé, J., Tumor promoting activity of n-alkalanes and l-alkanols, *Toxicol. Appl. Pharmacol.*, 9, 70, 1966.
57. Roe, F. J. C. and Peirce, W. E. H., Tumor promotion by citrus oil: tumors of the skin and urethral orifice in mice, *J. at. Cancer Inst.*, 24, 1389, 1960.
58. Roe, F. J. C. and Peirce, W. E. H., Tumor promotion by euphorbia lattices, *Cancer Res.*, 21, 338, 1961.
59. Gelhorn, A., The co-carcinogenic activity of cigarette tobacco tar, *Cancer Res.*, 18, 510, 1958.
60. Wynder, E. L. and Hoffman, D., A study of tobacco carcinogenesis. VIII. The role of acidic fractions as promoters, *Cancer*, 14, 1306, 1961.
61. Roe, F. J. C. and Walters, M. A., Some unsolved problems in lung cancer etiology, *Prog. Exp. Tumor Res.*, 6, 126, 1965.
62. Van Duuren, B. L., Sivak, A., Segal, A., Orris, L., and Langeseth, L., The tumor promoting agents of tobacco leaf and tobacco smoke condensate, *J. Nat. Cancer Inst.*, 37, 519, 1966.
63. National Cancer Institute Workshop on tumor promotion and cofactors in carcinogenesis, *Cancer Res.*, 37, 3461, 1977.
64. Luria, S. E., Viruses, cancer cells, and the genetic concept of virus infection, *Cancer Res.*, 20, 677, 1960.
65. Burnet, F. M., Cancer — a biological approach, *Br. Med. J.*, 1, 799, 841, 1957.
66. Pound, A. W. and Bell, J. R., The influence of croton oil stimulation on tumor initiation by urethan in mice, *Br. J. Cancer*, 16, 690, 1962.
67. Pound, A. W. and Withers, H. R., The influence of some irritant chemicals and scarification on tumor initiation by urethan in mice, *Br. J. Cancer*, 17, 460, 1963.
68. Marquardt, H., Cell cycle dependence of chemically induced malignant transformation *in vivo*, *Cancer Res.*, 34, 1612, 1974.
69. Jones, P. A., Benedict, W. F., Baker, M. S., Mondal, S., Rapp, U., and Heidelberger, C., Oncogenic transformation of C3H/10T1/2 Clone 8 mouse embryo cells by halogenated pyrimidine nucleosides, *Cancer Res.*, 36, 101, 1976.
70. Jones, P. A., Baker, M. S., Bertram, J. S., and Benedict, W. F., Cell cycle-specific oncogenic transformation of C3H/10T1/2 Clone 8 mouse embryo cells by 1-β-D-arabinofuranosylcytosine, *Cancer Res.*, 37, 2214, 1977.
71. Bertram, J. S. and Heidelberger, C., Cell cycle dependency of oncogenic transformation induced by N-methyl-N'-nitro-N-nitrosoguanidine in culture, *Cancer Res.*, 34, 526, 1974.
72. Berenblum, I. and Armuth, V., Effect of colchicine injection prior to the initiating phase of two-stage skin carcinogenesis in mice, *Br. J. Cancer*, 35, 615, 1977.

73. **Ames, B. N., Durston, W. E., Yamasaki, E., and Lee, F. D.,** Carcinogens are mutagens: a simple test system combining liver homogenates for activation and bacteria for detection, *Proc. Nat. Acad. Sci. U.S.A.,* 70, 2281, 1973.

74. **Brookes, P. and Lawley, P. D.,** Evidence for the binding of polynuclear aromatic hydrocarbons to nucleic acids of mouse skin. Relation between carcinogenic power and their binding to deoxyribonucleic acid, *Nature (London),* 202, 781, 1964.

75. **Goshman, L. M. and Heidelberger, C.,** Binding of tritium-labeled polycyclic hydrocarbons to DNA of mouse skin, *Cancer Res.,* 27, 1678, 1967.

76. **Brookes, P. and Heidelberger, C.,** Isolation and degradation of DNA from cells treated with tritium-labeled, 7,12-Dimethylbenz[a]anthracene: studies on the nature of the binding of the carcinogen to DNA, *Cancer Res.,* 29, 157, 1969.

77. **Kuroki, T. and Heidelberger, C.,** The binding of polycyclic aromatic hydrocarbons to the DNA, RNA and proteins of transformable cells in culture, *Cancer Res.,* 31, 2168, 1971.

78. **Miller, J. A.,** Carcinogenesis by chemicals: an overview — G. H. A. Clowes Memorial Lecture, *Cancer Res.,* 30, 559, 1970.

79. **Abell, C. W. and Heidelberger, C.,** Interaction of carcinogenic hydrocarbons with tissues. VIII. Binding of tritium-labeled hydrocarbons to the soluble proteins of mouse skin, *Cancer Res.,* 22, 931, 1962.

80. **Tasseron, J. G., Diringer, H., Frohwirth, N., Mirvish, S. S., and Heidelberger, C.,** Partial purification of soluble protein from mouse skin to which carcinogenic hydrocarbons are specifically bound, *Biochemistry,* 9, 1636, 1970.

81. **Kuroki, T. and Heidelberger, C.,** Determination of the h-protein in transformable and transformed cells in culture, *Biochemistry,* 11, 2116, 1972.

82. **Pitot, H. C. and Heidelberger, C.,** Metabolic regulatory circuits and carcinogenesis, *Cancer Res.,* 23, 1694, 1963.

83. **Jacob, F. and Monod, J.,** On the regulation of gene activity, Cold Spring Harbor, *Symp. Quant. Biol.,* 26, 193, 1961.

84. **Miller, E. C. and Miller, J. A.,** The presence and significance of bound aminoazodyes in the livers of rats fed p-dimethylaminoazobenzene, *Cancer Res.,* 7, 468, 1947.

85. **Berenblum, I. and Shubik, P.,** A new quantitative approach to the study of the stages of chemical carcinogenesis in the mouse skin, *Br. J. Cancer,* 1, 383, 1947.

86. **Berenblum, I.,** The anticarcinogenic action of dichlorodiethyl sulphide (mustard gas), *J. Pathol. Bacteriol.,* 34, 731, 1931.

87. **Van Duuren, B. L. and Melchionne, S.,** Inhibition of tumorigenesis, *Prog. Exp. Tumor Res.,* 12, 55, 1969.

88. **Shubik, P.,** Studies on the promoting phase in the stages of carcinogenesis in mice, rats, rabbits, and guinea pigs, *Cancer Res.,* 10, 13, 1950.

89. **Raick, A. N., Thummn, K., and Chivers, B. R.,** Early effects of 12-0-Tetradecanoyl-phorbol-13-acetate on the incorporation of tritiated precurosrs into DNA and the thickenss of the interfollicular epidermis and their relation to tumor promotion in mouse skin, *Cancer Res.,* 32, 1562, 1972.

90. **Paul, D. and Hecker, E.,** On the biochemical mechanism of tumorigenesis in mouse skin, *Z. Kresbsforsch.,* 73, 149, 1969.

91. **Baird, W. M., Sedgwick, J. A., and Boutwell, R. K.,** Effects of phorbol and four diesters of phorbol on the incorporation of tritiated precursors with DNA, RNA and protein in mouse epidermis, *Cancer Res.,* 31, 1434, 1971.

92. **Yuspa, S. H., Ben, T., Patterson, E., Michael, D., Elgio, K., and Hennings, H.,** Stimulated DNA synthesis in mouse epidermis cell cultures treated with 12-0-tetradecanoyl-phorbol-13-acetate, *Cancer Res.,* 36, 4062, 1976.

93. **Peterson, A. R., Mondal, S., Brankow, D. W., Thon, W., and Heidelberger, C.,** Effects of promoters on DNA synthesis in C3H/10T1/2 mouse fibroblasts, *Cancer Res.,* 37, 3223, 1977.

94. **Bertsch, S. and Marks, F.,** Lack of an effect of tumor-promoting phorbol esters and of epidermal, G_1 Chalone on DNA synthesis in the epidermis of newborn mice, *Cancer Res.,* 34, 3283, 1974.

95. **Cleaver, J. E.,** Defective repair replication of DNA in xeroderma pigmentosum, *Nature,* 218, 652, 1968.

96. **Guadin, D., Gregg, R. S., and Yielding, K. L.,** DNA repair inhibition: a possible mechanism of action of co-carcinogens, *Biochem. Biophys. Res. Commun.,* 45, 400, 1971.

97. **Gaudin, D., Gregg, R. S., and Yielding, K. L.,** Inhibition of DNA repair by co-carcinogens, *Biochem. Biophys. Res. Commun.,* 48, 945, 1972.

98. **Cleaver, J. E. and Painter, R. B.,** Absence of specificity in inhibition of DNA repair replication by DNA-binding agents, co-carcinogens and steroids in human cells, *Cancer Res.,* 35, 1773, 1975.

99. Poirier, M. C., Decicco, B. T., and Lieberanan, M. W., Nonspecific inhibition of DNA repair synthesis by tumor promoters in human diploid fibroblasts damaged with N-Acetoxy-2-acetylaminofluorene, *Cancer Res.*, 35, 1392, 1975.

100. Krieg, L., Kuhlmann, I., and Marks, F., Effect of tumor promoting phorbol esters and acetic acid on mechanisms controlling DNA synthesis and mitosis (chalones) and on the biosynthesis of histidine rich protein in mouse epidermis, *Cancer Res.*, 34, 3135, 1974.

101. Marks, F. and Rebien, W., Cyclic 3′-5′-AMP and theophylline inhibit epidermal mitosis in G_2 phase, *Naturwissenschaften*, 59, 41, 1972.

102. Voorhees, J. J., Duell, E. A., and Kelsey, W. H., Dibutryl cyclic AMP inhibition of epidermal cell division, *Arch. Dermatol.*, 105, 384, 1972.

103. Marks, F., Grimm, W., and Krieg, L., Distrubance by tumor promoters of epidermal growth control (Chalone mechanism), Hoppe-Seyler's, *Z. Physiol.Chem.*, 353, 1070, 1972.

104. Sivak, A., Cell membrane function and the control of cell division, in vitro, *Cancer Res.*, 8, 440, 1973.

105. Estensen, R. D., Hadden, J. W., Haddox, M. K., and Goldberg, N. D., Tumor Promoter (phorbol myristate acetate): Effects on Membrane Structure and Function in Mouse 3T3 Cells and Human Lymphocytes, Cold Spring Harbor Symp.: Control of Proliferation in Animal Cells, May 20-27, 1973.

106. Raick, A. N., Ultrastructural, histological, and biochemical alterations produced by 12-0-tetradecanoyl-phorbol-13-acetate on mouse epidermis, *Cancer Res.*, 33, 269, 1973.

107. Paul, D., Effects of carcinogenic agents on the biosynthesis of nucleic acids in mouse skin, *Cancer Res.*, 29, 1218, 1969.

108. Baird, W. M., Melera, P. W., and Boutwell, R. K., Acrylamide gel electrophoresis studies of the incorporation of cytidine-3H into mouse skin RNA at early times after treatment with phorbol esters, *Cancer Res.*, 32, 781, 1972.

109. Sivak, A. and Van Duuren, B. L., RNA synthesis in cell culture by a promoter, *Cancer Res.*, 30, 1203, 1970.

110. Hennings, H., Bowden, G. T., and Boutwell, R. K., The effect of croton oil pretreatment on skin tumor initiation in mice, *Cancer Res.*, 29, 1773, 1969.

111. Scribner, J. D. and Boutwell, R. K., Inflammation and tumor promotion, Selective protein induction in mouse skin by tumor promoters, *Eur. J. Cancer*, 8, 617, 1972.

112. Berenblum, I., The two stage mechanism of carcinogenesis in biochemical terms, in *The Physiopathology of Cancer*, Vol. 1, 3rd ed., S. Karger, Basel, 1974, 393.

113. Traut, M., Kriebich, G., and Hecker, E., Über die proteinbildung carcinogener kohlwasserstoffe und cocarcinogener phorbolester, in *Aktuelle Problem ausdem Gebiet der Cancerologie*, Vol. 3, Springer-Verlag, Berlin, 1971, 91.

114. Potter, V. R., Enzyme regulation in cancer cells, in *Proc. 10th Int. Cancer Cong.*, 1, 725, 1971.

115. Greenstein, J. P., *The Biochemistry of Cancer*, 2nd ed., Academic Press, New York, 1954.

116. O'Brien, T. G., Simsiman, R. C., and Boutwell, R. K., Induction of the polyamine-biosynthetic enzyme in mouse epidermis and their specificity for tumor promotion, *Cancer Res.*, 35, 2426, 1975.

117. Unkeless, J. C., Tobia, A., Ossowski, L., Quigley, J. P., Rifkin, D. B., and Reich, E., An enzymatic function associated with transformation of fibroblasts by oncogenic viruses. I. Chicken embryo fibroblast cultures transformed by avian RNA tumor viruses, *J. Exp. Med.*, 137, 85, 1973.

118. Pollack, R., Risser, R., Conlon, S., and Rifkin, D., Plasminogen activator production accompanies loss of anchorage regulation in transformation of primary rat embryo cells by SV40 virus, *Proc. Nat. Acad. Sci. U.S.A.*, 71, 4792, 1974.

119. Ossowski, L., Unkeless, J. C., Tobia, A., Quigley, J. P., Rifkin, D. B., and Reich, E., An enzymatic function associated with transformation of fibroblasts by oncogenic viruses. II. Mammalian fibroblast cultures transformed by DNA and RNA tumor viruses, *J. Exp. Med.*, 137, 112, 1973.

120. Jones, P., Benedict, W., Strickland, S., and Reich, E., Fibrin overlay methods for detection of a single transformed cell and colonies of transformed cells, *Cell*, 8, 323, 1975.

121. Mott, D. M., Fabisch, P. H., Sani, B. P., and Sorof, S., Lack of correlation between fibrinolysis and the transformed state of cultured mammalian cells, *Biochem. Biophys. Res. Commun.*, 61, 621, 1974.

122. Lang, W. E., Jones, P. A., and Benedict, W. F., Relationship between fibrinolysis of cultured cells and malignancy, *J. Nat. Cancer Inst.*, 54, 173, 1974.

123. Wolf, B. A. and Goldberg, A. R., Rous-sarcoma-virus-transformed fibroblasts having low levels of plasminogen activator, *Proc. Nat. Acad. Sci. U.S.A.*, 73, 3613, 1976.

124. Troll, W., Klassen, A., and Janoff, A., Tumorigenesis in mouse skin: inhibition by synthetic inhibitors of protease, *Science*, 169, 1211, 1970.

125. **Hozumi, M., Ogawa, M., Sugimura, T., Takeuchi, T., and Umezawa, H.,** Inhibition of tumorigenesis in mouse skin by leupeptin, a protease inhibitor from actinomycetes, *Cancer Res.,* 32, 1725, 1972.

126. **Troll, W., Rossman, T., Katz, J., Levitz, M., and Sugimura, T.,** Proteinase in tumor promotion and hormone action, in *Protease and Biological Control,* Vol. 2, Reich, E., Rifkin, D. B., and Shaw, E., Eds., Cold Spring Harbor, 1975, 977.

127. **Weissmann, G., Troll, W., Van Duuren, B. L., and Sessa, G.,** Studies on lysosomes X. Effects of tumor promoting agents upon biological and artificial membrane systems, *Biochem. Pharmacol.,* 17, 2421, 1968.

128. **Wigler, M. and Weinstein, I. B.,** Tumor promoter induced plasminogen activator, *Nature (London),* 259, 1232, 1976.

129. **Wigler, M., Ford, J. P., and Weinstein, I. B.,** Glucocorticoid inhibition of the fibrinolytic activity of tumor cells, *Proteases and Biological Control,* Reich, E., Rifkin, D. B., and Shaw, E., Eds., Cold Spring Harbor, 1975, 849.

130. **Vassalli, J. D., Hamilton, J., and Reich, E.,** Macrophage plasminogen activator: modulation of enzyme production by anti-inflammatory steroids, mitotic inhibitors and cyclic nucleotides, *Cell,* 8, 275, 1976.

131. **Levine, L. and Hassid, A.,** Effect of phorbol-12,13-diesters on prostaglandin production and phospholipase activity in canine kidney (MDCK) cells, *Biochem. Biophys. Res. Commun.,* in press.

132. **Levine, L.,** Chemical carcinogens stimulate canine kidney (MDCK) cells to produce prostaglandin, *Nature (London),* 268, 447, 1977.

133. **Tam, S., Hong Su-Chen, L., and Levine, L.,** Relationships among the steroids of anti-inflammatory properties and inhibition of prostaglandin production and arachidonic acid release by transformed mouse fibroblasts, *J. Pharmacol. Exp. Ther.,* 203, 162, 1977.

134. **Suss, R., Kinzel, V., and Kreibich, G.,** Co-carcinogenic croton oil factor A-1 stimulates lipid synthesis in cell cultures, *Experimentia,* 27, 46, 1971.

135. **Rohrschneider, L. R., O'Brien, D. H., and Boutwell, R. K.,** The stimulation of phospholipid metabolism in mouse skin following phorbol ester treatment, *Biochim. Biophys. Acta,* 280, 57, 1972.

136. **Driedger, P. E. and Blumberg, M.,** The effect of phorbol diesters on chicken embryo fibroblasts, *Cancer Res.,* 37, 3257, 1977.

137. **Mondal, S., Lillehaug, J. R., Boreiko, C., Brankow, D. W., and Heidelberger, C.,** Effects of a Tumor Promoting Phorbol Esters on the Morphology, Growth and 2-Deoxy-D-glucose Uptake of 10T1/2 Cells, Cold Spring Harbor Symp.'' Biologic Effects of Phorbol Esters in Cell Culture Systems'', 1978, in press.

138. **Weinstein, I. B., Wigler, M., and Pietrapaolo, C.,** The Action of Tumor Promoting Agents in Cell Culture, in Cold Spring Harbor Symp. Quant. Biol. on Origin of Human Cancer, 1977, in press.

139. **Weinstein, I. B., Wigler, M., and Pietrapaolo, C.,** The Action of Tumor Promoting Agents in Cell Culture, in Cold Spring Harbor Symp. Quant. Biol. on Origin of Human Cancer, 1977, in press.

140. **Lillehaug, J. R., Mondal, S., and Heidelberger, C.,** Effects of phorbol esters on 2-deoxy-D-glucose uptake by C3H/10T1/2 mouse embryo cells, *Proc. Am. Assoc. Cancer Res.,* p. 194, 1978.

141. **Kuroki, T. and Yamakawa, S.,** Kinetics of uptake of 2-deoxy-D-glucose and 2-amino isobutyric acid in chemically transformed cells, *Int. J. Cancer,* 13, 240, 1974.

142. **Siddiqi, M. and Iype, T.,** Studies on the uptake of 2-deoxy-D-glucose in normal and malignant rat epithelial liver cells in culture, *Int. J. Cancer,* 15, 773, 1975.

143. **Ord, M. G. and Stocken, L. A.,** Phosphate and thiol groups in histone f3 from rat liver and thymus nuclei, *Biochem. J.,* 102, 631, 1967.

144. **Raineri, R., Simsiman, R. C., and Boutwell, R. K.,** Stimulation of the phosphorylation of mouse epidermal histones by tumor promoting agents, *Cancer Res.,* 33, 134, 1973.

145. **Balmain, A., Alonso, A., and Fischers, J.,** Histone phosphorylation and synthesis of DNA and RNA during phases of proliferation and differentiation induced in mouse epidermis by tumor promoter 12-0-tetradecanoyl-phorbol-13-acetate, *Cancer Res.,* 37, 1548, 1977.

146. **Fambrough, D. M., Fujimura, F., and Bonner, J.,** Quantitative distribution of histone components in the pea plant, *Biochemistry,* 7, 575, 1968.

147. **Fukuyama, K., Seki, N., Nishita, K., and Epstein, W. L.,** Studies of Histone in Differentiated and Undifferentiated Epidermal Cells, Joint meeting, Society for Investigative Dermatology and European Society for Dermatological Research, Amsterdam, June 9 to 13, 1975, 16.

148. **Cohen, R., Pacifici, M., Rubinstein, N., Biehl, J., and Holtzer, H.,** Effect of tumor promoter on myogenesis, *Nature (London),* 266, 538, 1977.

149. **Rovera, G., O'Brien, T., and Diamond, L.,** Tumor promoters inibit spontaneous differentiation of murine erythrolukemia cells in culture, *Proc. Nat. Acad. Sci. U.S.A.,* 74, 2894, 1977.

150. Yamasaki, H., Fibach, E., Nudel, U., Weinstein, I. B., Rifkind, R., and Marks, P., Tumor promoters inhibit spontaneous and induced differentiation of murine erythroleukemia cells in culture, *Proc. Nat. Acad. Sci. U.S.A.*, 74, 3451, 1977.

151. Diamond, L., O'Brien, T., and Rovera, G., Inhibition of adipose conversion of 3T3 fibroblasts by tumor promoters, *Nature,* 269, 247, 1977.

152. Hershko, A. V., Mamont, P., Shields, R., and Tomkins, G. M., Pleiotypic response, *Nature, (New Biol.),* 232, 206, 1971.

153. Kreibich, G., Hecker, E., Süss, R., and Kinzel, V., Phorbol ester stimulates choline incorporation, *Naturwissenschaften,* 58, 323, 1971.

154. Kubinski, H., Strangstalien, M. A., Baird, W. M., and Boutwell, R. K., Interaction of phorbol esters with cellular membranes *in vitro, Cancer Res.,* 33, 3103, 1973.

155. Sivak, A., Induction of cell division: role of cell membrane sites, *J. Cell. Physiol.,* 80, 167, 1972.

156. Keibich, G., Süss, R., and Kinzel, V., On the biochemical mechanism of tumorigenesis in mouse skin. V. Studies of the metabolism of tumor promoting and non tumor promoting phorbol derivatives *in vivo* and *in vitro, Z. Krebsforsch.,* 81, 135, 1974.

157. Diamond, L., O'Brien, S., Donaldson, C., and Shimizu, Y., Growth stimulation of human diploid fibroblasts by the tumor promoter, 12-0-tetradecanoyl-phorbol-acetate, *Int. J. Cancer,* 13, 721, 1974.

158. Segal, A., Van Duuren, B. L., and Mate, U., The identification of phorbol myristate acetate as a new metabolite of phorbol myristate acetate in mouse skin, *Cancer Res.,* 35, 2154, 1975.

159. Trosko, J. E., Chang, C., Yotti, L. P., and Chu, E. Y. H., Effect of phorbol myristate acetate on the recovery of spontaneous and ultraviolet-light induced 6-thioguanine and ouabain-resistant Chinese hamster cells, *Cancer Res.,* 37, 188, 1977.

160. Laukas, G. R. Jr., Baxter, C. S., and Christian, R. T., Effects of tumor promoting agents on mutation frequencies in cultured V79 Chinese hamster cells, *Mutat. Res.,* 45, 153, 1977.

161. Fisher, P. B., Weinstein, I. B., Effenberg, D., and Ginsberg, H. S., Interaction between adinovirus, a tumor promotor, and chemical carcinogens in transformation of rat embryo cell culture, *Proc. Nat. Acad. Sci. U.S.A.,* 75, 2311, 1978.

162. American Cancer Society and National Cancer Institute (Sponsors), Symposium: nutrition in the causation of cancer, *Cancer Res.,* 35, 3231, 1975.

163. Toward a less harmful cigarette, *Nat. Cancer Inst. Monogr.,* p. 28, 1968.

164. Rusch, H. P., Kline, B. E., and Baumann, C. A., The influence of caloric restriction and of dietary fat on tumor formation with ultraviolet light, *Cancer Res.,* 5, 431, 1945.

165. Boutwell, R. K., Brush, M. K., and Rusch, H. P., The stimulating effect of dietary fat on carcinogenesis, *Cancer Res.,* 9, 741, 1949.

166. Mondal, S. et al., unpublished data.

Chapter 6

TUMOR IMMUNOLOGY AND CHEMICAL CARCINOGENESIS

Darwin O. Chee and Rishab K. Gupta

TABLE OF CONTENTS

* This study was supported in part by funds from the City of Hope National Medical Center, Duarte, California; grants 1-R26-CA22374-01A1, 1-R01-CA23047-01, CA12582 and CB64076PQ from the National Cancer Institute, National Institutes of Health, Bethesda, Maryland; Medical Services, Veterans Administration Hospital; California Institute for Cancer Research of the University of California, Los Angeles; and the Cancer Research Coordinating Committee.

I. INTRODUCTION

It has recently become apparent that there is a gradual increase in the incidence of cancer in man. The most likely explanation for this phenomenon is the increasing dependence of man on technology and its by-products as civilization evolves from a primitive to a more sohpisticated and complex form. The rapid progress of science and technology without the corresponding understanding of disposal of industrial wastes and the social and dietary habits of modern man expose him to a greater risk of contracting cancer. Today it is generally accepted that 70 to 90% of cancers in man are caused by environmental and societal factors, specifically chemicals[1] (see Chapter 1 for discussion). The great majority of these chemicals are not carcinogens per se, but are precarcinogens which must be activated by the body to proximate (ultimate) carcinogens which directly initiates the process of carcinogenesis[2] (see Chapter 2 for details).

It is debatable if the body has an homeostatic mechanism to destroy a cell or a small cluster of cells that have the rudiments of a neoplasm. Ehrlich conceived the immune system as a homeostatic surveillance system against nascent neoplasm and enunciated this hypothesis at the turn of the century.[3] But the collective evidence to support this thesis is untenable and at present, the immunological surveillance hypothesis is in a state of polemic.[4,5]

During the early 1900s investigators believed that tumors of experimental animals were rejected via tumor specific antigens. But it soon became obvious that the host rejected the tumor on the basis of histocompatibility antigens; for example, the H-2 system in mice and the HLA system in man. The era between the early 1900s and the early 1940s was a dark age for tumor immunology.

The advent of inbred (syngeneic) strains of laboratory animals, mostly through the endeavors of Snell,[6] reawakened a renaissance in tumor immunology. In the 1940s and 1950s investigators demonstrated the existence of tumor specific antigens on 3-methylcholanthrene-induced tumors.[7-9] But it remained for Prehn and Main in 1957 to perform the definitive and crucial experiment.[10]

These investigators demonstrated conclusively in syngeneic strains of mice that transplantable 3-methylcholanthrene-induced tumors possess tumor specific transplantation antigens (TSTA) and that these TSTA could evoke protective immunity in the host. Most important, they showed that the control skin graft from another member of the same inbred strains of mice in which the tumor was induced, was accepted. Subsequently, Klein and his collaborators demonstrated tumor immunity in the autochthonous host of 3-methylcholanthrene-induced mouse sarcoma and thereby excluded the possibility of residual heterozygosis.[11] These experiments in basic tumor immunology were major contributions because they implied that human cancer, if induced by chemical carcinogens, possibly could be prevented or effectively treated by a cancer vaccine.

II. IMMUNE RESPONSE

This section of the chapter focuses on the immune response of the host and its relationship to the tumor. The theme will be developed that oncogenesis disrupts the constancy of host's physiology and that the host in turn marshals one of its homeostatic mechanisms, the immune response, to counteract this instability by attempting to eradicate the tumor by interaction with the TSTA and return the *milieu interieur* of the host to its initial steady state. It must always be remembered, however, that central to the immune response and the eventual interactions of the products of the immune response, both cellular and humoral, are the TSTA of the tumor.

A. Ontogeny of the Immune System

The bone marrow is the hemopoietic organ in adults. It produces the precursor cell from which various blood and lymphoid cells are derived. In the chicken, bone marrow stem cells with pluripotential properties enter the circulation and migrate to either one of two lymphoid organs, the thymus or bursa of Fabricius. A population of bone marrow stem cells that sojourn to the thymus are destined to become T-lymphocytes under the maturing influence of the thymus. It is largely unknown at the present time the mechanism whereby the thymus converts pluripotential bone marrow stem-cells into T-lymphocytes. An important factor appears to be thymosin which is produced by the thymus.[12,13] It appears that the environment of the thymus in addition to thymosin and perhaps other thymic factors are responsible for causing differentiation of the immature bone marrow stem-cell to T-lymphocytes.

Bone marrow stem-cells that circulate to the bursa of Fabricius instead of the thymus, differentiate into B-lymphocytes under the influence of the bursa. Mature B-lymphocytes are called plasma cells. The bursal equivalent in mammals has not been discovered to date.

There is a dichotomy in function of the T- and B-lymphocytes. The T-lymphocytes are involved in protection against viral and mycobacterial infections, delayed hypersensitivity reactions, allograft and tumor rejections. The function of the B-lymphocytes is the production of antibodies for protection against microorganisms. B-cells generally require the cooperation of T-cells as "helper" cells to facilitate antibody production or as "suppressor" cells to inhibit antibody synthesis. Thus the dissociation between the T and B systems of lymphocytes is not absolute for cooperation occurs between the two types of lymphocyte population. The topic on compartmentalization and cooperation of T- and B-lymphocytes has been extensively reviewed.[14]

B. Immune Response to a Tumor

The immune response to a tumor can be compared to a reflex arc of the nervous system. As a tumor sheds its TSTA into the lymphatic and blood circulation system, the TSTA are transported (afferent arm) to the central component of the immune response where they are processed by lymphoid cells of the immune system. Amplification of T-cells specific for the TSTA occurs resulting in a subpopulation of T-cells that can specifically interact with the TSTA. Subpopulations of B-cells are also stimulated by the TSTA to divide, mature, and synthesize the various classes of antibodies specific for the TSTA. Both cellular (T-cells) and humoral (antibodies) factors are transported via the lymphatic/blood circulation system (efferent arm) to the target — the tumor. Depending on the relative balance between cellular and humoral factors, the strength of the immune response, and the antigenic strength of the TSTA on the tumor, the immunological factors may either destroy or enhance the growth of the tumor either by humoral factors (blocking factors) that nullify cellular immunity[15] or by cellular factors that stimulate tumor growth.[16]

A large body of evidence supports the proposition that allograft and tumor rejections are mediated by lymphoid cells and not by serum.[17-20] Transfer of tumor immunity from an immunized mouse to a nonimmunized mouse of the same syngeneic strain (adoptive transfer) was accomplished by lymphoid cells but not by serum.[18-23] Subsequent experiments with neonatally thymectomized mice and rats implicated that the T-lymphocytes were responsible for tumor destruction.[20,21] In addition, T-lymphocytes from immunized laboratory animals have been shown by in vitro assays to kill allogeneic target cells.[24-26]

C. Blocking Factors

In 1964, Moller demonstrated that inoculation with hyperimmune serum, containing antibodies specific for the TSTA of chemically induced mouse sarcomas could cause accelerated tumor growth in syngeneic animals.[27] However, serum blocking factors in an autochthonous system were first described by the Hellstroms in 1969. These investigators showed, by the colony inhibition assay, that the sera of mice bearing tumors, induced by the Moloney virus abrogated (blocked) cellular cytotoxicity.[15] This observation was corroborated by other laboratories by a variety of in vitro techniques in lower species and man.[28-30]

The exact nature of serum blocking factors is ill defined. Evidence exists that circulating free antigen[31,32] or circulating free antibody[15,27,33] could effectively abolish the effector function of sensitized lymphocytes. The product of the interaction of antigen and antibody, the antigen-antibody complex, has also been demonstrated to abrogate in vitro cell-mediated immunity.[33-36] Free antibody, presumably, blocks at the target level (tumor cells) by interacting with the TSTA on the tumor cells and thereby preventing sensitized T-lymphocytes from destroying the tumor cells. Free antigen blocks by binding to sensitized T-lymphocytes and inhibiting them to react with and destroy the tumor. Antigen-antibody complexes block when the antigen portion of an antigen-antibody complex interacts with the surface of sensitized lymphocytes having complementary steric configuration to the TSTA and neutralizes (blocks) the sensitized lymphocytes from interacting with the TSTA on the tumor cell. Antigen-antibody complex could also block sensitized lymphocytes from interacting with the tumor cells if the antibody portion of the complex attaches to the TSTA of the tumor cell. It can be envisaged that since antigen-antibody complex blocks both at the effector and target levels, it is perhaps a more potent blocker than either free antigen or antibody.

The postulated mechanism of enhancement of tumor growth is interference by circulating antigen, antibody or/and antigen-antibody complexes of T-lymphocytes to interact with the TSTA on the membranes of tumor cells. Since the sensitized T-lymphocytes are inhibited from interacting with the TSTA on the tumor to destroy the tumor, growth of the tumor is unrestricted (enhanced).

Experimental data have been consistent with the assumption that serum blocking factors play an important role in enhancement of tumor growth.[20] Therefore, serum blocking factors should be seriously considered as one of the escape mechanisms that thwart the host's immune system from destroying the tumor.

D. Immunogenetics

In the early part of this century, pioneers in transplantation immunology established that a genetic system in the mouse, designated the H-2 complex, controlled the expression of the major barrier to transplantation of foreign tissues (reviewed by Klein[37] and Snell[38]). These scientists demonstrated that the H-2 complex coded for the major histocompatibility antigens (H-2 antigens) and that differences of the H-2 antigens between donor and recipient resulted in the most rapid rejection of a graft.

The surprising discovery by McDeitt and Seal in 1965[39] that an immune response (Ir) gene in the mouse was autosomal dominant that controlled antibody production of a synthetic peptide antigen laid the foundation for modern immunogenetics. Subsequently, other Ir genes were found and shown to be closely linked to the major histocompatibility complex (MHC), that is, the H-2 complex in the mouse.[40,41] The exact location of these Ir genes was mapped to a new region, the I region of the H-2 complex between the K and S regions[42] of the 17th chromosome.[43] Similar MHC linked Ir genes that control immune responses were found in guinea pigs.[44] It is widely assumed that Ir genes in humans will map close to the HLA-D locus but definitive data are lacking.

Pertinent to this chapter were the studies by Lilly[45,46] which showed that susceptibility of mice to the Gross leukemia virus was genetically linked to the H-2 system. Resitance to leukemogenesis to the Gross virus was found to be dominant, and this gene, Rgv-1 (resistance to Gross virus-1),[45] was postulated to function as an Ir gene controlling the immune response to leukemia TSTA.[47] Recently, Meruelo et al.[48] provided the first data which suggested that the ability to recognize the TSTA and develop cell mediated immunity to an AKR tumor was genetically linked to and controlled by the H-2 system.

A significant association between the HLA system and an enormous variety of diseases including cancer has been found,[47,49] suggesting the involvement of Ir genes in malignancy. However, Ir genes have not been clearly defined in humans so the role of immunogenetics in human cancer awaits future research.

E. Immunosurveillance

The genesis, evolution, and progression of a tumor from a single cell to an overt malignant tissue requires several steps.[2,15] Selective pressures by homeostatic forces probably weed out many potential tumor cells from becoming blatant neoplasms. It is possible that the immune response plays a major role in preventing precancerous lesions from emerging into overt manifestations of clinical cancer. This idea was originally conceived by Ehrlich[3] and extended by Thomas[50] who suggested that the raison d' etre for the thymus-derived lymphocytes is the allograft (homograft) reaction. It was subsequently modified by Burnett[51] into the immunological surveillance theory and championed by Good and Finstad.[52] Implicit in the immunosurveillance hypothesis is that the homograft rejection is the price the species pays for its survival against neoplasia. Since the homograft rejection has an immunological basis[53] involving Ir genes[39,41] mapped in the H-2 complex of the mouse,[42] investigators have attempted to explain the immune surveillance hypothesis in immunogenetic terms by postulating that Ir genes control immunological resistance to nascent tumors.[54,55]

F. Immunostimulation

Contrary to the immunosurveillance hypothesis, Prehn and Lappe[16] have proposed that an immune reaction may stimulate rather than inhibit tumor growth. The immunostimulation hypothesis proposes that many tumors in their progression from inception to frank malignancy pass through a stage of lymphodependency. This occurs when a cluster of primary neoplastic cells reaches a critical mass and excites the lymphoreticular system to stimulate them to grow. The collective data support the immunostimulation hypothesis.[56] In addition, the immunostimulation hypothesis provides a unitarian hypothesis to explain some preplexing phenomena in immunobiology. These include the often observed intense lymphoid infiltration of early neoplasms,[57-59] the "sneaking through" phenomenon,[60,61] "enhancement" of tumor growth,[62] and "concomitant immunity."[63]

G. Measurements of Immune Response

1. In Vivo Assays

a. Inhibition of Tumor Growth

The classical procedure of assessing tumor immunity in syngeneic strains of laboratory animals is to induce a tumor by an oncogenic agent, such as a chemical carcinogen or oncogenic virus, excise the tumor and challenge the animal with varying dosages of the tumor cells 7 to 10 days postexcision of the tumor. Instead of allowing the animal to develop immunity to the tumor during tumor induction, an animal could be immunized directly with syngeneic tumor cells, followed 7 to 10 days by a challenge dose of varying numbers of tumor cells. The dose of tumor cells which fail to grow in the immunized animal is a measure of the amount of immunity the animal has engendered against the tumor.

In vivo tumor immunity in man was measured by Southam et al.[64] who injected varying numbers of autologous tumor cells in the arm of cancer patients and observed for inhibition of tumor growth. The largest number of tumor cells that failed to grow was a measure of tumor immunity. Moral and ethical reasons prohibit this type of assay to be performed routinely in humans.

b. Delayed Cutaneous Hypersensitivity Response

Challenge injection of an antigen into the skin of an individual who has been sensitized to the antigen results in an area of erythema, induration, and edema at the site of injection. These are the hallmarks of the delayed cutaneous hypersensitivity response. This skin reaction to an antigen has been widely accepted as a reflection of cell mediated immunity.

Instead of using live autologous tumor cells to assess the immune status of cancer patients, extracts of tumor cells prepared by a variety of procedures and presumably containing tumor-associated antigens (TAA) have been used as skin test antigens. Since the cancer patient has been exposed to his own tumor and thus has been sensitized to the TAA, delayed cutaneous hypersensitivity response to TAA in the tumor extract would constitute an anamnestic response and the TAA in the tumor extract is designated a recall antigen. Several microbial antigens listed in Table 1 also have been used as recall antigens in skin testing cancer patients to evaluate their immune status.

Primary immune capacity of cancer patients has been evaluated by sensitizing them with a neoantigen such as 2, 4-dinitrochlorobenzene or keyhole limpet hemocyanin (Table 1) then skin testing them with a challenge dose of the neoantigen.

2. In Vitro Assays

The definitive transplantation techniques used in basic tumor immunology in syn-

TABLE 1

Antigens Used for Skin Testing

Neoantigens	Dinitrochlorobenzene (DNCB)
	Keyhole limpet hemocyanin (KLH)
Recall antigens:	Monilia
	Mumps
	Pure protein derivative (PPD)
	Trichophyton
	Varidase (Streptokinase-streptodor-nase)
Tumor extracts:	Preparations by a variety of techniques

geneic strain of laboratory animals are forbidden in the study of tumor immunology in man. While in vivo assays employing tumor autographs[64] and skin test antigens for delayed cutaneous hypersensitivity response have been used to measure the immune parameters of cancer patients[65] and to search for TSTA on human tumors,[66] most investigations in human tumor immunology have been conducted with in vitro assay. Several ingenious in vitro assays have been developed to investigate the immunology of neoplasia in lower species and man.

The ultimate goal of the cancer immunologist is to understand the immune response in the host-tumor relationship so that a rational approach to immunotherapy can be achieved. But before such a goal can be attained, it is imperative to establish unequivocally that human tumors possess TSTA and that the cancer patient can develop effective immunity to his tumor engendered by the TSTA.

a. Cellular Assays

In vitro cellular assays were developed under the rationale that cell mediated immunity is the *modus operandi* by which a host rejects its tumor. Some of the most widely used in vitro cellular assays are listed in Table 2.

Lymphocytotoxicity — The lymphocytotoxicity assay is based on the assumption that lymphocytes from cancer patients are sensitized to the antigens of the tumor harbored by the cancer patient and in a vis-a-vis confrontation of patients' lymphocytes and tumor target cells in vitro the lymphocytes will destroy the tumor cells.

Lymphoblastogenesis — When lymphocytes are exposed to an antigen or mitogen in vitro, they are stimulated to undergo blastogenesis and can incorporate analogues of DNA nucleotides such as tritiated thymidine. This is the principle of the lymphoblastogenesis assay. It measures the proliferative capacity of lymphocytes. Allogeneic lympyocytes or autologous intact tumor cells ("stimulator" cells) also have been employed to trigger blastogenesis of cancer patients' lymphocytes ("responder" cells).

Leukocyte migration inhibition assay — Exposure of sensitized lymphocytes to an antigen stimulates them to synthesize and release soluble substances (lymphokines). One of these lymphokines, macrophage/leukocyte migration inhibition factor, inhibits macrophages (monocytes) or polymorphonuclear (PMN) leukocytes to migrate on glass or plastic surfaces. This is the princple of the leukocyte migration inhibition (LMI) test.

Leukocyte adherence inhibition assay — One disadvantage of the leukocyte migration inhibition assay is that it required 18 to 24 hr for optimum incubation time. For this reason, Halliday and Miller[94] devised the leukocyte adherence inhibition assay which entailed only 1 hr incubation period. Two explanations have been proposed for

TABLE 2

In Vitro Cellular Assays Used for Measurement of Immune Response to Tumors
and/or Detection of Tumor Associated Antigens

Assay	Application	Ref.
Lymphocytotoxicity	Different histologic types of solid neoplasms, and leukemia in lower species and man	67—72
Lymphoblastogenesis	Leukemia, Burkitt's lymphoma sarcoma and melanoma in man	73—81
Leukocyte migration inhibition	Animal tumors, melanoma, carcinomas in man	82—93
Leukocyte adherence inhibition	Animal tumors, melanoma and carcinomas in man	94—104
Antibody dependent cellular cytotoxicity	Animal tumors, various histologic types of cancer in man	105—117

the mechanism of the leukocyte adherence inhibition. Halliday and his associates[94,103] suggested that lymphokines released by respondent lymphocytes, upon interaction with antigen inhibit the adherence of indicator PMN leukocytes implying that two cell types are involved in the leukocyte adherence inhibition (LAI) assay. Holan et al.[96] and Grosser et al.[104] provided evidence that peripheral blood monocytes reacted directly with antigen and lost its property of adherence to glass.

Antibody-dependent cellular cytotoxicity assay — The antibody-dependent cellular cytotoxicity (ADCC) assay was first described by Moller in 1965 whereby nonimmune lymphoid cells destroyed murine 3-methylcholanthrene induced tumor cells in vitro.[105] Through the work of Perlmann et al.[106] and MacLennan's group[107] the mechanism of antibody-dependent cellular cytotoxicity has been elucidated. A non-T-lymphocyte[108] has been shown to be cytotoxic for target cells only if this lymphocyte termed K (Killer) or N (Null) cell lacking both T- and B-cell properties[109] is "armed" by antibody predominantly, if not, exclusively of the IgG class.[110] The K-cell is nonimmune but has the receptor for the Fc portion of the IgG antibody molecule.[111] Cytolysis of target cells by antibody-dependent cellular cytotoxicity does not require complement. In vitro target cells destruction by nonimmune K-cells in concert with humoral antibody have recently been found in human systems.[112,113] The antibody-dependent cellular cytotoxicity assay has been applied in both experimental animal models[114,115] and in studies in human tumor immunology.[116,117]

b. Humoral Assays

Although it has been over 20 years since the existence of TSTA has been demonstrated in tumors of experimental animals,[7-11] definitive evidence for the presence of TSTA on human tumors is lacking at the present time. This has been attributed to the weak antigenicity of human tumors, and the limitation of using in vitro transplantation techniques to discover TSTA on human tumors. Because cellular in vitro assays have led to confusion on the specificity of tumor-associated antigens on human tumors[69,118,119] and because "nonspecific" and "irrelevant" antibodies can be absorbed from immune sera, many investigators have been attracted to serological methods to define the antigenic specificity of human tumors. Tumor associated antigens have been detected and/or defined by numerous in vitro assays including those listed in Table 3.

Complement-dependent antibody cytotoxicity assay — Antibodies in combination with complement have the capacity to destroy target cells in vitro. This is the basis of

TABLE 3

In Vitro Humoral Assays Used for Measurement of Immune Response and/or Detection of Tumor Associated Antigens or Antibodies

Assay	Ref.
Complement-dependent antibody cytotoxicity	120—125
Complement fixation	126—134
Mixed hemadsorption	149, 150
Immune adherence	135—139
Immunofluorescence	140—146
Antiglobulin consumption	147, 148
Immunoprecipitation	149—154
Radioimmunoassay	155—158

the complement-dependent antibody cytotoxicity assay. Visual assays have been used in human tumor immunology but target cells prelabled with radioisotopes have increased the sensitivity and quantification of the complement-dependent antibody cytotoxicity (CDCC) assay. Besides its use in definition of human tumor antigen, the complementdependent antibody cytotoxicity has been used to monitor the clinical course of melanoma patients.[123.125]

Complement fixation test — The complement fixation (CF) test is a very sensitive serologic test and is useful when small quantities of antigen or antibody are available. Intact cells, insoluble or soluble antigens can be employed in this assay. Extracts of tumor cells prepared by the 3 M KCl procedure which have been antigenic in other immunologic assays have not been active in the complement fixation test.[133] Controls for anticomplementary activity of the antigen and antiserum must be included in the complement fixation test. A variation of the complement fixation test is the complement consumption assay which has been used to detect the presence of immune complexes in cancer patients' sera.[134]

Immune adherence test — Immune adherence (IA) is an agglultination reaction between a cell bearing antigen-antibody-complement complex and an indicator cell, usually human red blood cell. In this assay, target cells are mixed with antiserum, incubated, washed, and then mixed with complement. After appropriate incubation, the indicator cells are added. The receptor for C3b on the indicator cells combines with antigen-antibody-complement complex on the target ceils. The reaction is observed under light microscope.

Immunofluorescence test — The immunoflourescence test is one of the most widely used serological assays for the demonstration of TAA. In the direct immunofluorescence method, the fluorescein-labeled antibody is reacted with the antigen. After an appropriate incubation time, excess antibody is washed off and the reaction is read under an ultraviolet microscope. In the indirect immunofluorescence method unlabeled primary antibody is reacted with the antigen, then fluorescein-conjugated antiglobulin, a second antibody specific for the primary antibody, is reacted with the primary antibody. Both viable and nonviable (frozen sections or acetone fixed smears) cells can be employed in the indirect immunofluorescence test for the detection of cell surface and cytoplasmic antigens.

Antiglobulin consumption assay — The antiglobulin consumption assay is a variation of the indirect immunofluorescence test whereby the second antibody is labeled with ^{125}I instead of fluorescein. The extent of reaction is assessed by the amount of labeled ^{125}I-antibodies that have reacted with the first antibodies which in turn have reacted with the TAA of the tumor target cells. Thus, instead of examining the cells under an ultraviolet microscope, radioactivity is counted and the assay can be quantitated.

Mixed hemadsorption assay — The mixed hemadsorption test is used to demonstrate the interaction between an antibody and cell surface associated antigen. Tumor target cells are reacted with human serum, washed, and allowed to react with xenogeneic antiserum (bridging antibody). After washing, the target cells are mixed with sheep erythrocytes sensitized with monkey or baboon antiserum and the reaction (hemadsorption) is determned under light microscope. This assay detects membrane antigen and is considered by some to be more sensitive than the immunofluorescence test.

Immunoprecipitation — The Ouchterlony or immunoprecipitation test has been used to detect soluble TAA from extracts of tumor cells. The test is performed by allowing antibodies and soluble TAA to diffuse into an agar gel from wells opposite each other. Precipitin lines form at points where antibody and antigens react at optimal proportions. The immunoprecipitin test is useful in resolving a mixture of soluble antigens in a preparation.

Radioimmunoassay — The radioimmunoassay (RIA) developed by Yalow and Berson[183] in 1960 for the assay of insulin in the sera of diabetic patients is an extremely sensitive serological assay which can detect nanogram to picogram quantities of antigen. In this technique, antigen is usually radiolabeled with ^{125}I and is reacted with sufficient antibody to bind 40 to 70% of the labeled antigen. The mixtures are incubated for an appropriate period of time (usually 4 days) at 4°C during which time unlabeled and labeled antigens compete stoichiometrically for binding to antibody. Bound and free antigens are then separated by several techniques such as paper chromatoelectrophoresis, double antibody precipitation, or adsorption of the antigen to charcoal or talcum powder. The radioactivity of bound and free labeled antigen is determined by gamma counter and the ratios of the bound to free (B to F) antigen computed. The B to F ratios are plotted against antigen concentration to obtain a "standard curve." The concentration of antigen in an unknown sample is derived by comparing the B to F ratio of the unknown with the standard curve. Prerequisites for the development of radioimmunoassay systems are highly purified antigen and functionally monospecific antiserum.

III. ANTIGENS ASSOCIATED WITH TUMORS

A. Antigens of Chemically Induced Tumors

Two defined classes of antigens are expressed by tumors induced by chemical oncogens. One class of tumor antigens are the TSTA which are present on the membrane of carcinogen-induced tumors and are involved in the rejection of the tumor by immunological reactions. These tumor antigens are also referred to as tumor rejection antigens.

The second class of tumor antigens expressed by chemically induced tumors are fetal antigens. Two categories of fetal antigens have been described, a fetal antigen present on the cell membrane of the tumor cell and a fetal antigen secreted by the tumor cell.

1. Tumor Specific Transplantation Antigen

The most significant characteristic of the TSTA expressed by chemically induced tumors is their great diversity. Each tumor possesses a TSTA that is unique and individual. If a chemical carcinogen is applied at several different sites on the same tissue of an animal, the resultant tumors will express TSTA that are specific for each tumor. This phenomenon was first observed by Prehn and Main[10] and has withstood the test of time. Although occasional reports have been published to the contrary.[159-161] as a general rule, the uniqueness of TSTA on chemically induced tumors, defined operationally by immunization transplantation-rejection procedure,[7-11] is still valid. Since infection by an endemic virus of the animal colony used for such studies may impart cross-reacting immunogens to the chemically induced tumors,[162,163] any attempt to refute the idea that the TSTA on chemically induced tumors are individual must be done with "clean" colonies of experimental animals. However, a recent paper by Hellstrom et al., using transplantation techniques, suggests that chemically induced tumors express a minor common weak TSTA in addition to the major strong TSTA.[161]

a. Effect of Different Classes of Chemical Carcinogens

The immunogenicity of tumors induced by chemical oncogens depends on the class of chemical carcinogens. Tumors induced by polycyclic hydrocarbons generally express strong TSTA. But large variations in antigenic potency exist between tumors in the same and different species.[162] The polycyclic hydrocarbons that have been most studied are 3-methylcholanthrene, dibenz[a,h]anthracene, 7,12-dimethylbenz[a]anthracene, benzo[a]pyrene and dibenzo[a,i]pyrene. The amino dyes, 4-dimethylaminoazobenzene, and O-aminoazotoluene, and the simple nitrosamines, dimethylnitrosamine and diethylnitrosamine, also have been shown to impart relatively potent immunogens on the tumors they,induced.[162] Contrary to these compounds, the aromatic amine, 2-acetylaminofluorene-induced tumors failed to demonstrate consistently strong TSTA.[162]

b. Effect of Dose of Chemical Carcinogen

An inverse relationship was found between the concentration of carcinogen and tumor latency (time interval between application of the carcinogen and detection of gross tumor). The stronger the dose of the carcinogen, the shorter was the latent period of tumor induction,[164] that is tumors that were induced by a high concentration of carcinogen had a short latent period. Conversely, tumors that were induced by a low dose of oncogen had a long latency. However, a direct relationship was observed between the strength of the tumor antigen and the dose of the carcinogen. The higher the dose of the chemical oncogen the stronger was the TSTA expressed by the tumors induced by the chemical oncogen.[20]

An important question which is relevant to human tumors is the relationship of antigenic strength to latency. Since human tumors are notoriously weakly antigenic and have a long latent period of 15 to 20 years, it was a significant observation by Bartlett,[165] in murine models, that tumors with a short latent time possessed strong tumor antigens. Thus an inverse relationship was observed between the antigenic strength of the tumor and the latent period.

The weak antigenicity of human tumor could be explained by invoking the assumption that most human tumors are induced by low levels of carcinogens which have a long latency and thus are weakly antigenic.[164] Alternatively, human tumors may express low antigenicity because they might have been induced by classes of chemical oncogens, such as the aromatic amines,[162] that do not apparently confer strong immunogenicity on the tumors they induce.

2. Fetal Antigens

The existence of embryonic or fetal antigens on the membrane of chemically induced tumors was first conclusively demonstrated by Brawn in 1970 who showed inhibition of colony formation of 3-methylcholanthrene induced tumor cells in culture by lymph node cells from multiparous mice.[182] This finding was corroborated by Baldwin et al.[183] who found that the serum or lymph node cells from rats bearing 3-methylcholanthrene induced sarcomas were cytotoxic to the sarcoma cells by the microcytotoxicity test.

Membrane immunofluorescence reactions on the rat sarcoma cells with serum from multiparous rats provided evidence that the cytotoxicity was due to embryonic antigens on the membrane of the rat sarcoma cells. Similar results were obtained with 4-dimethylaminoazobenzene induced rat hepatomas.[184]

In contrast to the TSTA which are individually specific for each tumor, the embryonic or fetal antigens are cross-reacting.[162] Furthermore, the fetal antigens expressed on the plasma membrane of chemically-induced tumors have not been consistently shown to participate in tumor regression as the TSTA. But, the collective data on embryonic antigens on virus-induced tumors suggest that these embryonic antigens could elicit protective immunity.[161]

Another type of embryonic antigen synthesized by chemically induced tumors are the α-fetoprotein (AFP) which are present in normal embryonic serum, but which are absent in normal adult serum. These embryonic serum proteins are secreted by hepatomas induced by O-aminoazotoluene in mice[185] and by diethylnitrosamine and 4-dimethylaminoazobenzene in rats.[186,187] Since immunodiffusion studies established a line of identity between the α-fetoprotein in embryonic serum and adult serum of animals carrying hepatomas, it could be argued that chemical oncogens derepressed inactive genes coding for the synthesis of α-fetoproteins which were active during embryogenesis.

B. Antigens of Virus-Induced Tumors

It is axiomatic that viruses cause tumors in experimental animals. Each virus-induced tumor that has been tested for the presence of TSTA has been shown to possess TSTA. In 1961 Sjogren et al.[217] demonstrated the presence of TSTA on tumors in mice induced by the polyoma virus. In contrast to the TSTA on tumors induced by chemical carcinogens which are noncross-reacting, TSTA expressed by tumors induced by an oncogenic virus were cross-reacting.[217] Subsequent experiments by other investigators corroborated this observation and further showed that the cross-reacting TSTA on virus-induced tumors were independent of the histologic types of tumor and species, but was dependent on the oncogenic virus.[218] For instance, tumors induced by polyoma virus do not share TSTA that are induced by SV-40 virus or adenovirus 12. However, minor cross-reacting TSTA with tumor induced by the Friend, Moloney, and Rauscher groups of RNA-viruses have been reported.[219]

Two alternative mechanisms have been proposed to explain the existence of TSTA on virus induced tumors. The virus genome integrates *in toto* or in part with the host cell genome and codes for a viral antigen, the TSTA, on the transformed tumor cell. Alternatively, after the viral genes becomes integrated with the host cell genome, they derepress dormant host cell genes to code for the TSTA. This latter explanation on the mechanism of induction of TSTA on the tumor cell by the virus assumes that normal cells contain the genes coding for the TSTA and implies that TSTA are embryonic or fetal antigens. Recent data support this concept.[220,221]

Common TSTA on virus-induced tumors have practical importance in cancer immunotherapy. If human tumors share cross-reacting tumor antigens within histologic types,[173] the development of a cancer vaccine with human tumor cells would be easier than a tumor vaccine prepared from tumors that express unique TSTA. In the former case, one approach would be to screen and select the strongest antigenic tumor cell line for the production of a tumor cell vaccine. In the latter case, the logistics of designing a cancer vaccine for each cancer patient is impractical and may even be impossible since the biopsied specimens from many cancer patients are sometimes too small to provide an adequate supply of cells for a tumor cell vaccine.

The antigenic strength of the TSTA on tumors induced by oncogenic virus is at least comparable to those expressed on chemical carcinogen-induced tumors. The spectrum of antigenic strengths of virus induced tumors mimic those of chemically induced tumors ranging from no detectable antigenicity to very strong antigenicity. Most tumors induced by oncogenic virus are strongly immunogenic. But even with the minority of virus-induced tumors which are weakly antigenic, or nonantigenic, their immunogenicity can be strengthened by further infection with oncogenic or nononcogenic viruses.[222-224]

C. Antigens of Spontaneous Tumors

Naturally-occurring or "spontaneous" tumors are defined as neoplasms that appear sporadically and infrequently without known causative agents. Tumors, intentionally induced by chemical, viral, or physical oncogens obviously do not comply with this definition. Tumors that occur with high incidence in certain mouse strains, such as leukemia in AKR mice and mammary adenocarcinoma in C_3H mice, caused by vertical transmission of an oncogenic virus, are also excluded from this definition of spontaneous tumors. If these criteria of spontaneous tumor are accepted, then there is a profound difference in the immunogenicity between tumors "artificially" induced by chemical, viral, or physical agents and spontaneous tumors. Whereas most artificially induced tumors are strongly immunogenic,[225] almost all spontaneous tumors are weakly immunogenic[226,227] to nonimmunogenic.[10,228-230] However, a few chemically-induced tumors are nonimmunogenic[10,60,165,231] and a rare spontaneous tumor is strongly antigenic.[232] Again a spectrum of immunogenicity as displayed by artificial tumors is exhibited by natural tumors. But the immunogenicity of these two types of tumors are inversely related. At one end of the spectrum are most artificial tumors that contain high immunogenicity and most natural tumors that express nonimmunogenicity while at the opposite end of the spectrum the converse exists.

Since tumors induced by low concentrations of 3-methylcholanthrene possessed little or no immunogenicity, Prehn[164] proposed that spontaneous tumors may arise because of exposure to low levels of carcinogens present in the environment. This proposition is consistent with the observation that human tumors express weak antigenicity and with the concept that 70 to 90% of cancers in man are induced by environmental factors.[1]

D. Relationship of Tumor Antigens to Carcinogensis

An interesting question which has heuristic appeal as well as practical importance is whether the events leading to the conversion of a normal cell to a neoplastic cell are mutually exclusive from the events that are involved with the induction of the tumor antigen when a normal cell is transformed by a chemical carcinogen to a neoplastic cell. If the oncogenic process is mutually linked to the antigen-inducing process, or even if the tumor antigen is a by-product or is incidental to the process of carcinogenesis,[161,164,233] the tumor antigen could be exploited for early diagnosis of cancer and for screening of potential chemical carcinogens because the expression of the tumor antigen has been shown to occur simultaneously with or soon after oncogenesis.[16,234,235] If carcinogenesis is conjointly linked to induction of the tumor antigen, this would imply that the tumor antigen is essential to maintain the malignant state and it may be possible to devise chemotherapeutic agents which could inhibit synthesis of the tumor antigen perhaps resulting in perturbation of the neoplastic state or death of the cancer cell.

E. Relationship of Immunogenetics to Carcinogenesis

An important observation in chemical carcinogensis was observed by Kouri et al.[236] These investigators found that tumorigenic susceptibility of different strains of mice is not totally associated with aryl hydrocarbon hydroxylase inducibility. For example, tumorigenic susceptibility to 3-methylcholanthrene has been observed in the order C_3H > C57B1/6 > DBA/2 but aryl hydrocarbon hydroxylse inducibility is C57B1/6 > C_3H > DBA/2 in these three strains of mice.[237] This lack of correlation between tumorigenic susceptibility and aryl hydrocarbon hydroxylase inducibility suggests that other genetic predisoposing parameter(s), including the immune response, might account for this inconsistency. Since the aryl hydrocarbon hydroxylase enzyme system, which is induced by, and which metabolizes polycyclic aromatic hydrocarbons to proximate carcinogens, is under strict genetic control (discussed in Chapter 2), this raises the question if *Ir* genes control recognition of TSTA in different syngeneic strains of mice exhibiting different tumorigenic susceptibility to polycyclic aromatic hydrocarbons. This should be a fertile area of research in tumor immunology and immunogenetics.

On the other hand, in studies of viral oncogenesis, although MHC has been found to influence tumor incidence and latency, tumorigenic susceptibility or resistance did not involve *Ir* genes but genes that control inheritance of oncogenic viruses.[238] Therefore, it appears that susceptibility or resistance to oncogenesis is a product of complex interactions between genetic and environmental factors involving both immunologic and nonimmunologic mechanism.

F. Antigens of Human Tumors

As mentioned previously, a wide variety of in vitro procedures have been explored to discover TSTA on human tumors. Although the data are consistent with the hypothesis that human tumors possess TAA, unequivocal evidence for the existence of TSTA on human tumors has been lacking. The definition and classification of TAA on human tumor cells may not only be important academically, but also practically in terms of developing a diagnostic and/or prognostic test for cancer and perhaps for designing a cancer vaccine. Unfortunately, no uniform consensus of laboratory evidence, using the various in vitro assays described above, has emerged at the present state of the art to define and classify human tumor antigens systematically. The available data suggest that human melanomas and sarcomas express at least three categories of membrane TAA: (1) an individual TAA distinct for each tumor; (2) a common TAA specific for each histologic type; (3) a common TAA that is shared by fetal tissues.

1. Individual and Histologic Specific Tumor Antigens

A tumor antigen unique for each tumor obtained from melanoma patients was reported by Lewis[123] using the complement-dependent antibody cytotoxicity assay and membrane immunofluorescence test. Bodurtha and his collaborators[125] corroborated this finding with the complement-dependent antibody cytotoxicity assay and like Lewis et al.[124] found a correlation with the presence of cytotoxic antibody in the sera of melanoma patients with good prognosis and the absence of cytotoxic antibody with poor prognosis. Recently, Carey et al.[150] using the mixed hemadsorption assay, in agreement with Lewis et al.[123,124] and Bodurtha et al.,[125] concluded that human malignant melanoma expressed an autologous membrane specific melanoma antigen. In contrast to these data, Morton et al.,[166] Oettgen et al,[167] Muna et al.,[168] and recently Leong et al.[169] were unable to find a unique antigen on melanoma cells by the immunofluorescence test. These authors, however, described a cross-reacting common melanoma membrane antigen. This discrepancy could be attributed to the patient populations studied by these different groups of investigators and perhaps human malignant melanoma possesses both unique and cross-reacting melanoma antigens.[170] Individual[171,172] and cross-reacting[171-173] melanoma antigens also have been demonstrated by the lymphocytotoxicity assay. Recently, The et al.[174] and Siebert et al.[175] could not detect either an individual or cross-reacting melanoma specific membrane antigen but found a membrane associated antigen on melanoma cells that cross-reacted with 6 to 12 week old fetal cells. In addition, Grimm et al.[176] demonstrated a tumor antigen in the spent medium of a human malignant melanoma that was adapted to grow in serum-free chemically defined medium[177] that transcends histologic type. Autologous membrane antigen has been demonstrated on human osteogenic sarcoma;[178] however, cross-reacting sarcoma specific antigen have also been reported.[122,173-180] Furthermore, similar to the human melanoma system, a fetal antigen has been demonstrated on human sarcoma cells in culture.[181] Future research will doubtlessly uncover the antigenic systems of other histologic types of human tumors and elucidate the relationship of these antigens to one another and to the immune response of the cancer patient.

2. Oncofetal Antigens
a. Carcinoembryonic Antigen

Perhaps the most publicized and controversial oncofetal antigen is carcinoembryonic antigen (CEA) described by Gold and Freedman in 1965.[188] Originally, these authors proposed that CEA was an antigen shared by human colon carcinoma and embryonic epithelium arising from endodermally derived digestive system, gut, pancreas, and liver throughout the first two trimesters of gestation. Subsequent research by other investigators, however, have provided evidence that CEA is a misnomer. First, CEA has been found not only in cancerous colorectal tissues, but also has been detected on normal tissues.[189-195] A recent study indicated that the epithelium of the small intestine manufactured equivalent amounts of CEA to that of colorectal cancer, but, whereas some CEA from colorectal carcinoma entered the bloodstream, most of the CEA from the normal small intestine were shed in the lumen of the gut and excreted into the feces.[195] Second, CEA has been found not only in fetal tissue, but in adult tissue[189-195] indicating CEA is not solely an embryonic antigen. Third, CEA may not be antigenic in man;[196-198] however, it is in other species.[199,200] Xenoantisera to CEA have been raised in other species to develop a RIA for the detection of CEA in the sera of patients with colorectal cancer.[199] But because the concentration of CEA is elevated in the sera of patients with a variety of neoplastic and nonneoplastic diseases,[189-195, 200] the value of the RIA test to CEA has been shown to have very little diagnostic value. Monitoring of CEA levels by RIA, however, may be useful as a prognostic indicator for colon cancer patients postsurgically.[201]

b. α-Fetoprotein

Unlike CEA which is located in the glycocalyx surrounding the cell membrane,[202] AFP is a serum protein secreted from the cell. Historically, AFP was first reported by Bergstrand and Czar in 1956[203] who observed in human fetal serum a protein that migrated between albumin and α-globulin on paper electrophoresis. The highest concentration of this serum protein was found in the sera of human fetuses between 12 and 14 weeks of gestation. In 1963, Abelev et al.[185] isolated an identical alpha migrating protein in the sera of pregnant or newborn mice and in the sera of mice bearing transplanted hepatocellular carcinomas. They named this protein embryonal α-globulin. Pertinent to human tumor immunology was the important finding by Tatrainov[204] that although AFP was not usually detected in normal serum 5 weeks after birth and thereafter, it was found in the sera of patients with hepatocellular carcinoma. AFP was found in the sera of patients with teratocarcinomas, pancreatic, gastric, lung carcinomas, and even with leukemia and myeloma.[205] The presence of AFP also has been recorded in patients with other clinical states, including viral hepatitis[206] and ataxia telangectasia.[207] Sensitive immunoassays, including enzyme immunoassay, radioimmunoassay, immunofluorescent probes and immunoelectrophoresis to detect minute quantities of AFP have recently been developed.[208]

c. Brain Oncofetal Antigen

One of the most recent additions to the group of oncofetal antigens was the brain oncofetal antigen described by Irie et al.[209] These investigators showed by the IA test the existence of a membrane antigen on human tumor of various histologic types obtained from biopsied specimens or tissue culture cells. This antigen was found to cross-react with human fetal brain tissue and thus was designated oncofetal antigen (OFA). Its highest concentration was detected in second trimester human fetal brain tissue. Since OFA was absent on normal biopsied skin but was present on fibroblasts of skin grown in tissue culture, OFA probably represents a phenotypic expression of genes active during embryogenesis that are repressed in adult life but are derepressed in oncogenesis. Anti-OFA antibodies have been isolated from melanoma sera by affinity chromatography and characterized by absorption with human fetal brain cells.[210]

d. Other Oncofetal Antigens

Several other oncofetal antigens have been reported by various investigators. Edynak and co-workers[211] described a common fetal antigen in 75 to 95% of human carcinomas, sarcomas, and leukemias. The antigen was found in the extracts of 75% benign tumors but not in extracts of 172 normal or nonneoplastic diseased tissues. Fetal sulfoglycoprotein found in gastric cancer,[212-214] α_2 H-globulin present in 81% of sera from children with tumors,[215] α-oncofetal antigen associated with melanoma and colon, breast and endometrial carcinomas,[216] and the fetal antigen recently described by The et al.[174] are four other oncofetal antigens that have been described to a growing list of fetal antigens expressed by human neoplasms.

IV. CANCER IMMUNOTHERAPY IN ANIMAL MODELS

Table 4 lists a variety of immunotherapeutic procedures that have been tested in experimental animals. Most of these procedures, however, were performed by the immunization-challenge technique which simulates cancer immunoprophylaxis more than immunotherapy. It is important to distinguish between cancer immunoprophylaxis and immunotherapy. The former entails procedures that evoke the immune system to prevent a nidus of cancer cells to become clinically manifest. The latter involves manipulation of the immune system to destroy an established tumor.

It may appear, at first glance, that the approaches to immunoprophylaxis and immunotherapy are identical. Yet the literature is replete with successful implementation of immunoprophylactic procedures but very few successes have been reported with curing the host of its established tumor by immunotherapy. Perhaps the failure of current modalities of cancer immunotherapy is that it mimics the methods used in immunoprophylaxis. It may well be that novel avenues and principles must be developed before immunotherapy can become fruitful.

Most important, however, will be the direction that future research in tumor immunology pursues. If one of the ultimate goals of the tumor immunologist is to develop

TABLE 4

Immunotherapeutic Modalities Tested in Animal Models

Modality	Definition	Agent	Ref.
Specific:			
a. Active	Elicitation of tumor immunity by an animal when injected by a vaccine composed of intact, fragments or extracts of tumor cells	Live tumor cells	239—241
		Irradiated tumor cells	240—243
		Tumor cells coupled to bis-diazobenzene	244
		Tumor cells treated with dinitrophenyl aminocaproate, iodoacetate, iodoacetamie, N-ethylaleimide	245—247
		Neuraminidase treated tumor cells	248—251
Passive:			
a. Adoptive therapy	Transfer of immunity by donors lymphoid cells or their extracts from a syngeneic, allogeneic or xenogeneic animal to the recipient	Immune syngeneic lymphocytes	252—253
		Unsensitized allogeneic lymphocytes	254—255
		Sensitized allogeneic lymphocytes	253—255
		Immune xenogeneic lymphocytes	256
		Immune RNA	260—264
b. Serotherapy	Injection of hyperimmune sera produced in a syngeneic, allogeneic or zenogeneic animal into the tumor-bearing host	Anti-El-4 leukemia	268—269
		Anti-lymphoma	270
		Anti-sarcoma	271—273
		Antibody coupled to ^{131}I, drugs, enzymes or toxins	274
Nonspecific			
a. Active	Potentiation of the reticuloendothelial system by the injection of agents such as intact or subcellular fractions of microorganisms	Gram-positive bacilli	243
		Gram-negative bacilli	243
		Gram-negative cocci	275
		BCG	276—279
		BCG-MER	280—281
		BCG cell wall	282
		Corynebacterium parvum	289—290
		Synthetic ribonucleotides	291—293
		Plant products (Glucan, lantinan, pachymaran)	294—296

basic principles in tumor immunobiology that will lead to a rational approach to cancer immunotherapy, then the tumor immunologist must address himself to the real issue, namely, investigating the immunology of spontaneous tumors or tumors with weak antigenicity induced by low levels of chemical carcinogens.[164] This becomes apparent when it is recognized that the wealth of information that has been accumulated with studies conducted with highly antigenic tumors induced by chemical or viral oncogens, has yielded penurious utilitarian returns in immunotherapy of human neoplasms.

A. Specific Immunotherapy

Tumor cell either untreated[239-241] or treated by a number of different procedures including irradiation,[240-243] or coupling to bis-diazobenzene,[244] modification by chemicals,[245-247] and exposure to Vibrio Cholera neuraminidase to increase immunogenicity[248-251] have been reported to be effective vaccines. In one case complete regression of established tumors was reported.[249]

Adoptive transfer of tumor immunity with immunocompetent cells have been demonstrated with syngeneic lymphoid cells.[252,253] Transfer of specific tumor immunity from one animal to another was accomplished with unsensitized[254,255] or sensitized allogeneic lymphoid cells.[253-255] Even immune xenogeneic lymphocytes were capable of imparting specific tumor immunity in the recipient.[256] However, immunotherapy was most effective when it was preceded by chemotherapy to reduce the tumor load.[248,255,257-259]

Recently, it was demonstrated that RNA extracted from sensitized lymphocytes could transfer transplantation immunity in rabbits.[260] This work was subsequently extended to tumor immunity by Alexander et al.,[261] who found RNA extracted from sheep immunized with sarcomas induced by benzypyrene caused temporary tumor regression following foot pad injection. This observation was substantiated by Pilch et al.[262] and by Paque et al.[263] Additionally, Schlayer and his collaborators,[264] observed specific tumor regression after administration of xenogeneic immune RNA (I-RNA) in combination with unsensitized syngeneic peritoneal exudate cells and TSTA preparation. A major advantage of I-RNA immunotherapy is that allogeneic and even xenogeneic I-RNA could be used. This has important application in human immunotherapy since appropriately immunized animals could provide a source of I-RNA.

Serotherapy have been found to be effective in animal models.[265] Antibodies in the donor's serum in the presence of recipient's complement may directly kill the recipient's tumor cells or the antibodies may confer specificity and cytotoxicity to recipient's thymus-independent nonimmune lymphoid cells carrying Fc receptors.[111,266,267] Effective treatment with serotherapy have been observed with murine leukemia,[268,269] lymphoma,[270] and sarcoma.[271-273] One modification of serotherapy entails the coupling of radioactive isotopes, chemical drugs, enzymes or toxins to antibodies specific for the tumor in order to concentrate these agents at the target cell level when injected into tumor bearing animals. Some positive results have been recorded.[274]

B. Nonspecific Immunotherapy

Several agents have been tested for their ability to potentiate the lymphoreticular system under the premise that a heightened activity of the reticuloendothelial system would render the animal refractory to a tumor. Vaccines prepared from Gram positive and Gram negative bacteria have been used.[243-275] The most promising bacteria currently being used in cancer immunotherapy are Bacillus Calmette-Guerin (BCG) and *Corynebacterium parvum* (*C. parvum*).

BCG is a live, virulent strain of *Mycobacterium tuberculosis bovis* isolated and attenuated by Calmette and Guerin at the Pasteur Institute and has been used throughout the world except in the U.S. as an immunoprophylaxis measure against tuberculosis. Old et al.[276] were the first to use BCG to treat animal tumors. Subsequently, other investigators have used BCG,[277-279] extract of BCG[280,281] or cell wall of the BCG organisms[282] in antitumor therapy with varying degrees of success. The methanol extract residue of Weiss and his co-workers[280] and BCG cell wall attached to oil droplets[282] have been devised to circumvent the side effects of BCG.

Guinea pig models have been utilized to simulate clinical cancer in man to study the efficacy of BCG-immunotherapy in the prevention of recurrence. BCG-immunotherapy was administered adjunctive to surgery in an effort to reduce the incidence of recurrence.[282-284] The collective data suggests that surgical adjunctive BCG-immunotherapy might be beneficial if metastatic disease is microscopic but is ineffective if metastatic tumor deposits are palpable.

A paradoxical effect of BCG-immunotherapy has been demonstrated on the growth of tumor. Depending on the dose, route, schedule, animal species, and type of tumor, BCG-immunotherapy has been shown to either reduce or accelerate the growth of a tumor.[285-287] Similar observations with BCG cell wall have been recorded.[288] Therefore, caution should be exercised in the use of BCG in the treatment of human cancer.

In contrast to BCG vaccine, *C. parvum*-vaccine is prepared from killed *C. parvum* organisms. Intra-tumor injection of *C. parvum* has been shown to cause regression of established tumors.[289] The antitumor effect of *C. parvum* appears to be activation of macrophages and stimulation of antibody production.[290]

Synthetic ribonucleotides such as polyinosinic-polycytidylic acid[291-293] and some plant products including gluca,[294] lantinan,[295] and pachymanan[296] have been demonstrated to inhibit tumor growth in murine model systems. These compounds, especially the polynucleotide complexes which induce interferon, may eventually find application in a clinical setting.

V. CLINICAL TRIALS OF CANCER IMMUNOTHERAPY

Surgery is the most effective single treatment for cancer. Both the insidious and metastatic nature of cancer precludes curing all cancer patients by surgical procedures. Thus most cancer patients who visit the oncology clinic already have progressive disease that defy the two conventional local treatments, surgery and radiotherapy. Yet, sobering as it is, surgery and radiation therapy, either singly or in combination, are responsible for more than 95% of all cancer cured in the United States and throughout the world.[297] The remaining 5% of all cancer cured is by chemotherapy, a systemic modality of cancer treatment. The major disadvantages of chemotherapy are that most chemotherapeutic agents are immunosuppressive and they lack specificity, that is, they are toxic to both cancer cells and normal cells.

Immunotherapy, a systemic modality of cancer therapy, promises to be an effective treatment for cancer. However, the cancer patient's immune system is capable of destroying only small numbers of tumor cells, from 1 to 10 million, but not 100 million or more.[64] Thus the philosophy has been perpetuated that the most rational approach for the treatment of cancer is surgery, radiotherapy, or/and chemotherapy to reduce the tumor burden, if possible below 100 million tumor cells, followed by adjunctive immunotherapy.[297]

With this preface in mind, this section of the chapter will survey only those clinical trials of cancer immunotherapy that have been based on the approach of immunotherapy against minimum tumor burden. Selection of such clinical trials are obviously biased, but comprehensive reviews of immunotherapy are available.[298-303]

A. Specific Immunization

No objective, control and randomized clinical trial with active-specific immunotherapy that indicate a definite benefit has been reported to date. Vaccines composed of tissue culture allogeneic tumor cells in addition to BCG in malignant melanoma[304] and skeletal and soft tissue sarcomas[305] are in progress but preliminary data suggests only a minimum benefit. However, the full impact of specific active immunization against cancer awaits the availability of a vaccine(s) composed of strong tumor immunogens free of inhibitory substances.

B. Nonspecific Immunization

The rationale for nonspecific immunotherapy was based on an empirical observation by Coley in 1891 who noticed that a patient with a recurrent inoperable spindle-cell sarcoma of the tonsil and glands of the neck experienced a seven year regression after two bouts with erysipelas.[306] This prompted the development of Coley's toxins which consisted of a combination of living or heat-killed streptococcus and *Bacillus prodigiosus* in varying proportions. Impressive regressions and long-term cures occurred when

Coley's toxins were injected directly into a tumor or were given intralesionally. Unfortunately, recent preparations of Coley's toxins have not been as effective.

Although the exact mode of action of Coley's toxins is unknown, it has been assumed that it had a generalized effect of potentiating the immune system in addition to the pyrogenic effect of the bacterial toxins. Therefore, agents that have been known or suspected to augment the immune responses have been used in cancer immunotherapy.

Two successful clinical trials with BCG-immunotherapy led to a more extensive use of adjuvant BCG therapy. Mathé[277] reported a prolonged survival time in patients with acute leukemia who were treated with BCG adjunctive to chemotherapy. Morton and his colleagues[278] injected BCG directly into metastatic nodules of patients with malignant melanoma and observed regression of 90% of the injected lesions and 20% regression of uninjected nodules at distant sites from the BCG inoculation.

It is known from the natural history of human malignant melanoma that patients with disease seemingly limited to metastatic deposits in the skin and subcutaneous tissues harbor subclinical disseminated disease to internal organs of the body. The results of Morton et al.[307] which showed that 15 to 20% of the patients who experienced regression of uninjected metastaitc tumor nodules and survived from 1 to 7 years following BCG-immunotherapy, inferred that BCG-immunotherapy was successful in eradicating small metastatic tumor growths in parenchymal organs.

In view of this logic, studies were undertaken to assess the efficacy of BCG-immunotherapy adjunctive to surgical resection of regional lymph node metastases in malignant melanoma (Stage II). Approximately 80% of patients with Stage II malignant melanoma will have recurrent disease 5 years postsurgery because of subclinical disseminated disease. However, 64% of the 126 patients treated with postoperative adjuvant BCG-immunotherapy[308] remained disease-free for 2 years after surgery as compared with 36% treated by operation alone (p < 0.05).[307] These results exemplify the effectiveness of BCG vaccination in conjunction with surgery.

Postoperative BCG-immunotherapy have also been used in patients with a variety of neoplasms including lung, colon, and breast carcinomas.[301] The results have been optimistic to warrant continued clinical trials of BCG-immunotherapy adjunctive to conventional modality of cancer therapy.

Clinical trials with other nonspecific immunotherapeutic agents such as *C. parvum*, 2-4-dinitrochlorobenzene, and levamisole are currently underway. Since mechanism of action of these agents are different, each acting on different components of the lymphoreticular system, yet each providing some beneficial effect to the cancer patient, perhaps therapy with an agent or combination of agents that optimally stimulate the entire reticuloendothelial system may achieve maximum tumor regression.

C. Adoptive Transfer of Immunity

Adoptive immunotherapy with lymphoid cells or fractions of lymphoid cells have been used in cancer patients. Sumner and Foraker[309] reported a favorable response of a melanoma patient who was transfused with whole blood from another patient who had undergone complete remission.

Cross-immunization followed by cross-transfusion[310,311] is another method of adoptive immunotherapy that has been tried. In this procedure, two patients matched for blood and histologic tumor type were transplanted with each other's tumor. When the patients became immunized to the transplanted tumor, each was transfused with peripheral lymphocytes from the other paired patient. The low response rate of 15 to 20% and the logistic problem have discouraged wide scale use of this technique. Similar reasons have prevented more clinical trials of adoptive immunotherapy with thoracic duct lymphocytes from healthy siblings as donors for cancer patients.[311,312]

Adoptive immunotherapy with transfer factor[314] and immune RNA[315] are currently being investigated clinically. Since transfer factor appears to be species specific, it must be prepared from the leukocytes of man. Immune RNA may be extracted from the leukocytes of man or from the lymph nodes of xenogeneic species, such as the sheep, after the animal has been immunized with human tumor cells. The results of the clinical trials with transfer factor and immune RNA are too preliminary to draw any firm conclusions.

D. Passive Transfer of Immunity

Cancer serotherapy has been relegated to a secondary role to adoptive (cellular) immunotherapy because of the pervasive thought in tumor immunology that humoral antibodies facilitate tumor growth.[15,27,33] Antiserum or fractions of the antiserum for passive transfer of immunity have been obtained from "cured" cancer patients or from heterologous species such as horse, sheep, pigs, or rabbits that have been immunized with cancer cells. Results of clinical trials with serotherapy have not been impressive. However, this approach to cancer therapy should be given more serious consideration because recent clinical trials suggest some benefit with this modality of cancer therapy.[265,316]

VI. CONCLUDING REMARKS

There is very little doubt that chemicals are potent etiological agents of human neoplasia. If this is accepted, there are only two approaches to the solution of the cancer problem — prevention and curative therapy.

Cancer prevention can be approached from several fronts that are not mutually exclusive. One method being researched actively at present is the development of a screening system for potential carcinogenic substances. If a chemical is found to be carcinogenic, obviously the public should be educated in avoiding contact with it (see Chapter 1 for discussion of this subject). In this context, social and dietary habits, and industrial activities may have to be modified. Similarly, since genetic factors may contribute to chemical oncogenesis in man, genetic counseling may become expedient in the repertoire of a clinical oncologist (see Chapter 7 for discussion). Research should also be directed in understanding the mechanism of action of these chemicals, including such parameters as metabolic activation and detoxification (discussed in Chapter 2).

Another approach to cancer prevention would be the development of a cancer vaccine(s). The major problem in the development of a specific vaccine for cancer is that tumor induced by chemical carcinogens, at least in lower species, possess unique tumor regression antigens specific for each tumor. Therefore, it is unlikely or even impossible to develop a vaccine for cancer in man if each human tumor expresses an individual tumor regression antigen. Even though the evidence suggests that human tumors of the same histologic type share common tumor specific antigens, the probability of developing a vaccine composed of tumor specific antigens from each organ site is small. Consideration, therefore, should be given to membrane oncofetal antigens. Since these tumor antigens transcend histologic types and have been demonstrated to be antigenic in man, they have the potential of fulfilling the role of universal tumor antigens for the development of a vaccine against all types of cancer in man. Two speculations in this regard require recognition. One is that since OFA are components of normal embryonic cells, it is conceivable that residual embryonic cells exist in the adult and perform an important function, for example, regeneration and repair of tissues, or that adult cells express subthreshold levels of OFA below the sensitivity of current in vitro assays. Therefore, active immunization with OFA may induce an autoimmune response. Alternatively, successful vaccination against cancer with OFA may not be possible because the species in its evolutionary history of phylogeny and ontogeny have developed a fail-safe homeostatic system for its survival against such an event. Perhaps the greatest utilitarian value of OFA could be their use in a diagnostic test for early cancer in man.

In regard to therapy, surgery is still the single most effective treatment for cancer. But since the cure rate of cancer by surgery alone is only about 30%, supplemental therapies to surgery are needed. Immunotherapy has the potential of fulfilling the deficiency of surgery. But cognizance of the limit of immunotherapy should be heeded. Only a small number of tumor cells can be eradicated by the immune system. However, the immune system is only one component of the reticuloendothelial system. Evidence indicates that the full potential of the reticuloendothelial has not been tapped. The inflammatory response may be an important homeostatic surveillance system against neoplasia,[317-319] and in conjunction with the immune system and the "magic bullet" of cancer chemotherapy which remains to be designed,[320] the present scourge of mankind may be exterminated.

ACKNOWLEDGMENT

We fully appreciate the typing of this chapter by Ms. Jeanie Grigsby and Ms. Betty Baker and for their helpful suggestions.

REFERENCES

1. **Higginson, J.,** in *Environment and Cancer,* 24th Symp. Fundamental Cancer Res., Williams & Wilkins, Baltimore, 1972, 69.
2. **Miller, E. C.,** Some current perspectives on chemical carcinogenesis in humans and experimental animals, Presidential address, *Cancer Res.,* 38, 1479, 1978.
3. **Ehrlich, P.,** Ueber den jetzigen stand der Karzinomforschung, in *Ned. Tijdschr. Geneesk.,* No. 5, 1909.
4. **Prehn, R. T.,** in *Immune Surveillance,* Smith, R. T. and Landy, M., Eds., Academic Press, New York, 1970, 451.
5. **Moller, G. and Moller, E.,** Considerations of some current concepts in cancer research, *J. Natl. Cancer Inst.,* 55, 755, 1975.
6. **Snell, G. D.,** Genetics of tissue transplantation, in *Biology of the Laboratory Mouse,* Green, E. L., Ed., McGraw-Hill, New York, 1966, 457.
7. **Gross, L.,** Intradermal immunization of C3H mice against a sarcoma that originated in an animal of the same line, *Cancer Res.,* 2, 327, 1943.
8. **Foley, E. J.,** Antigenic properties of methylcholanthrene-induced tumors in mice of the strain of origin, *Cancer Res.,* 13, 835, 1953.

9. **Baldwin, R. W.**, Immunity to methylcholanthrene-induced tumors in inbred rats following atrophy and regression of the implanted tumors, *Br. J. Cancer*, 9, 652, 1955.

10. **Prehn, R. T. and Main, J. M.**, Immunity to methylcholanthrene-induced sarcomas, *J. Nat. Cancer Inst.*, 18, 769, 1957.

11. **Klein, G., Sjogren, H. O., Klein, E., and Hellstrom, K. E.**, Demonstration of resistance against methylcholanthrene-induced sarcomas in the primary authochthonous host, *Cancer Res.*, 20, 1561, 1960.

12. **Goldstein, A. L., Asanuma, Y., Battisto, J. R., Hardy, M. A., Quint, J., and White, A.**, Influence of thymosin in cell-mediated and humoral immune responses in normal and immunologically deficient mice, *J. Immunol.*, 104, 359, 1970.

13. **Komuro, K. and Boyse, E. A.**, *In vitro* demonstration of thymic hormone in the conversion of precursor cells into lymphocytes, *Lancet*, 1, 740, 1970.

14. **Kate, D. H. and Benacerraf, B.**, The regulatory influence of activated T cells on B cell responses to antigen, *Adv. Immunol.*, 15, 1, 1972.

15. **Hellstrom, I. and Hellstrom, K. E.**, Studies on cellular immunity and serum-mediated inhibition in Moloney-induced mouse sarcomas, *Int. J. Cancer*, 4, 587, 1969.

16. **Prehn, R. T. and Lappe, M. A.**, An immunostimulation theory of tumor development, *Transplant. Rev.*, 7, 26, 1971.

17. **Michinson, N. A.**, Passive transfer of transplantation immunity, *Proc. Roy. Soc. London*, 142, 72, 1954.

18. **Winn, J. H.**, The immune response and the homograft reaction, *Nat. Cancer Inst. Monogr.*, 2, 113, 1959.

19. **Klein, E. and Sjogren, H. O.**, Humoral and cellular factors in homograft and isograft immunity against sarcoma cells, *Cancer Res.*, 20, 452, 1960.

20. **Hellstrom, K. E. and Hellstrom, I.**, Lymphocyte-mediated cytotoxicity and blocking serum activity to tumor antigens, *Adv. Immunol.*, 18, 209, 1974.

21. **Medawar, P. B.**, The immunology of transplantation, *Harvey Lect.*, 52, 114, 1957.

22. **Wagner, J. L. and Haughton, G.**, Immunosuppression by antilymphocyte serum and its effect on tumors induced by 3-methylcholanthrene in mice, *J. Nat. Cancer Inst.*, 46, 1, 1971.

23. **Ting, R. C. and Law, L. B.**, Thymic function and carcinogenesis, *Prog. Exp. Tumor Res.*, 9, 165, 1967.

24. **Cerottini, J. C., Nordin, A. A., and Brunner, K. T.**, Specific *in vitro* cytotoxicity of thymus derived lymphocytes sensitized to allo-antigens, *Nature London*, 228, 1308, 1970.

25. **Goldstein, P., Wigzell, H., Blomgren, H., and Svedmyr, E.**, Cells mediating specific *in vitro* cytotoxicity. II. Probable autonomy of thymus-process lymphocytes (T cells) for the killing of allogeneic target cells, *J. Exp. Med.*, 135, 890, 1972.

26. **Brunner, K. T., Plata, F., Vasudevan, D. M., and Cerottini, J. C.**, Lymphocyte-mediated cytotoxicity mechanisms and relationship to tumor immunity, in *Host Defense Against Cancer and Its Potentiation*, Mizuno, D., Ed., University of Tokyo Press, 1975, 43.

27. **Moller, G.**, Effect on tumor growth in syngeneic recipients of antibodies against tumor-specific antigens in methylcholanthrene-induced mouse sarcomas, *Nature London*, 204, 846, 1964.

28. **Bubenik, J., Perlmann, P., Helmstein, K., and Moberger, G.**, Cellular and humoral immune responses to human urinary bladder carcinomas, *Cancer*, 5, 310, 1970.

29. **Jagarlamoody, S. M., Aust, J. C., Tew, R. H., and McKhann, C. F.**, *In vitro* detection of cytotoxic cellular immunity against tumor-specific antigen by a radioisotopic technique, *Proc. Nat. Acad. Sci. U.S.A.*, 68, 1346, 1971.

30. **Yonemoto, R. H., Fujisawa, T., and Waldman, S. R.**, Effect of serum blocking factors on leukocyte adherence inhibition in breast cancer patients, *Cancer*, 41, 1289, 1978.

31. **Brown, R. J.**, *In vitro* desensitization of sensitized murine lymphocytes by serum factor (soluble antigen), *Proc. Nat. Acad. Sci. U.S.A.*, 68, 1634, 1971.

32. **Thomson, D. M. P., Steele, K., and Alexander, P.**, The presence of tumor-specific membrane antigen in the serum of rats with chemically induced sarcoma, *Br. J. Cancer*, 27, 27, 1973.

33. **Ran, M. and Witz, I. P.**, Tumor-associated immunoglobulins enhancement of syngeneic tumors by IgG_2-containing tumor eluates, *Int. J. Cancer*, 9, 242, 1972.

34. **Sjogren, H. O., Hellström, I., Bensal, S. C., and Hellström, K. E.**, Suggestive evidence that the "blocking antibodies" of tumor-bearing individuals may be antigen-antibody complexes, *Proc. Nat. Acad. Sci. U.S.A.*, 68, 1372, 1971.

35. **Baldwin, R. W., Price, M. R., and Robbins, R. A.**, Blocking of lymphocyte-mediated cytotoxicity for rat hepatoma cells by tumor-specific antigen-antibody complexes, *Nature London New Biol.*, 238, 185, 1972.

36. **Baldwin, R. W., Bowen, J. G., and Price, M. R.**, Detection of circulating hepatoma D23 antigen and immune complexes in tumor bearer serum, *Br. J. Cancer*, 28, 16, 1973.

37. **Klein, J.**, *Biology of the Mouse Histocompatibility-2 Complex,* Springer-Verlag, New York, 1975.
38. **Snell, G. D., Dausset, J., and Natenson, S.**, *Histocompatibility,* Academic Press, New York, 1976.
39. **McDevitt, H. O. and Sela, M.**, Genetic control of the antibody response, *J. Exp. Med.,* 122, 517, 1965.
40. **McDevitt, H. O. and Chenitz, A.**, Genetic control of antibody response. Relationship between immune response and histocompatibility (H-2) type, *Science,* 163, 1207, 1969.
41. **McDevitt, H. O. and Benacerraf, B.**, Genetic control of specific immune responses, *Adv. Immunoo.,* 11, 31, 1969.
42. **McDevitt, H. O., Deak, B. D., Schreffler, D. C., Klein, J., Stimpfling, J. H. and Snell, G. D.**, Genetic control of the immune response. Mapping of the Ir. T locus, *J. Exp. Med.,* 135, 1259, 1972.
43. **Schreffler, D. C. and David, C. S.**, The H-2 major histocompatibility complex and the I immune response region. Genetic variations, function and organization, *Adv. Immunol.,* 207, 125, 1975.
44. **Ellman, L., Green, I., Martin, W. J., and Benacerraf, B.**, Linkage between the poly-L-lysine gene and the locus controlling the major histocompatibility antigens in strain 2 guinea pigs, *Proc. Nat. Acad. Sci. U.S.A.,* 66, 322, 1970.
45. **Lilly, F.**, The inheritance of susceptibility to the Gross leukemia virus in Mice, *Genetics,* 53, 529, 1966.
46. **Lilly, F.**, The influence of H-2 type on Gross virus leukemogenesis in mice, *Transplant. Proc.,* 3, 1239, 1971.
47. **McMichael, A. and McDevitt, H.**, The association between the HLA system and disease, *Prog. Med. Genet.,* 2, 39, 1977.
48. **Meruelo, D., Deak, B., and McDevitt, H. O.**, Genetic control of cell-mediated responsiveness to an AKR tumor-associated antigen. Mapping of the locus involved to the I region of the H-2 complex, *J. Exp. Med.,* 146, 1367, 1977.
49. **Walford, R. L., Waters, H., and Smith, G. S.**, Histocompatibility systems and neoplasia, in *RNA Viruses and Host Genome in Oncogenesis,* Emmelot, P. and Bentvelzen, P., Eds., American Elsevier, New York, 1972, 255.
50. **Thomas, L.**, Reactions to homologous tissue antigens and relation to hypersensitivity, in *Cellular and Humoral Aspects of the Hypersensitivity State,* Lawrence, H. S., Ed., Hoeker, New York, 1959, 529.
51. **Burnett, F. M.**, *Immunological Surveillance,* Pergamon Press, Oxford, 1970.
52. **Good, R. A. and Finstad, J.**, Essential relationship between the lymphoid system, immunity and malignancy, *Nat. Cancer Inst. Monogr.,* 31, 41, 1969.
53. **Gorer, P. A.**, The genetic and antigenic basis of tumor transplantation, *J. Pathol. Bacteriol.,* 44, 691, 1937.
54. **Williams, R. M., Dorf, M. E., and Benaceraff, B.**, H-2 linked genetic control of resistance to histocompatibility tumors, *Cancer Res.* 35, 1586, 1975.
55. **Germain, R. N., Dorf, M. E., and Benaceraff, B.**, Inhibition of T-lymphocyte-mediated tumor-specific lysis by alloantisera directed against the H-2 serological specificities of the tumor, *J. Exp. Med.,* 142, 1023, 1975.
56. **Prehn, R. T.**, Immunostimulation of the lymphodependent phase of neoplastic growth, *J. Nat. Cancer Inst.,* 59, 1043, 1977.
57. **Black, M. M.**, Cellular and biologic manifestations of immunogenicity in precancerous mastopathy, *Nat. Cancer Inst. Monogr.,* 35, 73, 1972.
58. **Ioachim, H. L.**, The stromal reaction of tumors: an expression of immune surveillance, *J. Nat. Cancer Inst.,* 57, 465, 1976.
59. **Clark, W. H., Mastrangelo, M. J., and Ainsworth, A. M.**, Current concepts in the biology of human cutaneous malignant melanoma, *Adv. Cancer Res.,* 24, 267, 1977.
60. **Old, L. J., Boyse, E. A., Clarke, D. A., and Carswell, E. A.**, Antigenic properties of chemically induced tumors, *Ann. N. Y. Acad. Sci.,* 101, 80, 1962.
61. **Bonmassar, A., Menconi, E., and Goldin, A.**, Escape of small numbers of allogeneic lymphoma cells from immune surveillance, *J. Nat. Cancer Inst.,* 53, 475, 1974.
62. **Kaliss, N.**, Immunological enhancement and inhibition of tumor growth: Relationship to various immunological mechanisms, *Fed. Proc.,* 24, 1024, 1965.
63. **Bashford, E. F., Murray, J. A., and Halland, M.**, General results of propagation of malignant new growth, *Rep. Imperial Cancer Res. Fund,* 3, 262, 1908.
64. **Southam, C. M., Brunschwig, A., Levin, A. G., and Dixon, S.**, Effect of leukocytes on transplantability of human cancer, *Cancer,* 19, 1743, 1975.
65. **Herbergman, R. B.**, Existence of tumor immunity in man, in *Mechanisms of Tumor Immunity,* Green, I., Cohen, S., and McCluskey, R. T., Eds., John Wiley & Sons, New York, 1977, 175.
66. **Spitler, L. E.**, Delayed hypersensitivity skin testing, in *Manual of Clinical Immunology,* Rose, N. R. and Friedman, H., Eds., American Society for Microbiology, Washington, D.C., 1976, chap. 6.

67. Wigzell, H., Quantitative titrations of mouse H-2 antibodies using ^{51}Cr-labeled target cells, *J. Infect. Dis.*, 102, 60, 1965.

68. Cohen, A. M., Burdick, J. F., and Ketcham, A. S. Cell-mediated cytotoxicity: an assay using ^{125}I-iododeoxyuridine-labeled target cells, *J. Immunol.*, 107, 895, 1971.

69. Takasugi, M., Mickey, M. R., and Terasaki, P. I., Reactivity of lymphocytes from normal persons on cultured tumor cells, *Cancer Res.*, 33, 2898, 1973.

70. Rosenberg, E. B., McCoy, J. L., Green, S. S., Donnelly, F. C., Siwarski, D. F., Levine, P. H., and Herberman, R. B., Destruction of human lymphoid tissue-culture cell lines by human peripheral blood lymphocytes in ^{51}-Cr-release cellular cytotoxicity assays, *J. Nat. Cancer Inst.*, 52, 345, 1974.

71. Pierce, G. E. and DeVald, B. L., Effect of human lymphocytes on cultured normal and malignant cells, *Cancer Res.*, 35, 1830, 1975.

72. Brooks, C. G., Studies on the microcytotoxicity test. III. Comparison of [^{75}Se] selenomethionine with [^{3}H] proline, ^{51}NaCrO$_4$ and ^{125}I-iododeoxyuridine for pre-labeling target cells in long-term cytotoxicity test, *J. Immunol. Methods*, 22, 23, 1978.

73. Burk, M. W., Yu, S., Ristow, S. S., and McKhann, C. F., Refractoriness of lymph-node cells from tumour-bearing animals, *Int. J. Cancer*, 15, 99, 1975.

74. Senik, A., Gomard, E., Plata, F., and Levy, J. P., Cell-mediated immune reaction against tumors induced by oncornaviruses. III. Studies by mixed lymphocyte-tumor reaction, *Int. J. Cancer*, 12, 233, 1973.

75. Gutterman, J. U., Mavligit, G., McCredie, K. B., Freireich, E. J., and Hersh, E. M., Auto-immunization with acute leukemia cells: demonstration of increased lymphocyte responsiveness, *Int. J. Cancer*, 11, 521, 1973.

76. Dean, J. H., McCoy, J. L., Lewis, D., Appello, E., and Law, L. W., Studies of lymphocyte stimulation by intact tumor cell and solubilized tumor antigen, *Int. J. Cancer*, 16, 465, 1975.

77. Rosenberg, E. B., Herberman, R. B., Levine, P. H., Halterman, R. H., McCoy, J. L., and Wunderlich, J. R., Lymphocyte cytotoxicity to leukemia associated antigens in identical twins, *J. Int. Cancer*, 9, 648, 1972.

78. Golub, S. H., Svedmyr, E. A. J., Hewetson, J. F., Klein, A., and Singh, S., Cellular reactions against Burkitt lymphoma cells. III. Effector cell activity of leukocytes stimulated *in vitro* with autochthonous cultured lymphoma cells, *Int. J. Cancer*, 10, 157, 1972.

79. Gutterman, J. U., Rossen, R. D., Butler, W. T., Immunoglobulins on tumor cells and tumor-induced blastogenesis in human acute leukemia, *N. Engl. J. Med.*, 288, 169, 1973.

80. Mavligit, G. M., Amkus, U., Gutterman, J. U., and Hersh, E. M., Antigen solubilized from human solid tumors: lymphocyte stimulation and cutaneous delayed hypersensitivity, *Nature London New Biol.*, 243, 188, 1973.

81. Venky, F., Stjernsward, J., Klein, A., and Nilsonne, V., Serum-mediated inhibition of lymphocyte stimulation by autochthonous human tumors, *J. Nat. Cancer Inst.*, 47, 95, 1971.

82. Rich, A. R. and Lewis, M. R., The nature of allergy in tuberculosis as revealed by tissue culture studies, *Bull. Johns Hopkins Hosp.*, 50, 115, 1932.

83. George, M. and Vaughn, J. H., *In vitro* cell migrations as a model for delayed hypersensitivity, *Proc. Soc. Exp. Biol.*, 111, 514, 1962.

84. David, J. R., Al-Askari, S., Lawrence, H. S., and Thomas, L. J., Delayed hypersensitivity *in vitro*. I. The specificity of inhibition of cell migration, *J. Immunol.*, 93, 264, 1964.

85. Bloom, B. R. and Bennett, B., Mechanism of a reaction *in vitro* associated with delayed-type hypersensitivity, *Science*, 153, 80, 1966.

86. Sorborg, M. and Bendixen, G., Human lymphoycte migration as a parameter of hypersensitivity, *Acta Med. Scand.*, 181, 247, 1967.

87. Clausen, J. E., Tuberculin-induced migration inhibition of human peripheral leukocytes in agarose medium, *Acta Allergol.*, 26, 56, 1971.

88. Anderson, V., Bendexin, G., and Schiodt, T., An *in vitro* demonstration of cellular immunity against autologous mammary carcinoma in man, *Acta Med. Scand.*, 186, 101, 1969.

89. McCoy, J. L., Jerome, L. F., Dean, J. H., Cannon, G. B., Alford, T. C., Doering, T., and Herberman, R. B., Inhibition of leukocyte migration by tumor-associated antigens in soluble extracts of human breast carcinoma, *J. Nat. Cancer Inst.*, 53, 11, 1974.

90. McCoy, J. L., Jerome, L. F., Dean, J. H., Perlin, E., Oldham, R. K., Char, D. H., Cohen, M. B., Felix, E. L., and Herberman, R. B., Leukocyte migration by tumor-associated antigens in soluble extracts of human malignant melanoma, *J. Nat. Cancer Inst.*, 55, 19, 1975.

91. Boddie, A. W., Jr., Holmes, E. C., Roth, J. A., and Morton, D. L., Inhibition of human leukocyte migration in agarose by KCl extracts of carcinoma of the lung, *Int. J. Cancer*, 15, 823, 1975.

92. Chee, D. O., Boddie, A. W., Jr., Roth, J. A., Holmes, E. C., and Morton, D. L., Production of melanoma-associated antigen(s) by a defined malignant melanoma cell strain grown in chemically defined medium, *Cancer Res.*, 36, 1503, 1976.

93. **Chee, D. O., Holmes, E. C., and Morton, D. L.,** Decreased correlation between the agarose leukocyte migration inhibition assay and delayed cutaneous hypersensitivity response to purified protein derivative in cancer patients, *J. Nat. Cancer Inst.,* 60, 769, 1978.

94. **Halliday, W. J., and Miller, S.,** Leukocyte adherence inhibition. A simple test for cell-mediated tumor immunity and serum blocking factors, *Int. J. Cancer,* 9, 477, 1972.

95. **Waldman, S. R. and Yonemoto, R. H.,** The use of cryopreserved lymphocytes in the leukocyte adherence inhibition assay. Evaluation of specificity of responses in cancer patients, *Int. J. Cancer,* 21, 542, 1978.

96. **Holan, V., Hasek, M., Bubenik, J., and Chutna, J.** Antigen-mediated macrophage adherence inhibition, *Cell. Immunol.,* 13, 107, 1974.

97. **Grosser, N. and Thomson, D. M. P.,** Cell-mediated anti-tumor immunity in breast cancer patients evaluated by antigen-induced leukocyte adherence inhibition in test tubes, *Cancer Res.,* 35, 2571, 1975.

98. **Marti, J. H., Grosser, N., and Thomson, D. M. P.,** Tube leukocyte adherence inhibition assay for detection of anti-tumor immunity. II. Monocyte reacts with tumor antigen via cytophilic anti-tumor antibody, *Int. J. Cancer,* 18, 48, 1976.

99. **Grosser, N. and Thomson, D. M. P.,** Tube leukocyte (monocyte) adherence inhibition assay for the detection of anti-tumor immunity. III. "Blockage" of monocyte reactivity by excess free antigen and immune complexes in advanced cancer patients, *Int. J. Cancer,* 18, 58, 1976.

100. **Holt, P. G., Roberts, L. M., Fimmel, P. J., and Keast, D.,** The LAI microtest: a rapid and sensitive procedurȩ for the demonstration of cell-mediated immunity *in vitro, J. Immunol. Methods,* 8, 277, 1975.

101. **Leveson, S. H., Howell, J. H., Holyoke, E. D., and Goldrosen, M. H.,** Leukocyte adherence inhibition: an automated microassay demonstrating specific antigen recognition and blocking activity in two murine tumor systems, *J. Immunol. Methods,* 17, 153, 1977.

102. **Russo, A. J., Douglass, H. O., Jr., Leveson, S. H., Howell, J. H., Holyoke, E. D., Harvey, S. R., Chu, T. M., and Goldrosen, M. H.,** Evaluation of the microleukocyte adherence inhibition assay as an immunodiagnostic test for pancreatic cancer, *Cancer Res.,* 38, 2023, 1978.

103. **Maluish, A. E. and Halliday, W. J.,** Quantitation of anti-tumor cell-mediated immunity by a lymphokine-dependent *in vitro* method using small volumes of blood, *Cell. Immunol.,* 17, 131, 1975.

104. **Grosser, N., Marti, J. H., Proctor, J. W., and Thomson, D. M. P.,** Tube leukocyte adherence inhibition assay for the detection of anti-tumor immunity. I. Monocyte is the reactive cell, *Int. J. Cancer,* 18, 39, 1976.

105. **Moller, E.,** Contact induced cytotoxicity by lymphoid cells containing foreign isoantigens, *Science,* 147, 873, 1965.

106. **Perlmann, P., Perlmann, H., and Wigzell, H.,** Lymphocyte mediated cytotoxicity *in vitro:* induction and inhibition of humoral antibody and nature of effector cells, *Transplant. Rev.,* 13, 91, 1972.

107. **MacLennan, I. C. M.,** Antibody in the induction and inhibition of lymphocyte cytotoxicity, *Transplant. Rev.,* 13, 67, 1972.

108. **Van Boxel, J. A., Stobo, J. D., Paul, W. E., and Green, I.,** Antibody dependent lymphoid cell-mediated cytotoxicity. No requirement for thymus-derived lymphocytes, *Science,* 175, 194, 1972.

109. **Greenberg, A. H., Hudson, L., Shen, L., and Roitt, I. M.,** Antibody-dependent cell-mediated cytotoxicity due to a "null" lymphoid cell, *Nature,* 242, 111, 1973.

110. **Larsson, A. and Perlmann, P.,** Study of Fab and F (ab')2 from rabbit IgG for capacity to induce lymphocyte mediated target cell destruction *in vitro, Int. Arch. Allergy Appl. Immunol.,* 43, 80, 1972.

111. **MacLennan, I. C. M. and Harding, B.,** Non-T cytotoxicity *in vitro, Prog. Immunol.,* 3, 347, 1974.

112. **Bier, A. M., Chess, L., and Schlossman, S. F.,** Human antibody dependent cellular cytotoxicity. Isolation and identification of a subpopulation of peripheral blood lymphocytes which kill antibody coated autologous target cells, *J. Clin. Invest.,* 56, 1580, 1975.

113. **Nelson, D. L., Bundy, B. M., Pitchon, H. E., Blaese, R. M., and Strober, W.,** The effector cells in human peripheral blood and mediating mitogen induced cellular cytotoxicity and antibody-dependent cellular cytotoxicity, *J. Immunol.,* 117, 1472, 1976.

114. **Pollack, S., Heppner, G., Brown, R. J., and Nelson, K.,** Specific killing of tumor cells *in vitro* in the presence of normal lymphoid cells and sera from hosts immune to the tumor antigens, *Int. J. Cancer,* 11, 138, 1973.

115. **Pollack, S.,** Specific " arming" of normal lymph node cells by sera from tumor-bearing mice, *Int. J. Cancer,* 11, 138, 1973.

116. **Hellström, I., Hellström, K. E., and Warner, G. A.,** Increase of lymphocyte-mediated tumor-cell destruction by certain patient sera, *Int. J. Cancer,* 12, 348, 1973.

117. **Hakala, T. R. and Lange, P. .,** Serum induced lymphoid cell mediated cytotoxicity to human transitional cell carcinomas of the genitourinary tract, *Science,* 184, 795, 1974.

118. Heppner, G., Henry, E., Stolbach, L., Cummings, F., McDonough, E., and Calabresi, P., Problems in clinical use of the microcytotoxicity assay for measuring cell-mediated immunity to tumor cells, *Cancer Res.,* 35, 1931, 1975.

119. Golub, S. H., Host immune response to human tumor antigens in *Cancer,* Vol. 4, Becker, F. F., Ed., Plenum Press, New York, 1975, 259.

120. Gorer, P. A. and O'Gorman, P., The cycotoxic activity of isoantibodies in mice, *Transplant. Bull.,* 3, 142, 1956.

121. Bloom, E. T., Quantitative detection of cytotoxic antibodies against tumor-specific antigens of murine sarcomas induced by 3-methylcholanthrene, *J. Nat. Cancer Inst.,* 45, 443, 1970.

122. Bloom, E. T. Further definition by cytotoxicity tests of cell surface antigens of human sarcomas in culture, *Cancer Res.,* 32, 960, 1972.

123. Lewis, M. G., Possible immunological factors in human malignant melanoma in Uganda, *Lancet,* 2, 921, 1967.

124. Lewis, M. G., Ikonopison, R. L., Nairn, R. C., Phillips, T. M., Hamilton-Fairley, G., Bedenham, D. C., and Alexander, P., Tumor-specific antibodies in human malignant melanoma and their relationship to the extent of disease, *Br. Med. J.,* 3, 547, 1969.

125. Bodurtha, H. J., Chee, D. O., Lancuis, J. F., Mastrangelo, M. J., and Prehn, R. T., Clinical and immunological significance of human melanoma cytotoxic antibody, *Cancer Res.,* 35, 189, 1975.

126. Eilber, F. R. and Morton, D. L., Immunologic studies of human sarcomas. Additional evidence suggesting an associated sarcoma virus, *Cancer,* 2, 588, 1976.

127. Sethi, J. and Hirshaut, Y., Complement-fixing antigen of human sarcomas, *J. Nat. Cancer Inst.,* 57, 489, 1976.

128. Eilber, F. R. and Morton, D. L., Sarcoma specific antigens: detection complement fixation with serum from sarcoma patients, *J. Nat. Cancer Inst.,* 44, 651, 1970.

129. Morton, D. L., Eilber, F. R., Malmgren, R. A., and Wood, W. C., Immunological factors which influence response to immunotherapy in malignant melanoma, *Surgery,* 68, 158, 1970.

130. Gupta, R. K. and Morton, D. L., Suggestive evidence for *in vivo* binding of specific antitumor antibodies of human melanomas, *Cancer Res.,* 35, 58, 1975.

131. Gupta, R. K., Irie, R. F., and Morton, D. L., Antigens on human tumor cells assayed by complement fixation with allogeneic sera, *Cancer Res.,* 38, 2579, 1978.

132. Gupta, R. K. and Morton, D. L., Detection of cancer associated antigen(s) in urine of sarcoma patients, *J. Surg. Oncol.,* 1979, in press.

133. Gupta, R. K. and Chee, D. O., unpublished data.

134. Gupta, R. K. and Morton, D. L., Tumor related immune complexes in sera from melanoma patients, *Fed. Proc.,* 37, 1595, 1978.

135. Shiku, H., Takahashi, T., Oettgen, H. F., and Old, L. J., Cell surface antigens of human malignant melanoma. II. Serological typing with immune adherence assays and definition of two new surface antigens, *J. Exp. Med.,* 144, 873, 1976.

136. Cornain, S. J., de Vries, J. E., Collard, J., Vennegoor, C., Wingerden, I. W., and Rumke, P., Antibodies and antigen expression in human melanoma detected by the immune adherence test, *Int. J. Cancer,* 16, 981, 1976.

137. Macher, E., Muller, C., Sorg, G., Gossen, A., and Sorg, C., Evidence for cross-reacting membrane associated antigens as detected by immunofluorescence and immune adherence, *Behring Inst. Mitt.,* 56, 86, 1975.

138. Mirie, R. F., Irie, K., and Morton, D. L., Natural antibody in human serum to a neoantigen in human cultured cells grown in fetal bovine serum, *J. Nat. Cancer Inst.,* 52, 1051, 1974.

139. Irie, K. Irie, R. F., and Morton, D. L., Evidence for *in vivo* reaction to antibody and complement to surface antigens of human cancer cells, *Science,* 186, 454, 1974.

140. Morton, D. L., Malmgren, R. A., Holmes, E. C., and Ketcham, A. S., Demonstration of antibodies against human malignant melanoma by immunofluorescence, *Surgery,* 64, 233, 1968.

141. Morton, D. L. and Malmgren, R. A., Human osteosarcoma: immunologic evidence suggesting an associated infectious agent, *Science,* 162, 1279, 1968.

142. Priori, E. S., Wilbur, J. R., and Dmochowski, L., Immunofluorescence test on sera of patients with osteogenic sarcoma, *J. Nat. Cancer Inst.,* 46, 1299, 1971.

143. Reilly, C. A., Jr., Pritchard, D. J., Biskis, B. O., and Finkal, M. P., Immunologic evidence suggesting a viral etiology of human osteosarcoma, *Cancer,* 30, 603, 1972.

144. Moore, M., Witherow, P. J., Price, C. H. G., and Clough, S. A., Detection by immunofluorescence of intracytoplasmic antigens in cell lines derived from human sarcomas, *Int. J. Cancer,* 12, 428, 1973.

145. Mukherji, B. and Hirsant, Y., Evidence for fetal antigen in human sarcoma, *Science,* 131, 440, 1973.

146. Saxton, R. E., Irie, R. F., Ferrone, S., Pellegrino, J. A., and Morton, D. L., Establishment of paired tumor cell and autologous virus-transformed cell lines to define humoral immune responses in melanoma and sarcoma patients, *Int. J. Cancer,* 21, 299, 1978.

147. **Holmes, E. C. and Morton, D. L.,** Detection of antibodies against the mammary tumor virus with the antiglobulin consumption test, *J. Nat. Cancer Inst.,*42, 733, 1969.
148. **Holmes, E. C. and Morton, D. L.,** Demonstration by the antiglobulin consumption test with murine antisera of common antigens in tissues infected with the mammary tumor virus from different mouse strains, *J. Nat. Cancer Inst.,* 46, 253, 1971.
149. **Irie, K., Irie, R. F., and Morton, D. L.,** Detection of antibody and complement complexed *in vivo* on membranes of human cancer cells by mixed hemadsorption technique, *Cancer Res.,* 35, 1244, 1975.
150. **Carey, T. E., Takahashi, T., Resnick, L. A., Oettgen, H. F., and Old, L. J.,** Cell surface antigens of human malignant melanoma: mixed hemadsorption assay for humoral immunity to cultured autologous melanoma cells, *Proc. Nat. Acad. Sci. U.S.A.,* 73, 3278, 1976.
151. **Sarcione, E. J.,** Synthesis and sequential appearance of alpha fetoprotein in carcinogen-fed rats, in *Cancer,* Vol. 2, Anderson, N. A., Coggin, J. H., Jr., Cole, E., and Holleman, J. W., Eds., Oak Ridge National Laboratory, Oak Ridge, Tennessee, 1972, 323.
152. **Gold, P. and Freedman, S. O.,** Demonstration of tumor-specific antigens in human colonic carcinomata by immunological tolerance and absorption technique, *J. Exp. Med.* 121, 439, 1965.
153. **Kithier, I., Al-Sarvab, M., and Cejka, J.,** Tumor-specific antigen (CEA) in tumor extracts and urine from cancer patients, in *Cancer,* Vol. 2, Anderson, N. G. et al., Eds., Oak Ridge National Laboratory, 1972, 225, 233.
154. **Old, L. J.,** Cell surface antigens of human malignant melanoma. Mixed hemadsorption assay for humoral immunity to cultured autologous melanoma cells, *Proc. Nat. Acad. Sci. U.S.A.,* 13, 3278, 1976.
155. **Yalow, R. S. and Berson, S. A.,** Immunoassay of endogenous plasma insulin in man, *J. Clin. Invest.,* 39, 1157, 1960.
156. **Thomson, D. M. P., Drupey, J., Freedman, S. O., and Gold, P.,** The radio-immunoassay of circulating carcinoembryonic antigen of the human digestive system, *Proc. Nat. Acad. Sci. U.S.A.,* 64, 161, 1969.
157. **Moore, T. L., Kupchik, H. Z., Marcon, N., and Zamcheck, N.,** Carcinoembryonic antigen assay in cancer of the colon and pancreas and other digestive tract disorders, *Am.J. Dig. Dis.,* 16, 1, 1971.
158. **Ruoslathi, E. and Seppala, M.,** Studies of carcino-fetal proteins. III. Development of a radioimmunoassay for α-fetoprotein. Demonstration of α-fetoprotein in serum of healthy human adults, *Int. J. Cancer,* 8, 374, 1971.
159. **Reiner, J. and Southam, C.,** Further evidence of common antigenic properties in chemically induced sarcomas of mice, *Cancer Res.,* 29, 1814, 1969.
160. **Economore, G. C., Takeichi, N., and Boone, C. W.,** Common tumor rejection antigens in methylcholanthrene-induced squamous cell carcinomas of mice detected by tumor protection and a radioisotopic footpad assay, *Cancer Res.,* 37, 37, 1977.
161. **Hellström, K. E., Hellström, I., and Brown, J. P.,** Unique and common tumor specific transplantation antigens of chemically induced mouse sarcomas, *Int. J. Cancer,* 21, 317, 1978.
162. **Baldwin, R. W.,** Immunological aspects of chemical carcinogenesis, in *Cancer, A Comprehensive Treatise,* Vol. 1, Becker, F. F., Ed., Plenum Press, New York, 1975, 1.
163. **Prehn, R. T.,** Tumor progression and homeostasis, in *Adv. Cancer Res.,* Vol. 23, 1975, 203.
164. **Prehn, R. T.,** Relationship of tumor immunogenicity to concentration of the oncogen, *J. Nat. Cancer Inst.,* 55, 189, 1975.
165. **Bartlett, G.,** Effect of host immunity on the antigenic strength of primary tumors, *J. Nat. Cancer Inst.,* 49, 493, 1972.
166. **Morton, D. L., Malmgren, R. A., Holmes, E. C., and Ketcham, A. S.,** Demonstration of antibodies against human malignant melanoma by immune fluorescence, *Surgery,* 64, 233, 1968.
167. **Oettgen, H. F., Aoki, T., Old, L. J., Boyse, E. A., DeHaven, E., and Milts, G. M.,** Suspension culture of a pigment-producing cell line derived from a human malignant melanoma, *J. Nat. Cancer Inst.,* 41, 827, 1968.
168. **Muna, N. M., Marcus, S., and Smart, C.,** Detection by immunofluorescence of antibodies specific for human melanoma cells, *Cancer,* 23, 88, 1969.
169. **Leong, S. P. L., Sutherland, C. M., and Krementz, E. T.,** Immunofluorescent detection of common melanoma membrane antigens by sera of melanoma patients immunized against autologous or allogeneic cultured melanoma cells, *Cancer Res.,* 37, 4035, 1977.
170. **Nairn, R. C., Nind, A. P. P., Guli, E. P. G., and Davies, D. J.,** Anti-tumor immunoreactivity in patients with malignant melanoma, *Med. J. Aust.,* 1, 397, 1972.
171. **Fossati, G., Colnaghi, M. I., Della Porta, G., Cascinelli, N., and Veronesi, U.,** Cellular and humoral immunity against human malignant melanoma, *Int. J. Cancer,* 9, 567, 1972.
172. **De Vries, J. E., Rumke, P., and Bernheim, J. L.,** Cytotoxic lymphocytes in melanoma patients, *Int. J. Cancer,* 9, 567, 1972.

173. Hellström, I., Hellström, K. E., Sjorgren, H. O., and Warner, G., Demonstration of cell-mediated immunity to human neoplasms of various histologic types, *Int. J. Cancer*, 7, 1, 1971.

174. The, T. H., Huiges, H A., Schaffrodt Koops, H., Lamberts, H. B., and Nieweg, H. O., Surface antigens on cultured malignant cells as detected by membrane immunofluorescence method with human sera. Lack of tumor-specific reactions on melanoma cell lines, *Ann. N. Y. Acad. Sci.*, 254, 528, 1975.

175. Seibert, E., Sorg, C., Happle, R., and Macher, ., Membrane associated antigens of human malignant melanoma. III. Specificity of human sera reacting with cultured melanoma cells, *Int. J. Cancer*, 19, 172, 1977.

176. Grimm, E. A., Silver, H. K. B., Chee, D. O., Gupta, R. K., and Morton, D. L,. Detection of tumor-associated antigen in human melanoma cell line supernatants, *Int. J. Cancer*, 17, 559, 1976.

177. Chee, D. O., Boddie, W., Jr., Roth, J. A., Holmes, E. C., and Morton, D. L., Production of a melanoma-associated antigen(s) by a human malignant cell strain grown in chemically defined medium, *Cancer Res.*, 36, 1503, 1976.

178. Thorpe, W. P. and Rosenberg, S. A., Identification of tumor specific antigens on human osteogenic sarcoma, *Proc. Am. Assoc. Cancer Res.*, 19, 107, 1978.

179. Wood, W. C. and Morton, D. L., Microcytotoxicity test. Detection in sarcoma patients of antibody cytotoxic to human sarcoma cells, *Science*, 170, 1318, 1970.

180. Eilber, F. R. and Morton, D. L., Sarcoma-specific antigens: detection by complement fixation with serum from sarcoma patients, *J. Nat. Cancer Inst.*, 44, 651, 1970.

181. Thorpe, W. P., Parker, G. A., and Rosenberg, S. A., Expression of fetal antigens by normal human skin cells grown in tissue culture, *J. Immunol.*, 119, 818, 1977.

182. Brawn, J., Possible association of embryonal antigen(s) with several primary 3-methylcholanthrene-induced murine sarcomas, *Int. J. Cancer*, 6,,245, 1970.

183. Baldwin, R. W. and Embleton, M. J., Tumor-specific antigens in 2-acetylamino-fluorene-induced rat hepatomas and related tumors, *Isr. J. Med. Sci.*, 7, 144, 1971.

184. Baldwin, R. W. and Glaves, D., Solubilization of tumor-specific antigen from plasma membrane of an aminoazo-dye-induced rat hepatoma, *Clin. Exp. Immunol.*, 11, 51, 1972.

185. Abelev, G. I., Perova, S. D., Khramkova, N. I., Postnikova, E. A., and Irlin, I. S., Production of embryonal α-globulin by transplantable mouse hepatomas, *Transplantation*, 1, 174, 1963.

186. Stanislawski-Birencwaig, M., Fraissinet, C., and Grabar, P., Embryonic antigens in liver tumors in rats, *Arch. Immunol. Mer. Exp.*, 14, 730, 1966.

187. Baldwin, R. W. and Barker, C. R., Antigenic comparison of transplanted rate hepatomas originally induced by 4-dimethylaminoazobenzene, *Br. J. Cancer*, 21, 338, 1967.

188. Gold P. and Freedman, S. O., Specific carcinoembryonic antigens of the human digestive system, *J. Exp. Med.*, 122, 467, 1965.

189. Kupchik, J. Z. and Zamcheck, N., Carcinoembryonic antigen(s) in liver diseases. Isolation from human cirrhotic liver and serum and fom normal liver, *Gastroenterology*, 63, 95, 1972.

190. Khoo, S. K., Warner, N. L., Lie, J. T., and MacKay, I. T., Carcinoembryonic antigenic activity of tissue extracts: quantitative study of malignant and benign neoplasms, cirrhotic liver, normal adult and fetal organs, *Int. J. Cancer*, 11, 681, 1973.

191. Pusztaszeri, G. and Mach, J. P., Carcinoembryonic antigen (CEA) in nondigestive cancerous and normal tissues, *Immunochemistry*, 10, 197, 1973.

192. Von Kleist, S., Chavanel, G., and Burtin, P., Identification of a normal antigen that cross reacts with the carcinoembryonic antigen, *Proc. Natl. Acad. Sci. U.S..*, 69, 2492, 1972.

193. Burtin, P., von Kleist, S., Sabine, M. C., and King, M., Immunohistological localization of carcinoembryonic antigen and nonspecific cross-reacting antigen in gastrointestinal normal and tumoral tissues, *Cancer Res.*, 33, 3299, 1973.

194. Goldenberg, D. M., Sharkey, R. M., and Premus, F. J., Carcinoembryonic antigen in histopathology: immunoperoxidase staining of conventional tissue sections, *J. Nat. Cancer Inst.*, 57, 11, 1976.

195. Isaacson, P. and Judd, M. A., Carcinoembryonic antigen (CEA) in the normal human small intestine: a light and electron microscopic study, *Gut*, 18, 786, 1977.

196. Collatz, E., von Kleist, S., and Burtin, P., Further investigations of circulating antibodies in colon cancer patients: on the autoantigenicity of the carcinoembryonic antigen, *Int. J. Cancer*, 8, 298, 1971.

197. Lo Gerfo, P., Herter, F. P., and Bennett, S. J., Absence of circulating antibodies to carcinoembryonic antigen in patients with gastrointestinal malignancies, *Int. J. Cancer*, 9, 344, 1972.

198. MacSween, J. M., The antigenicity of carcinoembryonic antigen in man, *Int. J. Cancer*, 15, 246, 1975.

199. Thomson, D. M. P., Krupey, U., Freedman, S. O., and Gold, P., The radioimmunoassay of circulating carcinoembryonic antigen of the human digestive system, *Proc. Nat. Acad. Sci. U.S.A.*, 64, 161, 1969.

200. **Lo Gerfo, P., Krupey, J., and Hansen, H. J.**, Demonstration of an antigen common to several varieties of neoplasia, *N. Engl. J. Med.*, 285, 138, 1971.
201. **Mach. J. P., Jaeger, P., Bertholet, M. M., Ruegsigger, C. H., Loosli, R. M., and Pettavd, J.**, Detection of recurrence of large-bowel carcinoma by radio-immunoassay of circulating carcinoembryonic antigen (CEA), *Lancet*, 2, 535, 1974.
202. **Gold, P., Krupey, J., and Ansari, H.**, Position of the carcinoembryonic antigen of the human digestive system in ultrastructure of tumor cell surface, *J. Nat. Cancer Inst.*, 45, 219, 1970.
203. **Bergstrand, C. G. and Czar, B.**, Demonstration of new protein in serum from the human fetus, *Scand. J. Clin. Lab. Invest.*, 8, 174, 1956.
204. **Tartarinov, Y. S.**, Content of embryo-specific alpha-globulin in the blood of human fetus, newborn, and adult man in primary cancer of liver, *Vopr. Med. Khim.*, 11, 20, 1965.
205. **Sell, S. and Becker, F. F.**, Alpha-fetoprotein, *J. Nat. Cancer Inst.*, 60, 19, 1978.
206. **Silver, H. K., Deneault, J., Gold, P., Thompson, G. W., Shuster, J., and Freedman, S. A.**, Detection of $_1$-fetoprotein in patients with viral hepatitis, *Cancer Res.*, 34, 244, 1974.
207. **Waldman, T. A. and McIntrie, K. R.**, Serum alpha-fetoprotein levels in patients with ataxia-telangiectasia, *Lancet*, 2, 1112, 1972.
208. **Stein, G. S., Stein, J. L., and Thomson, J. A.**, Chromosomal problems in transformed and neoplastic cells: a review, *Cancer Res.*, 38, 1181, 1979.
209. **Irie, R. F., Irie, K., and Morton, D. L.**, A membrane antigen common to human cancer and fetal brain tissues, *Cancer Res.*, 36, 3510, 1976.
210. **Gupta, R. K., Silver, H. K. B., Reisfeld, R. A., and Morton, D. L.**, Isolation and characterization of antitumor tumor antibodies from cancer patients' sera by affinity chromatography, *Proc. Am. Cancer Res.*, 19, 133, 1978.
211. **Edynak, E. M., Old, L. J., Vrana, M., and Lardis, M. P.**, A fetal antigen associated with human neoplasia, *N. Engl. J. Med.*, 286, 1178, 1972.
212. **Hakkinen, I., Jarvic, O., and Gronross, J.**, Sulphoglycoprotein antigens in human alimentary canal and gastric cancer. An immunohistological study, *Int. J. Cancer*, 3, 572, 1968.
213. **Hakkinen, I., Korhonen, L. K., and Saxon, L.**, The time appearance and distribution of sulphoglycoprotein antigens in the human fetal alimentary canal, *Int. J. Cancer*, 3, 582, 1968.
214. **Hakkinen, I. and Vikari, S.** Occurrence of fetal sulphoglycoprotein antigen in the gastric juice of patients with gastric diseases, *Ann. Surg.*, 169, 277, 1968.
215. **Buffe, D., Rimbaut, C., Lemerle, J., Schweisguth, O., and Burtin, P.**, Presence of a ferroprotein of tissular origin, the $\alpha 2$ H-globulin, in sera of children with tumors, *Int. J. Cancer.*, 5, 85, 1970.
216. **Fritsche, R. and Mach, J. P.**, Identification of a new oncofetal antigen associated with several types of human carcinomas, *Nature*, 258, 734, 737, 1975.
217. **Sjorgren, H. O., Hellstrom, I., and Klein, G.**, Transplantation of polyoma virus-induced tumors in mice, *Cancer Res.*, 21, 329, 1961.
218. **Smith, R. T.**, Tumor-specific immune mechanisms, *N. Engl. J. Med.*, 278, 1207, 1968.
219. **Old, L. J. and Boyse, E. A.** Antigens of tumors and leukemias induced by virus, *Fed. Proc.*, 24, 1009, 1965.
220. **Ambrose, K. R., Anderson, N. G., and Coggin, J. H.**, Interruption of SV_{40} oncogenesis with human foetal antigen, *Nature London*, 233, 194, 1971.
221. **Coggin, J. H., Ambrose, K. R., Bellomy, B. B., and Anderson, N. G.** Tumor immunity in hamsters immunized with fetal tissues, *J. Immunol.*, 107, 526, 1971.
222. **Pasternak, G.**, Antigens induced by the mouse leukemia viruses, *Adv. Cancer Res.*, 12, 1, 1969.
223. **Kobayashi, H.**, An approach to the immunological regression of the tumor, *Acta Pathol. Japn.*, 20, 441, 1970.
224. **Boone, C. W. and Blackman, K.**, Augmented immunogenicity of tumor cell homogenates infected with influenza virus, *Cancer Res.*, 32, 1018, 1972.
225. **Stutman, O.**, Immunodepression and malignancy, *Adv. Cancer Res.*, 22, 261, 1975.
226. **Baldwin, R. W.**, Tumor-specific immunity against spontaneous rat tumours, *Int. J. Cancer*, 1, 257, 1964.
227. **Hammond, W. G., Fisher, F. C., and Rolley, R. T.** Tumor-specific transplantation immunity to spontaneous mouse tumors, *Surgery*, 62, 124, 1967.
228. **Revesz, L.**, Detection of antigenic differences in isologous host-tumor systems by pretreatment with heavily irradiated tumor cells, *Cancer Res.*, 20, 443, 1960.
229. **Peters, L. J.**, Enhancement of syngeneic murine tumour transplant ability by whole body irradiation — a nonimmunological phenomenon, *Br. J. Cancer*, 31, 293, 1975.
230. **Hewitt, H. B., Blake, E. R., Walder, A. S.**, A critique of the evidence for active host defense against cancer, based on personal studies of 27 murine tumours of spontaneous origin, *Br. J. Cancer*, 33, 241, 1976.

231. **Prehn, R. T.,** Tumor-specific immunity to transplanted dibenz a,h-anthracene-induced sarcoma, *Cancer Res.,* 20, 1641, 1960.
232. **Carswell, E. A., Wanebo, H. J., Old, L. J., and Boyse, E. A.,** Immunogenic properties of reticulum-cell sarcomas of SJL/J mice, *J. Nat. Cancer Inst.,* 44, 1281, 1970.
233. **Basambrio, M. A. and Prehn, R. T.** Antigenic diversity of tumors chemically induced within the progeny of a single cell, *Int. J. Cancer,* 10, 19, 1972.
234. **Lappé, M. A.,** Evidence for the antigenicity of papillomas induced by 3-methylcholanthrene, *J. Nat. Cancer Inst.,* 40, 823, 1968.
235. **Prehn, R. T. and Slemmer, G. L.,** The role of immunity as a homeostatic mechanism during onco-genesis, in *Endogenous Factors Influencing Host-Tumor Balance,* Wissler, R. W., Dao, T. L., and Wood, S., Eds., University of Chicago Press, Chicago, 1967, 185.
236. **Kouri, R. E., Salerno, R. A., and Whitmire, C. E.,** Relationships between aryl hydrocarbon hydrox-ylase inducibility and sensitivity to chemically induced subcutaneous sarcomas in various strains of mice, *J. Nat. Cancer Inst.,* 50, 363, 1973.
237. **Thomas, P. E., Kouri, R. E., and Hutton, J. J.,** The genetics of aryl hydrocarbon hydroxylase induction in mice: a single gene difference between C57BL/6 and DBA/2J, *Biochem. Genet.,* 6, 157, 192.
238. **Haughton, G. and Whitmore, H. C.,** Genetics, the immune response and oncogenesis, *Transplant. Rev.,* 28, 75, 2976.
239. **McKhann, D. G.,** The effect of X-ray on the antigenicity of donor cells in transplantation immunity, *J. Immunol.,* 92, 811, 1964.
240. **Kronman, B. S., Wepsic, H., and Churchill, W.,** Immunotherapy of cancer: an experimental model in syngeneic guinea pigs, *Science,* 168, 257, 1970.
241. **Eilber, F. R., Holmes, E., and Morton, D. L.,** Immunotherapy experiments with a methylcholan-threne-induced guinea pig liposarcoma, *J. Nat. Cancer Inst.,* 46, 803, 1971.
242. **Mathe, G., Ponillart, P., and Lapeyraque, F.** Active immunotherapy of L-1210 leukemia applied after the graft of tumor cells, *Br. J. Cancer.,* 23, 814, 1969.
243. **Ellman, L., and Green, I.,** L_2C guinea pig leukemia: immunoprotection and immunotherapy, *Cancer,* 28, 647, 1971.
244. **Czajkowski, N., Rosenblatt, M., and Cushing, F. R.,** Production of active immunity to malignant neoplastic tissue, *Cancer,* 19, 749, 1966.
245. **Martin, W., Wunderlich, J., Fletcher, F., and Inman, J. K.,** Enhance immunogenicity of chemically-coated syngeneic tumor cells, *Proc. Nat. Acad. Sci. U.S.A.,* 68, 469, 1971.
246. **Apffel, G. A., Arnason, B., and Peters, J. H.,** Induction of tumor immunity with tumour cells treated with iodoacetate, *Nature,* 209, 696, 1966.
247. **Prager, M. D., Derr, I., Swann, A., and Cotropia, J.,** Immunization with chemically modified lym-phoma cells, *Cancer Res.* 31, 1488, 1971.
248. **Bagshawe, K. D. and Currie, G.,** Immunogenicity of L-1210 murine leukemia cells after treatment with neuraminidase, *Nature,* 218, 1254, 1968.
249. **Simmons, R. L., Rios, A., and Kersey, J. H.,** Regression of spontaneous mammary carcinomas using direct injections of neuraminidase and BCG, *J. Surg. Res.* 12, 57, 1972.
250. **Bekesi, J. G., Robot, J. P., Walter, L., and Holland, J. F.** Stimulation of specific immunity against cancer by neuraminidase-treated tumor cells, *Behringwerk Mitt.,* 55, 309, 1974.
251. **Kollmorgen, G. M., Killion, J. J., Sansing, W. A., and Cantrell, J. L., Bundren, J. C., and LeFever, A. V.,** Immunotherapy with neuraminidase-treated cells and BCG, *Surgery,* 79, 202, 1976.
252. **Mikulska, Z., Smith, C., and Alexander, P.,** Evidence for an immunological reaction of the host against its own actively growing primary tumor, *J. Nat. Cancer Inst.,* 36, 29, 1966.
253. **Delorme, E. J. and Alexander, P.,** Treatment of primary fibrosarcoma in the rat with immune lym-phocytes, *Lancet,* 2, 117, 1964.
254. **Alexander, P.,** Immunotherapy of cancer: experiments with primary tumors and syngeneic tumor grafts, *Prog. Exp. Tumor Res.,* 10, 22, 1968.
255. **Vadlamudi, S., Padarathsingh, R., Bonmassar, E., and Goldin, A.,** Effect of combination treatment with cyclophosphamide and isogeneic or allogeneic spleen and bone marrow cells in leukemia (L1210—mice, *Int. J. Cancer,* 7, 160, 1970.
256. **Alexander, P., Delorme, E. J., and Hall, J. G.** The effect of lymphoid cells from the lympho of specifically immunized sheep on the growth of primary sarcomata in rats, *Lancet,* 1, 1186, 1966.
257. **Mihich, E.,** Combined effects of chemotherapy and immunity against leukemia L1210 in DBA/2 mice, *Cancer Res.,* 29, 848, 1969.
258. **Fefer, A.,** Adoptive chemoimmunotherapy of a Moloney lymphoma, *Int. J. Cancer,* 8, 364, 1971.
259. **Fass, L. and Fefer, A.,** Studies of adoptive chemoimmunotherapy of a Friend virus-induced lym-phoma, *Cancer Res.,* 32, 997, 1972.

260. **Mannick, J. A. and Eddahl. R. H.**, Transformation of nonimmune lymph node cells to state of transplantation immunity by RNA: a preliminary report, *Ann. Surg.*, 156, 356, 1962.
261. **Alexander, P., Delorme, E. J., Hamilton, L. D. G., and Hall, J. G.**, Effect of nucleic acids from immune lymphocytes of rat sarcomata, *Nature*, 213, 569, 1967.
262. **Pilch, Y. H., Fritze, D., and Kern, D.**, Immune RNA in the immunotherapy of cancer, *Med. Clin. North Am.*, 60, 567, 1967.
263. **Paque, R. E., Meltzer, M., Zbar, B., Rapp, H., and Dray, H.**, Transfer of tumor-specific delayed cutaneous hypersensitivity *in vitro* to normal guinea pig peritoneal exudate cells using RNA extracts from sensitized lymphoid tissues, *Cancer Res.*, 33, 3165, 1973.
264. **Schlager, S I., Paque, R. E., and Dray, W.**, Complete and apparently specific local tumor regression using syngeneic or xenogeneic tumor immune RNA extract, *Cancer Res.*, 35, 1907, 1975.
265. **Wright, P. W., Hellström, K. D., Hellström, I., and Bernstein, I. D.** Serotherapy of malignant disease, *Med. Clin. North Am.*, 60, 607, 1976.
266. **Pulmann, P., Perlmann, H., and Wigzell, H.**, Lymphocyte-mediated cytotoxicity *in vitro*: induction and inhibition by humoral antibodies and nature of effector cells, *Transplant. Rev.*, 13, 91, 1972.
267. **Lamon, E. W., Skurzak, A. M., Klein, E., and Wigzell, H.**, The lymphocyte response to primary Moloney sarcoma virus tumors in BALB/c mice. *J. Exp. Med.*, 137, 1472, 1973.
268. **Gorer, P. and Amos, D. B.**, Passive immunity of mice against C57BL leukosis EL-4 by means of 180 immune serum, *Cancer Res.*, 16, 338, 1956.
269. **Motta, R.**, Passive immunotherapy of murine leukemia. I. The production of antisera against leukemic antigens, *Eur. J. Clin. Biol. Res.*, 15, 161, 1970.
270. **Old, L., Stockert, E., Boyse, E. A., and Geering, G.**, A study of passive immunization against a transplanted G + leukemia with specific antiserum, *Proc. Soc. Exp. Biol. Med.*, 124, 63, 1967.
271. **Law, L. W., Ting, R., and Stanton, M.**, Some biologic, immunogenic, morphologic effects in mice after infection with a murine sarcoma virus: biologic and immunogenic studies, *J. Nat. Cancer Inst.*, 40, 1101, 1068.
272. **Bubenik, J., Turano, A., and Fadda, G.**, Prevention of carcinogenesis by murine sarcoma virus (Harvey) following injection of immune sera during the latent period, *Int. J. Cancer*, 4, 648, 1969.
273. **Fefer, A.**, Immunotherapy and chemotherapy of Moloney sarcoma virus-induced tumors in mice, *Cancer Res.*, 29, 2177, 1969.
274. **Motta, R.**, Passive immunotherapy of leukemia and other cancer, *Adv. Cancer Res.*, 14, 161, 1971.
275. **Yashphe, D. J.**, Immunological factors in nonspecific stimulation of host resistance to syngeneic tumors: a review, *Isr. J. Med. Sci.*, 7, 90, 1971.
276. **Old, L. J., Benaceraff, B., Clarke, D. A., Carswell, E. A., and Stockhert, E.**, The role of the reticuloendothelial system in the lost reaction to neoplasia, *Cancer Res.*, 21, 1281, 1961.
277. **Mathe, G., Amiel, J. L., Schwarzenberg, R., Schndier, M., Coltan, A., Schlumberger, J. R., Hayat, M., and deVassal, F.**, Active immunotherapy for acute lymphoblastic leukemia, *Lancet*, 1, 697, 1969.
278. **Morton, D. L., Eilber, F. R., Malmgren, R. A., and Wood, W. C.**, Immunological factors which influence response to immunotherapy in malignant melanoma, *Surgery*, 68, 158, 1970.
279. **Zbar, B., Bernstein, I. D., and Rapp, H. J.**, Suppression of tumor growth at the site of infection with living Bacillus Calmette-Guerin, *J. Nat. Cancer Inst.*, 46, 831, 1971.
280. **Weiss, D. W., Bonhag, R. S., and Leslie, P.**, Studies on the heterologous immunogenicity of methanol-insoluble fraction of attenuated tubercle bacilli (BCG). II. Protection against tumor isografts, *J. Exp. Med.*, 124, 1039, 1966.
281. **Mikulski, S. M. and Muggia, F. M.**, The biologic activity of MER-BCG in experimental systems and preliminary clinical studies, *Caner Treatment Rev.*, 4, 103, 1977.
282. **Zbar, B., Ribi, E., Meyer, T., Azuma, I., and Rapp, H. J.**, Immunotherapy of cancer: regression of established intradermal tumors after intralesional injection of Mycobacterial cell walls attached to oil droplets, *J. Nat. Cancer Inst.*, 52, 1571, 1974.
283. **Baldwin, R. W. and Pimm, M. V.**, BCG immunotherapy of local subcutaneous growths and postsurgical pulmonary metastases of a transplanted rat epithelioma of spontaneous origin, *Int. J. Cancer.*, 12, 420, 1973.
284. **Sparks, F. C., O'Connell, T. X., Lee, Y. T., and Breeding, J. H.**, BCG therapy given as an adjunct to surgery. Prevention of death from metastases from mammary adenocarcinoma in rats, *J. Nat. Cancer Inst.*, 53, 1825, 1974.
285. **Hanna, M. G., Jr., Peters, L. C., and Fidler, I. J.**, The efficacy of BCG-induced tumor immunity in guinea pigs with regional and systemic malignancy, *Cancer Immunol. Immunother.*, 1, 171, 1976.
286. **Chee, D. O. and Bodurtha, A. J.** Facilitation and inhibition of B16 melanoma by BCG in vivo and by lymphoid cells from BCG-treated mice in vitro, *Int. J. Cancer*, 14, 137, 1974.
287. **Sparks, F. C. and Breeding, J. H.**, Tumor regression and tumor enhancement from immunotherapy with Bacillus Calmette-Guerin (BCG) and neuraminidase, *Cancer Res.*, 34, 3262, 1974.

288. Wepsic, H. T., Harris, S., Sander, J. Alaimo, J., and Morris, H., Enhancement of tumor growth following immunization with Bacillus Calmette-Guerin cell walls, *Cancer Res.*, 36, 1950, 1976.

289. Likhite, V. V. and Halpern, B. N., Lasting rejection of mammary adenocarcinoma cell tumors in DBA/2 mice with intratumor injection of killed *Corynebacterium parvum, Cancer Res.*, 34, 341, 1974.

290. Woodruff, M. F. A., Dunbar, N., and Ghaffar, A. The growth of tumors in T-cell deprived mice and their response to treatment with *Corynebacterium parvum, Proc. Roy. Soc. London Ser. B*, 184, 97, 1973.

291. Levy, H., Law, L. W., and Rabson, A., Inhibition of tumor growth by polyinosinic-polycytidylic acid. *Proc. Nat. Acad. Sci. U.S.A.*, 62, 357, 1969.

292. Grelboin, H. V. and Levy, H., Polyinosinic-polycytidylic acid inhibits chemically induced tumoringenesis in mouse skin, *Science*, 167, 205, 1970.

293. Field, A., Tytell, A., Lampson, G., and Hilleman, M. R., Inducers of interferon and host resistance. II. Multistranded synthetic polynucleotide complexes, *Proc. Nat. Acad. Sci. U.S.A.*, 58, 1004, 1967.

294. Chihara, G., Hamuro, J., and Maeda, Y., Antitumor polysaccharide derived chemically from natural glucan (Pachyman), *Nature*, 225, 943, 1970.

295. Maeda, Y. and Chihara, G., Lantinan, a new immuno-accelerator of cell-mediated responses, *Nature*, 229, 634, 1971.

296. Hamura, J., Yamashita, Y., and Oshaka, Y., Carboxymethylpachymanan, a new water soluble polysaccharide with marked antitumor activity, *Nature*, 233, 486, 1971.

297. Morton, D. L. and Wells, S. A., Jr., Immunobiology and immunotherapy of nepolastic disease, in *Davis Christopher Textbook of Surgery, The Biological Basis of Modern Surgical Practice*, 11th ed., Sabiston, D. C., Jr., Ed., W. B. Saunders, Philadelphia, 1977, chap. 23.

298. Pilch. Y. H., Myers, G. H., Sparks, F. S. and Golub, S. H., Prospects for immunotherapy of cancer II. Current status of immunotherapy, *Curr. Prob. Surg.*, 1, 61, 1975.

299. Terry, W. D., Symposium on immunotherapy in malignant diseases, *Med. Clin. North Am.*, 60, 387, 1976.

300. Rosenberg, S. A. and Terry, W. D., Passive immunotherapy of cancer in animals and man, *Adv. Cancer Res.*, 25, 323, 1977.

301. Gutterman, J. U., Cancer systemic active immunotherapy today — prospects for tomorrow, *Cancer Immunol. Immunother.*, 2, 1, 1977.

302. Goodnight, J. E. and Morton, D. L., Immunotherapy for malignant disease, *Ann. Rev. Med.*, 29, 231, 1978.

303. Hersh, E. M., Mavligit, G. M., Gutterman, J. U., and Richman, S. P. Immunotherapy of human cancer, in *Cancer: A Comprehensive Treatise*, Vol. 6, Becker, F. F., Ed., Plenum Press, New York, 1977, 425.

304. Morton, D. L., Clinical trial comparing no further therapy to BCG or BCG plus allogeneic cells in stage II melanoma, in *Immunotherapy of Cancer: Present Status of Trials in Man*, Terry, W. D. and Windhorst, D., Eds., Raven Press, New York, 1978, in press.

305. Townsend, C. M., Jr., Eilber, F. R., Morton, D. L., Skeletal and soft tissue sarcomas: treatment with adjuvant immunotherapy, *J. Am. Med. Assoc.*, 236, 2187, 1976.

306. Coley, W. B., Treatment of bone sarcoma, *Cancer Rev.*, 4, 425, 1929.

307. Morton, D. L., Eilber, F. R., Holmes, E. C., Hunt, J. S., Ketcham, A. S., Silverstein, M. J., and Sparks, F. C., BCG immunotherapy of malignant melanoma: summary of a seven year experience, *Ann. Surg.*, 180, 635, 1974.

308. Eilber, F. R., Morton, D. L., Holmes, E. C., Sparks, F. C., and Ramming, K. P., Adjuvant immunotherapy with BCG in treatment of regional lymph node metastases from malignant melanoma, *N. Engl. J. Med.*, 294, 237, 1976.

309. Sumner, W. C. and Foraker, A. C., Spontaneous regression of human melanoma, clinical and experimental study, *Cancer*, 13, 79, 1960.

310. Nadler, S. H. and Moore, G. E., Clinical immunologic study of malignant disease, response to tumor transplants and transfer of lymphocytes, *Ann. Surg.*, 164, 482, 1966.

311. Krementz, E. T. and Samuels, M. T., Tumor cross-transplantation and cross-transfusion in the treatment of advanced malignant disease, *Bull. Tulane Univ. Med. Fac.*, 26, 263, 1967.

312. Yonemoto, R. H. and Terasaki, P. I., Cancer immunotherapy with HLA-compatible thoracic duct lymphocyte transplantation. A preliminary report, *Cancer*, 30, 1438, 1972.

313. Yonemoto, R. H., Adoptive immunotherapy utilizing thoracic duct lymphocytes, *Ann. N. Y. Acad. Sci.*, 277, 7, 1976.

314. Lo Buglio, A. F. and Neidhart, J. A., Transfer factor: a potential agent for cancer therapy, *Med. Clin. North Am.*, 60, 585, 1976.

315. **Ramming, K. P., de Kernion, J. B., and Pilch, Y. H.**, Immunotherapy of cancer with immune RNA: current status, in *Handbook of Cancer and Immunology,* Waters, H., Ed., Garland Publishers, New York, 1972.

316. **Oettgen, H. F.**, Immunotherapy of cancer, *N. Engl. J. Med.,* 297, 484, 1977.

317. **Keller, R.**, Cytostatic elimination of syngeneic rat tumor cells *in vitro* by nonspectifically activated macrophages, *J. Exp. Med.,* 138, 625, 1973.

318. **Fisher, B. and Saffer, E. A.**, Tumor cell cytotoxicity by granulocytes from peripheral blood of tumor-bearing mice, *J. Nat. Cancer Inst.,* 60, 687, 1978.

319. **Chee, D. O., Townsend, C. M., Galbraith, M. A., Eilber, F. R., and Morton, D. L.**, Selective reduction of human tumor cell populations by human granulocytes *in vitro, Cancer Res.,* 38, 4534, 1978.

320. **Apple, M. A.**, New anticancer drug design: past and future strategies, in *Cancer, A Comprehensive Treatise,* Vol. 5, Becker, F. F., Ed., Plenum Press, New York, 1977, 559.

Chapter 7

HOST—ENVIRONMENTAL INTERACTION AND CARCINOGENESIS IN MAN

Henry T. Lynch, Patrick M. Lynch, and Hoda A. Guirgis*

TABLE OF CONTENTS

*   We are deeply appreciative of the support received by the Council for Tobacco Research — U.S.A., Inc., Grants No. 941A and 1132; the Fraternal Order of Eagles Cancer Fund; and for the highly dedicated technical assistance provided by Mrs. Mary Bourque in the preparation of this manuscript.

INTRODUCTION

The fundamental mechanisms of carcinogenesis involve differential responses of the host to chemical and physical carcinogens. Therefore, the comprehension of those stochastic events at the interface of the genetic code and specific structural and physical characteristics of carcinogens should allow us to one day decipher crucial information about carcinogenesis at the molecular level. Consequently, the oft-quoted statement that "80 to 90% of all cancer is environmental" can be rather misleading in that it can readily be interpreted to imply that 80 to 90% of the many tumor types are solely induced by environmental agents, while the remaining 10 to 20% have no environmental basis. A more complete statement of the environmental role in carcinogenesis would emphasize the fact that while in a given population, the environment is the dominant etiologic agent in most occurrences of a given tumor type, the exogenous contribution at the individual level may actually range from practically none (as in familial retinoblastoma)[1] to practically all (such as in β-naphthylamine-induced bladder cancer in aniline dye workers).[2]

In the monograph series, *The Evaluation of Carcinogenic Risk of Chemicals to Man*, sponsored by the International Agency for Research on Cancer (IARC), a total of 368 chemicals were evaluated.[3,4] Of these, 26 chemicals or industrial processes showed a positive association between exposure and the occurrence of cancer in humans. In 221 chemicals, there was some evidence of carcinogenicity in at least one species of experimental animal. However, epidemiological studies and case reports evaluating their carcinogenic risk to humans either did not exist or were inconclusive.

Studies of chemical carcinogenesis in animals, as well as descriptive epidemiologic investigations of the subject in humans, consistently show nonuniform responses to a given carcinogen (i.e., cancer yield) not only between species, but within species. Even within highly inbred strains only relatively few of the animals exposed to controlled dosages of supposed carcinogens develop cancer, a factor which suggests the importance of the following: (1) variation in genetic susceptibility to cancer within membership of any highly inbred strain: (2) peculiarities in the interaction of genetic-environmental factors within a given host; (3) differences in delivery of the chemical (carcinogen) and the response to same in each given animal relevant to induction and/or enhancement (promotion) of tumor production; and finally (4) animal experimentation, utilizing the "pure" form of a given carcinogen, is in no way comparable to the actual experiences in man. Hence, any deductions made from carcinogenesis experiments in animals relevant to specific carcinogens must harbor serious limitations when extrapolations are given to humans. For example, uncontaminated asbestos (magnesium silicate) can be administered to animals via several routes and in quantifiable amounts.[5] In man the exposure will be to "dirty" compounds and mixtures involving polycyclic hydrocarbons, and other particulate matter, i.e., the shipyard where workers' experience exposure to oily products containing asbestos and myriad other substances. But in this context, the presence of asbestos *and* likely cocarcinogens still leads to only a relatively small fraction of the exposed population being afflicted with asbestos-related malignant neoplasm (mesotheliomas, bronchogenic carcinomas, colon cancer).

This particular frame of reference bearing on carcinogens and cancer occurrence has immediate implications for many human problems. For example, of the many thousands of fetuses exposed to diethylstilbesterol, only a miniscule number have developed clear-cell adenocarcinoma of the vagina or cervix. Of the millions of women on estrogen contraceptive agents and/or who have received estrogens for treatment of menopausal and postmenopausal problems, only a relatively small proportion developed endometrial carcinoma. Of the many individuals exposed to vinyl chloride in the plastic industries, only a fraction developed angiosarcoma of the liver. Of the millions of individuals who are heavy smokers, only a relatively small proportion develop bronchogenic carcinoma and other smoking-associated disorders. Thus a rather limited number of exposed humans develop the malignant neoplastic lesions generally associated with a specific carcinogen. The question is, "What characteristics of these cancer-affected individuals distinguishes them from the majority of their peers who have the same, or even greater, exposure to carcinogens, but who remain free of cancer?" We suggest, as have many others over the decades, that genetic factors exist which predispose certain individuals to the action of specific carcinogen(s), and that the resulting malignant neoplastic lesion is invariably a function of genetic and environmental (carcinogen) interaction.

In this chapter, we shall review the general methods and substantive findings of investigations which have attempted to grapple with the exceedingly complex matter of assessing host-environment interaction in carcinogenesis. Although reference will be made to experimental models involving infra-human species, primary attention will be devoted to variable genetic response to dietary, pharmacological, and other chemical agents in human cancer. Attention will also be given to biomarkers of cancer-susceptibility.

A. Animal Studies

Because of the difficulty in selecting and using a human population which responds uniformly to a given environmental insult, practically all existing information that purports to quantify genetic and environmental interaction in cancer has been gleaned from studies at the infra-human level, particularly studies of inbred strains of laboratory mice. Since C. C. Little first established the DBA strain of inbred mice in 1909, more than 70 strains of homozygous mice have been bred for studies of carcinogenesis. In certain of these strains such as BALB/C, we find a high incidence of mammary tumors and hepatomas. Conversely tumor resistance is manifested in C57 Black, in which only a few mammary or pulmonary tumors develop spontaneously.[6] Utilizing such strains as these, investigators are provided an invaluable resource for experiments which manipulate host and environmental factors.[7] Utilizing extreme caution, one might make certain extrapolations from these observations to carcinogenesis in man.

B. General Epidemiologic Methods of Assessing Genetic and Environmental Factors in Human Carcinogenesis

Traditionally, the environmental role in tumorigenesis involving a particular target organ in man has been demonstrated through the epidemiologic method of comparing cancer incidence (per person years of observation) in populations having high and low rates for the particular malignancy.[8] When substantial differences in incidence occur between populations, such variation is properly attributed to deleterious environmental agents which are present in high-risk areas and absent in low-risk areas. The figures quoted at the outset (80 to 90% of cancers are environmental) have been generated by first regarding the incidence in lowest risk to be of primarily nonenvironmental etiology; the environmentally-induced proportion is then construed to be the difference in rates between the highest risk areas and such low-risk geographies.[9,10] However, when there is substantial evidence of within-group variation (i.e., not all members of an exposed class develop the disease), as is almost invariably the situation in cancer epidemiologic studies, unifactorial etiologic models are clearly inadequate. In other words, demonstration of an association between a given carcinogen and its correlated malignancy on a population basis tells us only part of what we need to know about the sequence of events that comprise tumorigenesis at the individual level. One could postulate the action of additional, unknown deleterious agents which affect certain members of a class that is otherwise relatively homogeneous in its exposures. Differentially occurring protective agents could achieve the same effect. Of course variability in host-susceptibility, the main theme of this report, can also account for a significant fraction of such variability. Examples of this epidemiologic approach will be discussed subsequently.

The study of host-environmental interaction in humans can best be facilitated by utilizing populations at homogeneous genetic risk, since such populations most closely approximate the inbred animal models upon which some of our most specific information on mechanisms of genetic-environmental interaction in carcinogenesis have been based. The nearest we can come to the approximation of the animal model is through the study of identical twins. Indeed, twin registries have proven to be of great value to the cancer epidemiologist and geneticist.

Individuals at risk for simply inherited cancer predisposing traits, such as familial polyposis coli, xeroderma pigmentosum, and the multiple nevoid basal cell carcinoma syndrome, familial retinoblastoma, and others, also can be utilized for studies of host-environmental interaction. Unfortunately, retrospective study of such populations suffers from the limited recall of living patients as to specific environmental exposures and dietary practices which may have modified expression of the genes involved; sampling for the study of biomarkers in living relatives over more than three or four generations of a family is impossible, and the variable ages and environments of available subjects complicate interpretation of such data. More will be said of the role of family studies, a method our group has relied on heavily.

Another traditional approach to assessing host-environmental interaction has been to compare the frequency of cancer affected first-degree relatives in the families of a series of cancer patients with the families of age- and sex-matched groups of controls.[11] Such case-control studies have generally yielded significant familial aggregation only when limited to a particular histologic variety of cancer in the proband and relatives.[12] However, any such simple classification based on "cancer in the family" rightly suffers from the criticism that individuals with as many as two or three immediate family members with cancer merely experience a common detrimental environment to a greater extent than individuals having an absence of, or only one such family member affected. This criticism remains valid until the incidence of cancer in the family is so great that the generally implicated environmental factors or chance aggregation are clearly insufficient explanations of the cancer clustering. As such, family studies limited to first-degree relatives provide painfully little guidance as to the relative contributions of genetics and environment.

Declining cancer incidence with decreasing co-ancestry, (i.e., remoteness of kinship from the affected probands), in extended families of a series of cancer cases compared to control families, provides a more suitable basis for genetic analysis.[13] In order to establish a sufficiently large population for useful discrimination, one would necessarily have to extend all pedigrees to include at least second- or third-degree relatives and achieve a high degree of medical history verification, a formidable data-gathering task.

Such an example appears in the pedigree (Figure 1) of a kindred showing hereditary site-specific colon cancer (in the absence of polyposis). In the family there exists an approximately 50% excess of colon cancer risk in patients having an affected-parent versus those with an unaffected-parent.[14] More recent statistical analysis, according to Elston and Stewart's "maximum likelihood" method,[15] similarly supports an autosomal dominant mode of inheritance in the kindred. Such a pattern can really only be critically discerned and subjected to meaningful genetic analysis when occurring over multiple generations and in branches of the family geographically remote from one

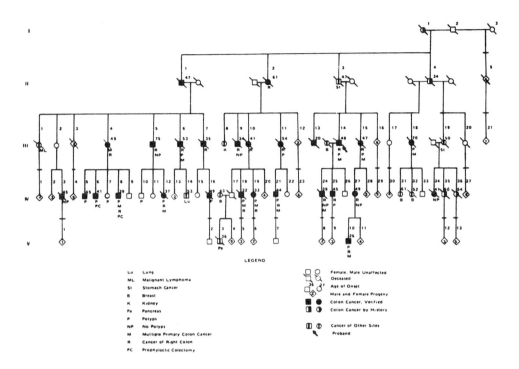

FIGURE 1. Pedigree of a Kindred exhibiting hereditary site-specific colon cancer in the absence of multiple polyposis.

another. However, even in this specific context of hereditary colon cancer, one must immediately discern problems of genetic heterogeneity (Table I). Indeed, in concert with the primary theme of our chapter, these colon cancer predisposing genotypes may have discrete susceptibilities to differing carcinogens. Therefore, the search for specific host-environmental interactions in hereditary colon cancer must take into consideration the particular genotype, i.e., Cancer Family syndrome, familial polyposis coli, Gardner's syndrome, Turcot's syndrome, and others, as described in the Table. One must then laboriously search for possible carcinogenic specificity in each of these clinical-genetic settings.

Unlike families which appear to be genetically susceptible to cancer, a complete lack of cancer through second-degree relatives would, given the obviously higher rate of nonoccurrence of cancer, fail to imply a cancer resistance. If anything, nonoccurrence of cancer suggests a favorable environment, rather than a lack of genetic susceptibility. Thus only an absence of cancer occurrences in a large family, all of whose environmental exposures are detrimental, would begin to suggest a bona fide genetic resistance to cancer. Because of this, little effort has been devoted to the identification of families at extremely low genetic risk for cancer of corresponding organs. This is surprising since the comprehension of cancer resistance could provide important clues to etiology.

We shall discuss several malignant neoplasms and cancer predisposing disorders in humans in an attempt to highlight those areas which might provide clues to genetic-environmental interactions.

C. Lung Cancer

Malignant neoplasms which show a sharp temporal progression in incidence provide an opportunity to study environmental carcinogens as they interact with variably susceptible hosts. Lung cancer is the most striking example of a once (turn of the century)

TABLE 1

Catalog of Hereditary Colon Cancer Predisposing Syndromes and/or Tumor Associations Showing Familial Aggregation in Certain Families

Syndrome	Mode of inheritance	Anatomical location & pathology of polyps or cancer or both	Associated clinical features
Familial polyposis coli	Autosomal dominant	Colon, adenomatous polyps	None
Gardner's syndrome	Autosomal dominant	Colon, adenomatous polyps; adenomatous polyps may occasionally be found in the small intestine and stomach	Soft-tissue (sebaceous cysts, fibromas) and bone lesions (osteomas of mandible, sphenoid, and maxilla), rare occurrences thyroid carcinoma and retroperitoneal sarcoma
Turcot's syndrome	Autosomal recessive	Colon and central nervous system; adenomatous polyps	None
Peutz-Jeghers' syndrome	Autosomal dominant	Entire gastrointestinal tract, except esophagus, harbors polyps which may show malignant degeneration (cancer issue remains controversial in spite of recent documentation); hamartomas of muscularis mucosa, ovarian tumors	Melanin spots of oral and vaginal mucosa and distal portions of fingers
Solitary polyps	Autosomal dominant	Colon	Predominant proximal location of colonic cancer
Ulcerative colitis	Possible autosomal dominant in certain families	Colon	Occasionally arthritis, systemic manifestations, and psychological aberrations
Juvenile polyposis coli	Autosomal dominant	Hamartomatous polyps of colon; increased occurrence of adenomatous polyps and adenocarcinoma in relatives; connective tissue abnormality	None
Cancer family syndrome	Autosomal dominant	Colon, Endometrium, other adenocarcinomas	Various adenocarcinomas, particularly of endometrium; multiple primary malignant neoplasms; early age at onset of cancer; proximal colonic excess of colon cancer

TABLE 1 (continued)

Catalog of Hereditary Colon Cancer Predisposing Syndromes and/or Tumor Associations Showing Familial Aggregation in Certain Families

Syndrome	Mode of inheritance	Anatomical location & pathology of polyps or cancer or both	Associated clinical features
Generalized gastrointestinal juvenile polyposis	Not established	Stomach, small and large bowel	None
Generalized gastrointestinal adenomatous polyposis	Possible autosomal dominant	Stomach, small and large bowel; adenomatous polyps	Desmoid reported
Cronkite-Canada syndrome	No known familial reports	Stomach, small and large bowel; adenomatous polyps	Skin pigmentation, atrophy of nails, hypoproteinemia
Familial combined breast & colon cancer	Possible autosomal dominant	Colon and breast	None

infrequent tumor, whose incidence has reached epidemic proportions in response to some rather specific agents. Nevertheless, its etiology appears to be exceedingly complex, as reflected by the ever-expanding array of environmental factors which have been implicated.

While cigarette smoking has for obvious reasons received primary attention in lung cancer research during the past several decades,[16,17] it is now becoming clear that lung cancer incidence rates vary with rural-urban differences, race (elevated risk in black men,[18] in Mexican-American,[19] and Chinese women[20]), migratory patterns, and even the socioeconomic and educational status of the patient[21] (each of which may of course reflect peculiar patterns of tobacco usage). Specific underlying occupational (environmental) factors must be given careful scrutiny.[22] Such agents as asbestos, chromium, nickel, inorganic arsenic, iron ore (hematite), wood dust, isopropyl alcohol, haloethers, mustard gas, radioisotopes, polycyclic aromatic hydrocarbons, and possibly vinyl chloride (known agent for liver angiosarcoma) provide examples of nontobacco related carcinogens.[23,24] Their role as promoters of tobacco's carcinogenic effect must be reckoned with, thus introducing problems of synergism in lung cancer etiology.[21,24,25] Latrogenic exposures such as to immunosuppressive agents and Thorotrast (a known agent in liver hemangioendothelioma) must also be integrated into an encompassing lung cancer carinogenesis model for this disease.[25]

As emphasized previously, not all people who smoke develop lung cancer or other tobacco-associated tumors such as carcinoma of the oral cavity, larynx, pharynx, esophagus, kidney, urinary bladder, and pancreas. Consequently, host responsiveness to carcinogens and their metabolites should be assessed in those individuals who do *not* develop malignant tumors but who smoke heavily and/or who are exposed to the other agents discussed above; the class comprising the other end of the susceptibility spectrum, nonsmokers with bronchogenic cancer, should be compared in terms of history of other carcinogenic exposures, presence or absence of chronic obstructive pulmonary disease (COPD), and inborn metabolic factors such as inducibility of arylhydrocarbon hydroxylase (AHH), discussed below.[26]

Preliminary evidence by Tokuhata and Lillienfeld[27] has shown an increased familial predisposition to lung cancer. Interestingly, this risk is increased multifold in cigarette smokers who have a positive family history of lung cancer. More recently, work of Kellerman et al.,[28] Guirgis et al.,[29] and Lynch et al.[30] have suggested that individuals who are high inducers of AHH and who are smokers, are more apt to develop lung cancer than are appropriately matched controls.

While the findings from these efforts are still preliminary, they do represent an attempt to assess gene-determined responses to environmental carcinogens (and their precursors) in those individuals who appear to be at high-risk for lung cancer. Should conclusive associations between a biomarker such as AHH inducibility and cancer susceptibility be established, then we will have identified specific high-risk individuals who should avoid cigarette smoking and other known pulmonary carcinogens.

In order to assess the role of COPD in lung cancer, van derWal et al.,[31] studied 150 lung cancer patients and control subjects (Control Group I) matched for sex, age, and home environment, but who were nonsmokers. They utilized an additional 100 control subjects (Control Group II) who were matched for cigarette smoking, in addition to the variables mentioned above. Of the patients with lung cancer, 96% manifested COPD compared with 34% of the first control group. Interestingly, only 28% of the second control group showed evidence of COPD. This difference was statistically significant (P <0.001). In addition, there was an excess of lung cancer among first-degree relatives of the lung cancer group compared to the control populations. The authors suggested that the increased frequency of lung cancer may be partly explained by the

TABLE 2

Lung Cancer Patients of 12 Pedigrees

Histology	Number	Mean Onset ± S.E.M.		
Adenocarcinoma	5	66.6	±	2.9
Oat Cell	2	59.0	—	—
Squamous	10	54.3	±	3.5
Undifferentiated	5	61.8	±	5.2
Unknown	7	64.6	±	2.8
Totals	29	60.5	±	2.2

nearly universal presence of COPD. The high frequency of a positive personal childhood history of COPD and family history of COPD in the lung cancer patients strongly suggested that there was an etiologic relationship between COPD and lung cancer, and that this association was not dependent solely on cigarette smoking. Furthermore, COPD was found with equal frequency on the bronchograms of light- and heavy smokers with lung cancer.

Our own team has conducted genetic studies on lung cancer probands and their families. These investigations were performed in accordance with protocols utilized routinely for our cancer genetic studies.[32] The sample contained 12 pedigrees ascertained through two first-degree relatives with histologically verified lung cancer, i.e., two lung cancer probands. Questionnaires designed for elucidation of genealogy, medical history, occupational exposures, and habit patterns, particularly cigarette smoking, were distributed to living probands and all available first- and second-degree relatives and their spouses. Whenever possible, interviews with key-relatives were conducted by epidemiology nurses. Primary medical documents from physician, hospital, and pathology laboratories were then reviewed for verification of medical history, with emphasis upon cancer of all anatomic sites and COPD.

The 12 pedigrees contain a total of 29 lung cancer patients. Table 2 shows the distribution of lung cancer by histology with descriptive statistics for each histologic type. The age of onset of lung cancer in these pedigrees is quite similar to population expectations. An analysis of the variation in age of onset of lung cancer among and within families showed a lack of correlation among siblings of the same families (intraclass correlation = 29.9%).

The cancer risk to family members is summarized according to closeness of genetic relationship (i.e., co-ancestry) to a lung cancer proband (Table 3). The two probands with lung cancer from each pedigree are excluded to provide a correction for ascertainment bias. First-degree relatives correspond to a co-ancestry of 1/4; second-degree relatives to a co-ancestry of 1/8; and third-degree relatives to a co-ancestry of 1/16.[13] Results are presented in terms of cumulative lifetime cancer risk,[33] all anatomic sites included (Table 4). Note that the cumulative cancer risk to first-degree relatives is significantly greater than that for second-degree relatives (P < 0.05). Cancer risk estimates for second- and third-degree relatives are in accord with population expectations.

The heterogeneous tumor spectrum among relatives of lung cancer probands from the 12 pedigrees is shown in Table 4 (a and b). Figures 2 to 5 are representative pedigrees of the 12 kindreds studied and exemplify a tumor spectrum consistent with genetic heterogeneity. No specific lesion appears to be predominant among male or female relatives except for the occurrence of four lung cancers among male first-degree relatives in Figure 3 (TLF-202). There was a decreasing frequency of COPD with more remote co-ancestry to probands (Table 5).

TABLE 3

Lifetime Cancer Risk to Relatives of Lung Cancer Probands Based Upon 12 Pedigrees

Sex	1st Degree			2nd Degree			3rd Degree		
	Total number	Number w/cancer	Risk (%)	Total number	Number w/cancer	Risk (%)	Total number	Number w/cancer	Risk (%)
Females	81	15	37 ± 8	91	8	27 ± 7%	80	6	29 ± 10
Males	74	14	42 ± 8	76	8	26 ± 8%	96	2	15 ± 7
Pooled	155	29	39 ± 6	167	16	26 ± 5%	176	8	19 ± 5

TABLE 4

Tumor Spectrum in Relatives of Lung Cancer Probands from 12 Pedigrees (2 Lung Cancer Probands Are Excluded per Pedigree)

Cancer site	1st Degree relatives	2nd Degree relatives	3rd Degree relatives
Female			
Breast	3	2	1
Colon	2	2	0
Cervix	2	0	0
Endometrium	2	0	0
Leukemia	0	0	2
Lung	0	1	0
Pancreas	2	0	0
Skin	2	0	1
Others	2	2	2
Total	15	7	6
Mean Onset ± S.E.M.	57.4 ± 2.8	62.1 ± 5.5	46.5 ± 9.7
Range	(45—81)	(43—85)	(7—73)
Male			
Colon	3	1	1
Larnyx/Pharnyx	1	1	1
Leukemia	1	0	0
Lung	4	0	0
Prostate	1	2	0
Skin	1	2	0
Others	3	2	0
Total	14	8	2
Mean Onset ± S.E.M.	62.7 ± 2.8	53.1 ± 6.6	85.0
Range	(43—83)	(20—75)	(82—88)

TABLE 5

Frequency of Chronic Obstructive Pulmonary Disease (COPD)[a] in Lung Cancer Probands and Relatives from 12 Pedigrees

Lung cancer probands			First-degree relatives			Second-degre (or less) relatives		
N	COPD	(%)	N	COPD	(%)	N	COPD	(%)
24	9	38	127	12	9	166	5	3

[a] COPD includes chronic bronchitis and emphysema.

D. Xeroderma Pigmentosum

Xeroderma pigmentosum (XDP) is an exceedingly rare, autosomal recessively inherited, chronically progressive, multi-system disease. The skin is the major cancer target. The most common malignant skin tumors are basal and squamous cell carcinomas, although malignant melanoma occurs in about 3% of these patients.[34] Patients with XDP often die within the first two decades of life as a result of metastases from multiple skin tumors.[35]

In 1968, Cleaver[36] demonstrated that the critical biochemical defect in XDP is the failure of excision-repair of ultraviolet damage to DNA in skin fibroblasts from patients with XDP, associated with a deficiency of UV-endonuclease, responsible for initiation of excision.[36-38] Subsequent studies have suggested that XDP may involve enzymatic defects in more than one system.[38] Thus a full understanding of the bio-

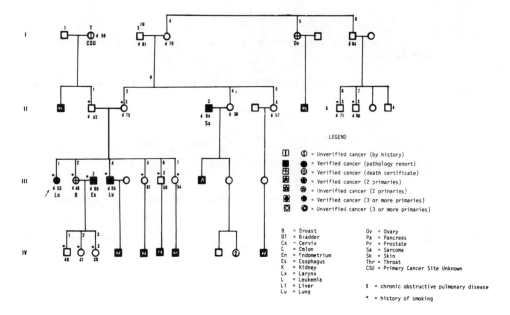

FIGURE 2.   Pedigree of a lung cancer-prone family (TLF-018).

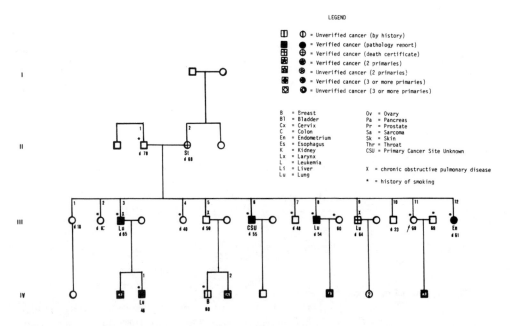

FIGURE 3.   Pedigree of a lung cancer-prone family (TLF-020).

chemistry of this disorder may be more complex than previously realized.[39] See Chapter 3 for further discussion of this repair complexity.

XDP provides a classical mechanism for the action of a specific carcinogen (UV-radiation) upon a clearly defined cancer-prone genotype. Each factor is a necessary, although neither a sufficient, agent in carcinogenesis. Consequently, if patients with XDP could meticulously avoid exposure to the carcinogenic effects of solar radiation, then the skin cancer incidence could be reduced quantitatively. That this is the case has been clearly evidenced by our observation of identical twin boys who manifested

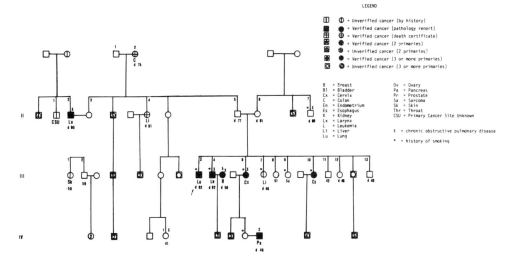

FIGURE 4. Pedigree of a lung cancer-prone family (TLF-024).

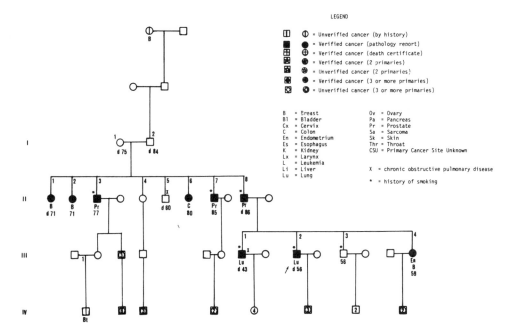

FIGURE 5. Pedigree of a lung cancer-prone family (TLF-227).

histologic, biochemical (DNA repair deficiency, complementation group C), and clinical evidence of xeroderma pigmentosum.[40] These twin boys have been protected virtually since birth from the effects of solar radiation. Each day an ester of para-aminobenzoic acid is applied topically for photo-protection. They wear long trousers, long-sleeved shirts, wide-brimmed hats and dark glasses. All of their physical activities such as swimming and tennis are accomplished at night under artificial lighting. As a result of a very considerate and empathetic family, they have adjusted extremely well psychologically to this regimen. Figure 6 shows the twins at age 8, and Figure 7 shows them again at age 16. They are now 19, are still being followed by Dr. Lynch, and continue to show a complete absence of skin cancer.

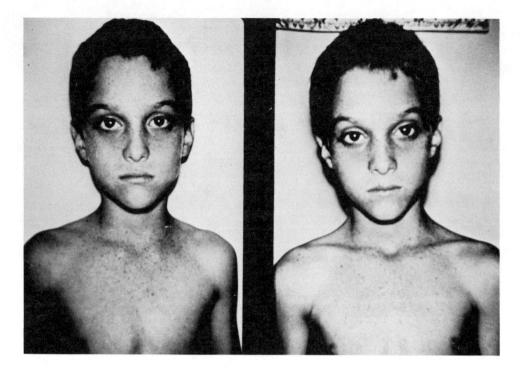

FIGURE 6.   Identical twin boys with xeroderma pigmentosum (XDP) at age 8.

It has been shown that cells from patients with XDP show variation in the excision defect; the extent of repair replication varies between 0% and 90% of normal.[41] Affected siblings are usually similar to each other in the degree of repair replication. Heterozygotes are generally indistinguishable from normal patients with respect to dimer excision and repair replication.[37] These observations clearly indicate that variation in the extent of dimer excision and repair replication in patients with XDP results from gene-determined biochemical differences; hence, genetic heterogeneity in patients with XDP is likely.[39]

Since cells from affected members of a particular family generally show the same degree of repair replication, it is likely that the level of repair is inherited as a distinct genetic trait. In vitro hybridization of cells from numerous patients with XDP has permitted study of genetic heterogeneity and has enabled complementation tests similar to those performed on microorganisms. This has resulted in the identification of five distinct complementation groups within the XDP syndrome.[41] These are now described as complementation groups A, B, C, D, and E. As noted, our identical twin brothers with XDP belong to complementation group C (5 to 20% repair).

Knowledge of these complementation groups could be used advantageously to determine whether there is a quantitative association between the percent of repair characterizing each group and the susceptibility to UV-radiation carcinogenesis. Therefore, in a disease such as XDP, heterogeneity exists and in this context it may also portend different responses to the same carcinogen, i.e., solar radiation. Such subtle differences in response to chemical and physical carcinogens, based upon enzymatic and other biochemical characters of the host, presumably occur not only in specific hereditary varieties of cancer, but also on a polygenic basis in the general population as well.

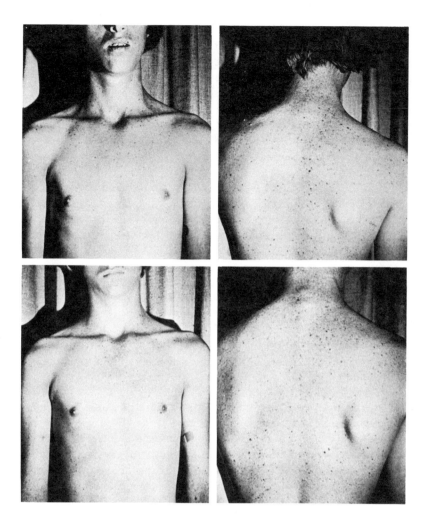

FIGURE 7. Same twins, age 16.

E. Breast Cancer

There are significant geographic variations in breast cancer incidence. Breast cancer is rare in the Orient.[42] Migrant studies have conclusively demonstrated that Japanese women who move to the United States assume higher rates of breast cancer, approaching those of the indigenous American population.[43] The age of onset of breast cancer in Japan is consistently earlier (premenopausal) than in the United States,[42] but Japanese migrants to the United States show an increase in the mean age of onset.[43] The premenopausal peak in Japanese women has been attributed to hormonal abnormalities dependent upon ovarian function, and the postmenopausal peak in the West has been in-part attributed to the Occidental diet. Based upon this, deWaard concluded that " . . . an increase in potency of a carcinogenic stimulus is in time capable of overcoming the postmenopausal leveling off trend [in age specific incidence rates] which is seen most clearly in populations following a nonwestern way of life."[9] The relatively discrete age-distributions between Japan and the United States, as hypothesized by deWaard et al,[9] is suggested to occur because there are two etiologically distinct types of breast cancer, whose age-distributions partially overlap between ages 40 and 50.

Because affected women from breast cancer-prone families in the United States have shown an early age of onset,[44] hormonal factors of the type investigated in Japanese women have come under increasing scrutiny. Indeed, our working hypothesis is that the defective mechanisms of ovarian hormone production are similar.

We consider breast cancer-prone families to be an excellent model for the study of those women who are already predisposed to premenopausal breast cancer but who may also live in an environment which increases risk for breast cancer. The questions immediately occur: "Do these genetic and environmental susceptibilities interact? If so, in what manner is their interaction expressed?" More testable questions include:

1. Given a suitable population of women at high-risk for premenopausal breast cancer (women from cancer-prone families) are their significant differences in estriol ratios (or other estrogen/androgen fractions) in women who are also at greater risk for "late onset" breast cancer, relative to high genetic risk women with a more favorable environment?
2. Do women manifesting dual liabilities (genetic risk and environmental risk) exhibit a higher rate of bilaterality of breast cancer and a higher rate of carcinoma of other anatomical sites than woman whose risk is of only one type?
3. Do such women exhibit an earlier age of onset?

Our own observation of earlier onset of breast cancer in contemporary daughters of breast cancer-affected mothers may be, in part, attributable to changing life-patterns of modern women.[45]

F. A Model for the Study of Environmental Modulation of Colon Cancer Expression in Genetically Susceptible Individuals

Spontaneous colon cancer is rare in wild, and in most inbred rat strains.[46] However, surveys of the incidence of spontaneous colonic tumors in rats have shown that when such tumors do occur, they tend to be clustered in the cecum and the proximal colon.[46] Rats subjected to such carcinogens as dinitrochlorobenzene and dimethylhydrazine develop tumors at a much higher rate.[47] Significantly, when tumors are chemically induced, the site-distribution begins to shift, favoring the distal colon and rectum.

This observation in the laboratory animal poses an interesting model for the study of colon tumorigenesis in man. Such a model suggests that there should exist an increase in the incidence rates, and a change in the site-distribution of colon cancer in man, as he moves from a pristine to a more carcinogenically hazardous environment. International comparisons of low and high colon cancer rate geographies have in fact shown such differences in rates and a shift in the site-distribution of colon cancer. For example, while the total incidence of colonic cancer in Africa and South America is quite low,[42] when such tumors do occur, they occur rather frequently in the proximal colon.[48] Consistent with the animal data on the frequency and site-distribution of chemically-induced colonic malignancy, geographic areas which exhibit the highest colon cancer rates in humans also show an excess of carcinoma of the distal colon.[42] This may be associated with the greater concentration of possible carcinogens in the distal colon through the reduced water content of the feces as the contents move toward the rectum, coupled with the enzymatic and microbiological conversion of carcinogens or their precursors to more active carcinogenic metabolites. More prolonged exposure of the colonic mucosa to possible carcinogens via reduced transit time, correlated with a western diet, has been another suggested variable; however, international studies suggest that the variation of food-fiber content, with which transit time is intimately related, is a more fruitful subject for investigation than transit time per se.[10,49]

Colon cancer-prone families evaluated by our group (and many others) constitute a most useful comparison group for scrutinizing the biological significance of the epidemiologic findings described above. It has been shown that pedigrees which show a vertically expressed excess of colon cancer (consistent with genetic etiology), exclusive of familial polyposis coli, also show early onset and a significant excess of proximal colonic cancer, relative to the American population as a whole.[14,50,51]

Given that dietary and other alleged environmental factors in colon tumorigenesis are "weak" carcinogens, requiring decades of chronic exposure to induce cancer, both the early age of onset and the more proximal location of colon cancer in families and in low-risk countries are inconsistent with a predominantly environmental etiology. This further reinforces the notion that a "stronger" agent such as genetic predisposition is needed to explain the cancer occurrences in families and perhaps in low-rate geographies as well.

Although the evidence in heritable colonic cancer suggests that very little additional environmental insult is required to initiate or promote colonic tumors, such colonic cancer-prone families provide an excellent opportunity to critically assess the effect of known environmental factors. For instance, starting with a class of individuals from cancer-prone families who are at approximately equal genetic risk (e.g., 50% risk to offspring of affected parents), one might further classify such individuals according to their environmental exposures. Hypotheses for testing host-environmental interaction include the following: (1) that genetically susceptible individuals who experience a less favorable environment [high dietary fat and animal protein, low fiber, etc.,] exhibit a more distal colonic expression than those with a more favorable dietary history; (2) that individuals at high-risk on both genetic and environmental grounds exhibit an earlier age of cancer onset and higher frequency of multiple primary colonic cancer, than those with "only" a genetic predisposition; and (3) that a sufficiently "protective" environment could forestall cancer occurrence altogether in an individual genetically predisposed, much like the phenylalanine-free diet that protects the phenolketonuric patient from mental retardation, or sunlight avoidance by the twins with XDP.

G. Other Familial Disorders with Specific Target Tissue Aberrations

1. Systemic Lupus Erythematosis

The relationship between host factors, chemicals, and carcinogenesis may relate to changes in differing bodily tissues which render them more susceptible to cancer induction through chemicals and/or other exogenous agents. Systemic lupus erythematosus is a familial disorder[52] where autoimmune manifestations of nephritis, arthralgia, and pigmentary eruptions of the skin may precede by several or more years the occurrence of lymphoma, malignant thymoma, and other associated malignant neoplasms. We support the suggestion that the target tissues in this disease may, in some as yet unknown manner, be rendered highly susceptible to the carcinogenetic effects of certain chemicals and/or oncogenic viruses.[32]

2. Celiac Disease (Non-tropical Sprue; Gluten-induced Enteropathy)

Celiac disease consists of a triad of intestinal malabsorption, abnormal small bowel structure, and gluten intolerance. These features comprise the main clinical characteristics of this familial precancerous disorder.[32] In the presence of specific pathological changes in the mucosa of the small bowel, evidence has suggested that in the absence of a gluten-free diet, such patients are more susceptible to cancer, including lymphomas of the small bowel.[53]

H. Drug Use, Genetics, and Cancer

When Garrod[54] described inborn errors of metabolism in 1902, he also suggested that some idiosyncratic drug reactions might be the result of genetically determined abnormalities in metabolic pathways. Approximately 50 years later, Haldane[55] continued to use this line of reasoning to explain idiosyncratic drug reactions. This entire issue has been addressed in even greater detail by Motulsky.[56]

The primary concern of pharmacogenetics centers around the study of the response to drugs by hosts of variable genotypic status. Although only a few of the many idiosyncratic drug reactions have been clearly ascribed to primary genetic factors, genetic differences in man may increasingly explain the pharmacologic significance of a variety of side effects and disease processes. The problem is that the busy physician seldom takes the time to inquire about the family history when he encounters idiosyncratic pharmacologic responses and they are thus incompletely recorded in the patient's files, and lack further investigation.

Clear examples of pharmacogenetic problems are now known to relate to the following: (1) Coumadin and its deficient anticoagulant effect (autosomal dominant); (2) inability to metabolize and inactivate succinylcholine chloride (autosomal recessive); (3) erythrocyte glucose-6-phosphate sensitivity in over 100 million people throughout the world: (4) slow and rapid metabolism of isoniazid (autosomal recessive trait) with susceptibility to isoniazid neuropathies and possibly to isoniazid hepatitis in slow metabolizers in the absence of Vitamin B_6 supplementation; and (5) drug sensitivity (barbiturates, griseofulvin, chlordiazepoxide, meprobamate) in patients with autosomal recessively inherited acute intermittent porphyria.

These examples have been mentioned in order to provide a rationale for scrutiny of drug-use patterns in patients with positive family histories of cancer in epidemiologic studies. For instance, increasing attention to the relationship between specific pharmacologic agents and cancer during the past decade has led to the recognition of an association between chronic estrogen usage and the development of endometrial carcinoma.[57] Indeed, evidence has disclosed that patients with Turner's syndrome, a cytogenetic abnormality (45XO karyotype), who have been treated with estrogens for secondary sexual development may be at inordinately high-risk for development of early onset endometrial carcinoma. In a study of 24 patients with gonadal dysgenesis who were receiving stilbesterol for at least 5 years, carcinoma of the endometrium developed in two and possibly three of these patients.[58] It was of interest that these tumors were of early onset and were of an unusual mixed or adenosquamous type.

Evidence of genetic susceptibility to endometrial carcinoma (in the Cancer Family syndrome) suggests that more attention should be given to the family history of this lesion in patients receiving estrogen therapy and/or who are on estrogen containing contraceptive agents, in order to discern whether they may be particularly vulnerable to carcinogenesis. Finally, patients prone to other familial endocrine dependent tumors, including carcinoma of the breast and ovary, should be evaluated for possible enhancement of carcinogenicity from estrogen usage.

Hoover and Fraumeni[59] list several varieties of drugs which are believed to be causally related to cancer in man (Table 6). These ivestigators stressed the fact that while few pharmacologic agents have been etiologically related to cancer, many drugs in clinical practice have not been critically scrutinized from the standpoint of pharmacogenetic carcinogenesis. Consequently, they urge epidemiologic evaluation of widely used drugs that either show clinical suspicion of a cancer hazard or are known to be carcinogenic in laboratory animals.

TABLE 6

Cancers Related to Drug Exposures in Man

Radioisotopes

Phosphorus (^{32}P)	Acute leukemia
Radium, mesothorium	Osteosarcoma and sinus carcinoma
Thorotrast	Hemangioendothelioma of liver

Immunosuppressive Drugs
(for renal transplantation)

Antilymphocyte serum	Reticulum cell sarcoma
Antimetabolites	(?) Other cancers (skin, liver, soft-tissue carcoma)
Corticosteroids	

Cytotoxic Drugs

Chlornapnazine	Bladder cancer
Melphalan	Acute myelomonocytic leukemia
Cyclophosphamide	

Hormones

Synthetic estrogens	
Prenatal	Vaginal and cervical adenocarcinoma (clear cell type)
Postnatal	Endometrial carcinoma (adenosquamous type)
Adrogenic-anabolic steroids (for aplastic anemia)	Hepatocellular carcinoma

Others

Arsenic	Skin cancer
Phenacetin-containing drugs	Renal pelvis carcinoma
? Diphenylhydantoin	Lymphoma
Coal tar ointments	Skin cancer
? Chloramphenicol	Leukemia
? Amphetamines	Hodgkin's disease

From Hoover, R. and Fraumeni, Jr., J. F., Jr., *J. Clin. Pharm.*, 15, 16, 1975. With permission.

II. CONCLUSIONS

The chain of etiologic events contributing to cancer is exceedingly complex and may vary significantly from one patient to another, even when the lesions appear to be identical. Carcinogenesis may be initiated almost at conception, as evidenced by congenital occurrences of Wilms' tumor, neuroblastoma, hepatoblastoma, and rhabdomyosarcoma. Malignant neoplasms detected at birth may be found in association with congenital skeletal, cardiac, or cytogenetic abnormalities, suggesting both carcinogenic and teratogenic effects of gene-carcinogen interaction.

Primary genetic events have been shown to predispose host tissues to the action of exogenous agents (hormones such as diethylstilbestrol, tumor specific antigens, other drugs, chemicals, radiation and oncogenic viruses) consistent with the germinal-somatic double mutation (two-hit) hypothesis as advanced by Knudson and others.[60-62] Modifications of this two-step mutational theory could readily explain a fraction of the other tumors of childhood, early youth, and later adult-life.

The several observations of premorbid pathogenetic processes which may contribute to the clinical evolution of cancer, suggest the following suppositions: (1) single gene-determined traits may strongly predispose to cancer in a small fraction of the population; polygenic-risk characterizes the gradually decreasing significance of genetic factors in the remaining bulk of the populace; (2) in accord with this reasoning, environmental carcinogenic agents may act in concert with the genotype at any or all phases in the disease evolution process, i.e., both in contributing to the primary disease(s) process (premorbid state), as well as to the ultimate malignant neoplastic transformation. As in the case of lung cancer, the carcinogen may contribute to the pathogenetic process resulting in COPD per se, or it may be restricted pathogenetically to a carcinogenic effect on a preexisting COPD state. Thus one could reason that a primary genetic event contributed to the COPD, rendering the tissue more vulnerable to carcinogenic action of certain agents which might otherwise have produced COPD themselves.

Host-environmental interaction in carcinogenesis may be modulated further by horizontally or vertically transmissible oncogenic factors (oncogenic virus?), and/or oncodevelopmental proteins. An "infectious" etiology in certain forms of cancer, i.e., Burkitt's lymphoma,[63] nasophryngeal carcinoma,[64] Hodgkin's disease,[65] osteogenic sarcoma,[66] and uterine cervical and prostatic carcinoma[67,68] is supported by geographic, racial, familial, connubial and time-space clustering data. With respect to connubiality, the Hodgkin's disease model of Vianna et al.[65] is of particular interest. Viral antibodies were elevated in Hodgkin's contacts who did not develop Hodgkin's disease, but who were nevertheless believed to participate in the "infectious" cycle as contacts for others who did develop Hodgkin's disease. Similar phenomena have also been documented in patients with neuroblastoma and their first-degree relatives through lymphocyte colony inhibition assays,[69] with comparable data observed in household contacts of patients with carcinoma of the breast and sarcoma.[70,71]

Findings from our own laboratories suggest the existence of communicable agents which lead to an elevation of CEA in spouses of high-risk patients from the Cancer Family syndrome. This has led us to an hypothesis for cancer etiology in which the cancer-prone genotype is acted upon by de-repressed oncogenes, activated oncogenic viruses, and putative transmission via respiratory or venereal route.[72] Figure 8 shows this schematic based upon data from high-risk patients and their spouses.

In contrast to our hypothesis for hereditary adult malignant neoplasms, as reflected in the Cancer Family syndrome, our model for certain occurrences of childhood cancer involves transplacental transmission of putative carcinogenic factors (oncogenic virus?, tumor specific antigens?) emanating from mothers with occult carcinoma of the breast (Figure 9) who also transmitted the SBLA* gene to their fetuses.[73] In other words, the subject fetuses, genetically primed for the development of cancer, were exquisitely sensitive to the action of transplacental agents (Figures 9 and 10). This genetic-environmental hypothesis for cancer is readily testable through amniocentesis and determination of specific genetic and immunologic parameters (immunologic alterations and deficiencies, viral antibodies, fetal proteins, cytogenetic aberrations, and tumor products) in both mother and fetus.

These contrasting etiologic hypotheses stress the wide range of variation in both age of expression and type of tumor in hereditary cancer and precancerous syndromes, and have specific relevance to the timing of the subsequent somatic (environmental) mutation.

Through the examples discussed herein we have emphasized the gaps that exist in

---

* Hereditary predisposition to sarcoma [S], brain tumors [B], leukemia, lymphoma, laryngeal, and lung cancer [L], and adrenal cortical carcinoma [A].

TARGET THEORY

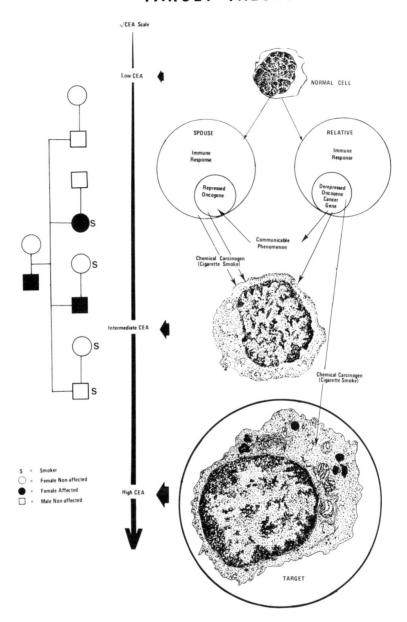

FIGURE 8.   Model for connubiality of CEA elevation in the Cancer Family syndrome.

our understanding of the intricate relationship between host factors and the physico-chemical agents in carcinogenesis. They have also raised questions which may be responded to through the implementation of existing laboratory, statistical, and clinical models for the study of these interactions. For example, one might reasonably consider the possibility that vigorous treatment during the precancerous state of the patient, such as through the use of steroids in systemic lupus erythematosus might lessen the risk for subsequent cancer. Pursuring this same line of reasoning, one might wonder about certain forms of dietary intervention in celiac disease or pharmacologic agents

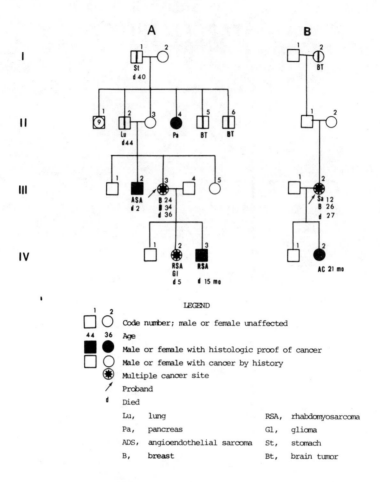

FIGURE 9.   Pedigrees of two kindreds exhibiting the SBLA syndrome.

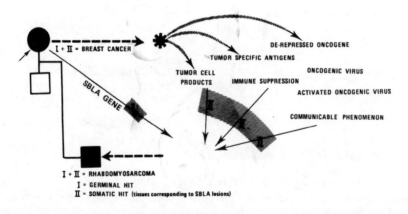

FIGURE 10.   Model of transplacental transmission of carcinogens within the SBLA syndrome.

such as ascorbic acid for polyp regression in patients with familial adenomatous polyposis coli. Finally, might early management of COPD, as through prompt treatment of pulmonary infections and restriction of cigarette smoking ultimately reduce the risk of lung cancer?

REFERENCES

1. Gordon, H., Family studies in retinoblastoma, *Birth Defects Orig. Artic. Serv.*, 19(10), 185 1974.
2. Case, R. A. M., Hosker, M. E., McDonald, D. B., et al., Tumors of the urinary bladder in workmen engaged in the manufacture and use of certain dye-stuff intermediates in the British chemical industry. Part I. The role of aniline, benzidine, α-naphthylamine and β-naphthylamine, *Br. J. Ind. Med.*, 2, 75, 1954.
3. Tomatis, L., Agthe, C., Bartsch, H., Huff, J., Montesano, R., Saracci, R., Walker, E., and Wilbourn, J., Evaluation of the carcinogenicity of chemicals: a review of the monograph program of the International Agency for Research on Cancer, *Cancer Res.*, 38, 877, 1978.
4. International Agency for Research on Cancer Monograph, *The Evaluation of Carcinogenic Risk*, Vol. 1, IARC Scientific Publishers, Lyon, France, 1977.
5. International Agency for Research on Cancer Monograph, *The Evolution of Carcinogenic Risk, Asbestos*, Vol. 14, IARC Scientific Publishers, Lyon, France, 1977.
6. Green, E. L., *Biology of the Laboratory Mouse*, 2nd ed., McGraw-Hill, New York, 1966.
7. Diwan, H. A. and Meier, H., Carcinogenic effect of a single dose of diethylnitrosamine in three unrelated strains of mice: genetic dependence of the induced tumor types and incidence, *Cancer Lett. Netherlands*, 1, 249, 1976.
8. Higgenson, J., Present trends in cancer epidemiology, in *Proc. Can. Cancer Res. Conf.*, 8, 40, 1969.
9. DeWaard, F., Nurture and nature in cancer of the breast and the endometrium, in *Host-environment Interaction in the Etiology of Cancer in Man*, Doll, R., Vodopija, I., and Davis, W., Eds., IARC Scientific Publishers, Lyon, France, 1973, 121.
10. Wynder, E. L. and Shigematsu, T., Environmental factors of cancer of the colon and rectum, *Cancer*, 20(9), 1520, 1967.
11. Deelman, H. T., Heredity & cancer, *Ann. Surg.*, 93, 30, 1931.
12. Woolf, C. M., A genetic study of carcinoma of the large intestine, *Am. J. Hum. Genet.*, 10, 42, 1958.
13. Falconer, D. W., *Introduction to Quantitative Genetics*, Ronald Press, New York, 1962.
14. Lynch, H. T., Harris, R. E., Bardawil, W. A., Lynch, P. M., Guirgis, H. A., Swartz, M. J., and Lynch, J. F., Management and control of hereditary site-specific colon cancer, *Arch. Surg.*, 112, 170, 1977.
15. Elston, R. C. and Stewart, I., A general model for the genetic analysis of pedigree data, *Hum. Heredit.*, 21, 523, 1971.
16. Doll, R. and Peto, R., Mortality in relation to smoking: 20 year's observations on male British doctors, *Br. Med. J.*, P. 1525, 1976.
17. Hammon, E. C., Smoking habits and air pollution in relation to lung cancer, in *Environmental Factors in Respiratory Disease*, Lee, H. K., Ed., Academic Press, New York, 1972.
18. Burbank, F. and Fraumeni, J. R., Jr., U.S. cancer mortality: non-white predominance, *J. Natl. Cancer Inst.*, 49, 649, 1972.
19. Buell, P. E., Mendez, W. M., and Dunn, J. E., Jr., Cancer of the lung among Mexican immigrant women in California, *Cancer*, 22, 186, 1968.
20. Fraumeni, J. F., Jr. and Mason, T. J., Cancer mortality among Chinese-Americans, 1950-69, *J. Natl. Cancer Inst.*, 52, 659, 1974.
21. Fraumeni, J. F., Jr., Respiratory carcinogenesis: an epidemiologic appraisal, *J. Nat. Cancer Inst.*, 55, 1039, 1975.
22. Blot, W. J. and Fraumeni, J. F., Jr., Geographic patterns of lung cancer: industrial correlations, *Am. J. Epidemiol.*, 103, 539, 1976.
23. Blot, W. J. and Fraumeni, J. F., Jr., Arsenical air pollution and lung cancer, *Lancet*, 2, 142, 1975.
24. Becklake, M. R., Asbestos-related diseases of the lung and other organs: their epidemiology and implications for clinical practice, *Am. Rev. Respir., Dis.*, 114, 187, 1976.
25. Doll, R., Strategy for detection of cancer hazards to man, *Nature*, 265, 589, 1977.
26. Mulvihill, J. J., Host factors in human lung tumors: an example of ecogenetics in oncology, *J. Nat. Cancer Inst.*, 57(1), 3, 1976.
27. Tokuhata, C. K. and Lillienfeld, A. M., Familial aggregations of lung cancer in humans, *J. Nat. Cancer Inst.*, 39, 289, 1963.
28. Kellerman, C., Shaw, and Luyten-Kellerman, M., Aryl-hydrocarbon hydroxylase inducibility and bronchogenic cancer, *N. Engl. J. Med.*, 289, 934, 1973.
29. Guirgis, H. A., Lynch, H. T., Mate, T. E., Harris, R. E., Wells, I., Caha, L., Anderson, J., Maloney, K., and Rankin, L., AHH activity in lymphocytes from lung cancer patients and normal controls., *Oncology*, 33, 105, 1976.
30. Lynch, H. T., Guirgis, H. A., Harris, R. E., and Swartz, M. J., Clinical, epidemiologic, and genetic considerations in lung cancer, in *Pulmonary Disease: Defense Mechanisms and Populations at Risk*, Clark, M. A., Ed., University of Kentucky Printers, Lexington, 1978.

31. van DerWal, A. M., Huizinga, E., Orie, N. G., et al., Cancer and chronic non-specific lung disease (CNSLD), *Scand. J. Respir. Dis.*, 47, 161, 1966.
32. Lynch, H. T., *Canceer Genetics*, Charles C Thomas, Springfield, Ill., 1975, 639.
33. Colton, T., *Statistics in Medicine*, Little, Brown, Boston, 1974.
34. Lynch, H. T., Anderson, D. E., Smith, J. O., Jr., et al., Xeroderma pigmentosum, malignant melanoma, and congenital ichthyosis: a family study. *Arch. Dermatol.*, 96, 625, 1967.
35. Pathak, M. A. and Epstein, J. H., Normal and abnormal reactions of man to light, in *Dermatology in General Medicine*, Fitzpatrick, T. B., et al., Eds., McGraw-Hill, New York, 1971.
36. Cleaver, J. E., Xeroderma pigmentosum: a human disease in which an initial state of DNA repair is defective, in *Proc. Nat. Acad. Sci. U.S.A.*, 63, 428, 1969.
37. Cleaver, J. E., DNA repair and radiation sensitivity in human (xeroderma pigmentosum) cells, *Int. J. Radiat. Biol.*, 18, 557, 1970.
38. Cleaver, J. E. and Bootsma, D., Xeroderma pigmentosum: biochemical and genetic characteristics, *Annu. Rev. Genet.*, to be published.
39. Cleaver, J. E., DNA damage and repair in light-sensitive human skin disease. *J. Invest. Dermatol.*, 54, 181, 1970.
40. Lynch, H. T., Frichot, B. C., III, and Lynch, J. F., Cancer control in xeroderma pigmentosum, *Arch. Dermatol.*, 113, 193, 1977.
41. Robbins, J. H., Kraemer, H. H., Lutzner, M. A., et al., Xeroderma pigmentosum: an inherited disease with sun sensitivity, multiple cutaneous neoplasms, and abnormal DNA repair, *Ann. Intern. Med.*, 80, 221, 1974.
42. Doll, R., Payner, P., and Waterhouse, J., Eds., Cancer incidence in five continents, II, in *International Union Against Cancer (UICC)*, Springer-Verlag, Basel, 1970.
43. Buell, P., Changing incidence of breast cancer in Japanese-Amercan women, *J. Nat. Cancer Inst.*, 51, 1479, 1973.
44. Lynch, H. T., Guirgis, H., Brodkey, F., Maloney, K., Lynch, P., Rankin, L., and Lynch, J., Early age of onset of familial breast cancer, *Arch. Surg.*, 111, 126, 1976.
45. Lynch, H. T., Mulcahy, G., King, M. C., Elston, R., Maloney, K., Rankin, L., Foley, J., and Lemon, H. M., New Developments in Breast Cancer Genetics, in Proc. 12th Ann. Mtg. of the Am. Society of Clin. Oncol., Toronto, May 4, to 8, 1976.
46. Miwa, M., Takenaka, S., Ito, K., Fujiwara, K., Tokunaga, A., Hozumi, M., Fujimura, S., and Sugimura, T., Spontaneous colon tumors in rats, *J. Natl. Cancer Inst.*, 56(3), 615, 1976.
47. Deschner, E. E. and Long, F. C., Colonic neoplasms in mice produced with six injections of 1,2-dimethylhydrazine, *Oncology*, 34(6), 255, 1977.
48. Correa, D. and Haenszel, W., Comparative international incidence and mortality, in *Cancer Epidemiology and Prevention*, Schottenfeld, D., Ed., Charles C Thomas, Springfield, Ill., 1975, 386.
49. Walker, A. R. P., Colon cancer and diet, with special reference to intakes of food and fiber, *Am. J. Clin. Nutr.*, 29, 1417, 1976.
50. Lynch, P., Lynch, H., Harris, R., Lynch, J., and Guirgis, H., Heritable colon cancer and solitary adenomatous polyps, in *Cancer Detection and Prevention*, Vol. 2, Nieburg, Ed., 1978.
51. Lynch, P. M., Lynch, H. T., and Harris, R. E., Hereditary proximal colonic cancer, *Dis. Colon Rectum*, 29(8), 661, 1977.
52. Block, S. R., Winfield, J. B., Lockshin, M. D., et al., Studies of twins with lupus erythematosus: a review of the literature and presentation of 12 additional sets, *Am. J. Med.*, 59, 533, 1975.
53. Harris, O. D., Cooke, W. T., Thompson, H., and Waterhouse, J. A. H., Malignancy in adult celiac disease and idiopathic steatorrhea, *Am. J. Med.*, 42, 899, 1967.
54. Garrod, A. E., The incidence of alkaptonuria — a study in chemical individuality, *Lancet*, 1, 161, 1902.
55. Haldane, J. B. S., *The Biochemistry of Genetics*, Allen and Unwin, London, 1954.
56. Motulsky, A. G., Pharmacogenetics, in *Progress in Medical Genetics 3*, Steinberg, A. G. and Bearn, A. G., Eds., Grune & Stratton, New York, 1964, 49.
57. Greenblatt, R. B., Estrogens and endometrial cancer — gross exaggeration or fact?, *Geriatrics*, 60, 1977.
58. Cutler, B. S., Forbes, A. P., Ingersol, F. M., etal., Endometrial carcinoma after stilbestrol therapy in gonadal dysgenesis, *N. Engl. J. Med.*, 287, 628, 1972.
59. Hoover, R. and Fraumeni, J. F., Drugs in clinical use which cause cancer, *J. Clin. Pharmacol.*, 15, 16, 1976.
60. Knudson, A. G., Mutation and cancer: sttistical study of retinoblastoma, in, *Proc. Natl. Acad. Sci. U.S.A.*, 68, 820, 1971.
61. Knudson, A. G. and Strong, L. C., Mutation and cancer: a model for Wilms' tumor of the kidney, *J. Natl. Cancer Inst.*, 48, 313, 1972.

62. Knudson, A. G. and Strong, L. C., Mutation and cancer: neuroblastoma and pheochromocytoma, *Am. J. Hum. Genet.*, 24, 514, 1972.
63. O'Connor, G. T., Persistent immunologic stimulation as a factor in oncogenesis, with special reference to Burkitt's tumor, *Am. J. Med.*, 48(3), 279, 1970.
64. de-The, G., Ho, H. C., Kwam, H. C., Desgrauges, C., and Favre, M. D., Nasopharyngeal carcinoma (NPC). I. Types of cultures derived from tumor biopsies and non-tumorous tissues of Chinese patients with special reference to lymphoblastoid transformation, *Int. J. Cancer*, 6, 189, 1970.
65. Vianna, N. J., Greenwald, P., and Davis, J. N. P., Extended epidemic Hodgkin's disease in high school students, *Lancet*, 1, 1209, 1971.
66. Morton, D. L. and Malgren, R. A., Human osteosarcomas: immunologic evidence suggesting an associated infectious agent, *Science*, 162, 1279, 1968.
67. Kessler, I. I., Lulcar, Z., Rawls, W. E., et al., Cervical cancer in Yugoslavia. I. Antibodies to genital herpesvirus in cases and controls, *J. Natl. Cancer Inst.*, 52(2), 369, 1974.
68. Singer, A., Reid, B., and Coppleston, M., A hypothesis: the role of a high-risk male in the etiology of cervical carcinoma, *Am. J. Obstet. Gynecol.*, 126, 110, 1976.
69. Hellstrom, K. E. and Hellstrom, I., Cellular immunity against tumor antigens, *Adv. Cancer Res.*, 12, 167, 1969.
70. Byers, V. S., Levin, A. S., Hacket, A. J., et al., Tumor-specific cell-mediated immunity in household contacts of cancer patients, *J. Clin. Invest.*, 55, 500, 1975.
71. Teynoso, G., Chu, T. M., Holyoke, D., et al., Carcinoembryonic antigen in patients with different cancer, *JAMA*, 220, 361, 1972.
72. Guirgis, H. A., Lynch, H. T., Harris, R. E., and Vandevoorde, J. P., Genetic and communicable effects on carccinoembryonic antigen expressivity in the cancer family syndrome, *Cancer Res.*, 38, 2523, 1978.
73. Lynch, H. T. and Guirgis, H. A., Childhood cancer and the SBLA syndrome, *Med. Hypotheses*, 5, 15, 1979.

INDEX

A

Mitomycin C, 7, 50, 73, 79
Mixed-function oxidases, 22—31, 35—36,
    45—46, 48
  general characteristics, 22—25
  genetic regulation, 25—31
Mixed hemadsorption assay, 159—160
3 M KCl procedure, 159
MMC, see Mitomycin C
MMS, see Methylmethane sulfonate
Moloney virus, 94, 102—103, 114, 154, 162
Monocytes, 157—158
Monooxygenases, 22—25, 27, 36—37, 42—43,
    45—48
  metabolism of, 23
  smoke-induced activity, 43
5(Morpholinomethyl)-3-[(5-nitrofurfurylidene)-
    amino]-2-oxazolidinone, 12
Mouse cell resistance, to xenotropic virus, 112
Mouse studies, see Murine headings; Rodent
    studies
Murine amphototropic viruses, 99
Murine B-tropic viruses, 112—113
Murine dual-tropic viruses, 103
Murine ecotropic viruses
  chemical carcinogenesis and, 116—117
  classification, 99
  dual-tropic forms, 103
  gene responsible for, 112
  host gene regulation, 105—106
  induced expression, 105—106, 108
  spontaneous expression, 104—108
Murine endogenous RNA viruses, inheritance of,
    94—120
  classification, 96, 99
  general discussion, 94—96, 119—120
  genetic regulation of virus expression, 104—114
  genetics of viral expression and disease states,
    114—118
  structure and composition, 96—101
  viral footprints in man, 119
  virogene expression, 100—104
Murine NB-tropic viruses, 112—113
Murine N-tropic viruses, 112—113
Murine xenotropic viruses
  chemical carcinogenesis and, 117—118
  classification, 99
  host gene regulation, 106
  human, 119
  induced expression, 110
  mouse cell resistance to, 112
  spontaneous expression, 108—110
Mustard gas, 5, 10, 192
Mutagens, mutagenesis, and mutagenicity
  exposure, uptake, and distribution studies,
    3—4, 13—15
  lesion repair studies, 70, 73, 77—78
  metabolism studies, 22—23, 30, 33, 45—49,
    51—54
  promoter studies, 133
ts Mutants, 104
Mutation, 22, 49, 68, 120, 133, 135, 142
  somatic, 68, 133

N

N, cell, see Null cell
N, -tropic viruses, 112—113
NADPH-cytochrome P-450 reductase, 24
NADPH-generating system, 48—49
α-Naphthoflavone, 36
β-Naphthoflavone, 26, 28, 36, 40
1-Naphthylamine, 5
2-Naphthylamine, 5, 10
β-Naphthylamine, 9, 186
NAT, see N-Acetyltransferase
Naturally occurring tumors, 163
NB-tropic viruses, 112—113
Neoantigens, 156—157
Neoplasia, 114, 119, 155, 157
Neoplastic transformation, 45, 47—48
Neuraminidase, 167
NIH cells, endogenous RNA virus studies,
    115—116
Nitro aromatics and heterocyclics, 22
4-Nitrobiphenyl, 12
Nitrofurans, 22
1[5-Nitrofurfurylidene)-amino]-2-
    imidazolidinone, 12
N [-4-(5-Nitro-2-furyl)-2-thiazolyl] acetamide, 12
4-Nitroquinoline-N-oxide, 114—115
4-Nitroquinoline-1-oxide, 71
Nitrosamides, 7
Nitrosamines, 7—9, 22, 35, 114—115, 161
N-Nitrosodiethylamine, 12
N-Nitrosodimethylamine, 12
N-Nitroso-di-n-butylamine, 12
Nitrosoethylurea, 12
Nitrosomethylurea, 12
N-Nitroso-N-methylurethane, 12
Nitrous compounds
Noncarcinogens, initiating effect, 131
Nongenetic tests, aryl hydrocarbon hydroxylase
    levels, 36—41
Nonresponsive reaction, AHH and TCDD, 40
Nonspecific antibodies, 158
Nonspecific immunotherapy, 167—170
Non-tropical sprue, 201
4NQO, see 4-Nitroquinoline-1-oxide
Nucleic acid antigens, 118
Nucleic acids, 96—99, 119, 134—135
Nucleoid, 96—100
Nucleotides, 70—71, 119, 157
Null cell, 158
Nutritional factors, see Diet; Food
NZB, mouse strain, RNA virus studies, 108—110,
    116—118
Nzv-1, gene, 106, 109
Nzv-2, gene, 106, 109

O

Occupational sources, chemical carcinogenesis, 3,
    5—14, 171, 186—187
OFA, see Oncofetal antigen